Biomechanical Basis of Orthotic Management

Biomechanical Basis of Orthotic Management

Edited by

P. Bowker BSc, PhD, CEng, MIMechE, MBES
School of Prosthetics and Orthotics, University College Salford, Salford, UK

D.N. Condie BSc, CEng, MIMechE, MBES
Tayside Rehabilitation Engineering Services, Dundee Limb Fitting Centre, Dundee, UK

D.L. Bader BSc, MSc, PhD, MBES
Department of Materials, Queen Mary College, University of London, London, UK

D.J. Pratt BSc, MSc, PhD, MInstP, CPhys, MBES
Trent Regional Centre for Orthotics, Derbyshire Royal Infirmary, Derby, UK

Consultant Orthopaedic Editor

W.A. Wallace FRCSEd, FRCSEd(Orth)
Department of Orthopaedic and Accident Surgery, Queen's Medical Centre, Nottingham, UK

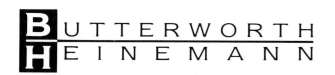

Butterworth-Heinemann Ltd
Linacre House, Jordan Hill, Oxford OX2 8DP

A member of the Reed Elsevier group

OXFORD   LONDON   BOSTON
MUNICH   NEW DELHI   SINGAPORE   SYDNEY
TOKYO   TORONTO   WELLINGTON

First published 1993

British Library Cataloguing in Publication Data
Biomechanical Basis of Orthotic Management
  I. Bowker, P.
  617.307

ISBN 0 7506 1380 7

Library of Congress Cataloguing in Publication Data
Biomechanical basis or orthotic management/edited by P. Bowker ...
  [et al.]; consultant orthopaedic editor.
    p.   cm.
  Includes bibliographical references and index.
  ISBN 0 7506 1380 7
  1. Orthopedic apparatus.   2. Human mechanics.   I. Bowker, P.
  (Peter)
  [DNLM: 1. Orthothic Devices.   2. Biomechanics.   WE 26 B615 1993]
  RD755.B53   1993
  617.3'07—dc20
  DNLM/DLC
  for Library of Congress   93–7836
                                                              CIP

Typeset by TecSet Ltd, Wallington, Surrey

Printed and bound in Great Britain by The Bath Press, Avon

Contents

Contributors

D.L. Bader BSc, MSc, PhD, MBES
Department of Materials and IRC in Bio-
medical Materials, Queen Mary and Westfield
College, University of London, London, UK

G. Bardsley BEng, PhD, MBES
Tayside Rehabilitation Engineering Services,
Dundee Limb Fitting Centre, Dundee, UK

P. Bowker BSc, PhD, CEng, MIMechE,
MBES
School of Prosthetics and Orthotics, University
College Salford, Salford, UK

D. Carus BSc(Eng), CEng, MIMechE, AKC
Dundee Institute of Technology, Dundee, UK

A. P. Chase MPhil, DipOTC, LBIST
Nuffield Orthotics and Rehabilitation En-
gineering, Nuffield Orthopaedic Centre, NHS
Trust, Oxford, UK

D.N. Condie BSc, CEng, MIMechE, MBES
Tayside Rehabilitation Engineering Services,
Dundee Limb Fitting Centre, Dundee, UK

P. Convery MSc
National Centre for Training and Education in
Prosthetics and Orthotics, University of
Strathclyde, Glasgow, UK

G.R. Johnson BSc, PhD, CEng, FIMechE,
MBES
Department of Mechanical Materials and
Manufacturing Engineering,
University of Newcastle Upon Tyne,
Newcastle Upon Tyne, UK

J. Lamb LBIST
Tayside Rehabilitation Engineering Services,
Orthotic Department, Dundee Royal Infirm-
ary, Dundee, UK

B. McHugh BEng, PhD, CEng, MIMechE
National Centre For Training and Education in
Prosthetics and Orthotics
University of Strathclyde, Glasgow, UK

C. B. Meadows BSc, PhD, CEng, MIMechE,
MHSM
Bioengineering Centre, Princess Margaret
Rose Hospital, Edinburgh, UK

J. C. Peacock MCSP, LBIST
J. C. Peacock and Son Ltd
Newcastle Upon Tyne, UK

M.J. Pearcy BSc, PhD, CEng, MBES
Department of Orthopaedic Surgery and
Trauma, Royal Adelaide Hospital, Adelaide,
Australia

D.J. Pratt BSc, MSc, PhD, MInstP, CPhys,
MBES
Orthotics and Disability Research Centre,
Trent Regional Centre for Othotics
Derbyshire Royal Infirmary, Derby, UK

J. Stallard BTech, CEng, FIMechE, MBES
Orthotic Research and Locomotor Assessment
Unit, The Robert Jones and Agnes Hunt
Orthopaedic Hospital, Oswestry, Shropshire,
UK

D. R. Tollafield DPodM, BSc, FPodA
Nene College, School of Health and Life
Sciences (Podiatry), Northampton, UK

W.A. Wallace FRCSEd, FRCSEd(Orth)
Department of Orthopaedic and Accident
Surgery, Queen's Medical Centre,
Nottingham, UK

Acknowledgements

We would like to thank all those who have contributed in so many ways to the production of this book, and in particular its many authors; our colleagues in the Tayside Orthotic Service, in the Trent Regional Centre for Orthotics and in the Salford School of Prosthetics and Orthotics — especially Gillian Young and Norah Virtue; and both past and present staff at Butterworth–Heinemann. We would also like to acknowledge the contribution of David Begg, from whom, many years ago, most of us learnt what an orthosis is.

1

Introduction and anatomical terminology

Peter Bowker, Dan Bader, David Condie, David Pratt and W.A. Wallace

1.1 Introduction

1.1.1 What is an orthosis?

The International Standards Organisation has defined an orthosis (plural: orthoses) as:

An externally applied device used to modify the structural or functional characteristics of the neuro-musculo-skeletal system.

During physical activity the body is subjected to an external system of forces and moments. Normally these forces are resisted or controlled by forces generated in the tissues of the body so that a normal, functional pattern of motion is generated. In a pathological situation, however, one or more of these tissues may be impaired and thus be unable to perform its normal role. In this case more normal function may be restored by using an orthosis to modify the system of external forces and moments acting across one or more of the joints of the body. In this way, orthoses compensate for the inadequacy of the body's tissues.

Sometimes the sole purpose of an orthosis will be to relieve forces or moments from pathological skeletal structures. For example, a weight-bearing knee-ankle-foot orthosis will reduce the pressure in a diseased joint or the stress in a weakened bone. More commonly, however, the effect of the orthosis may be to modify the motion which occurs at a joint, for example to prevent giving way of the joint resulting from weakened muscles or to resist the action of spastic muscles. The mechanisms through which the orthoses achieve these various functions are discussed in detail in Chapter 3.

1.1.2 Prescribing an orthosis

Successful orthotic prescription requires a detailed analysis of the patient's physical and functional status, followed by careful consideration of their requirements. The orthotic objectives must be realistic otherwise the fitting will be unsuccessful and the patient disappointed.

Orthoses must not be looked upon as a substitute for effective and appropriate surgery. In some cases a combination of surgical and orthotic management may produce the optimum result. For example, a Duchenne muscular dystrophy patient with a severe scoliosis may benefit from a spinal fusion thus permitting the patient to be positioned satisfactorily in a seat/wheelchair system. In contrast for other patients, such as an elderly person with cardiovascular insufficiency, major surgery requiring a general anaesthetic and an extended rehabilitation programme may be contraindicated if the condition is not life threatening. In such cases the benefit which can be gained from the use of an external support system is to be preferred. These considerations will be discussed in more detail in the individual chapters of the book dealing with specific types of orthoses.

1.1.3 Orthotic prescription – a compromise

As orthoses function through the application of mechanical forces to the musculoskeletal system, their success depends on a thorough understanding of biomechanical principles and their correct application to the particular pathology being managed. It is the purpose of this book to address these topics in detail. However, the ultimate success or failure of an orthotic prescription depends also on a number of other factors. These principally relate to the fact that the orthosis is an externally worn device, whose weight, bulk and perhaps most of all appearance are of very great importance to the user. Sometimes therefore, even after careful discussion with the patient, and after adopting the most cosmetic style of orthosis or developing ingenious designs utilizing state of the art materials, it may still be necessary to compromise biomechanical effectiveness in order to make the orthosis acceptable. Better a partly effective compromise solution which is used than a technically brilliant one which lies in the cupboard under the stairs.

1.2 Anatomical terminology

An understanding of the gross anatomy of the skeleton, and particularly the motions which occur at the different joints of the body, is essential to the understanding of biomechanics. The relevant anatomy of the various regions of the body will be considered in the subsequent chapters. However, it is useful to define here the basic terms relating to the body planes and the body segment movements.

1.2.1 Description of position

Figure 1.1 shows the human figure positioned in the *standard anatomical position* intersected by three imaginary perpendicular 'mid-planes'. The *sagittal* plane divides the body into symmetrical right and left halves, the *coronal* plane is the vertical plane at right-angles to the sagittal plane, which divides the body into front and back sections, and the *transverse* plane is the horizontal plane which divides the body into upper and lower sections. Whilst the diagram shows only 'mid-planes', the three terms are used to refer to any plane parallel to the appropriate mid-plane.

Positions within the body are described in relation to the three perpendicular planes. In relation to the sagittal plane, positions towards the mid-plane are referred to as *medial*, and those further away from the mid-plane are termed *lateral*; relative to the coronal plane, positions towards the front of the body are *anterior* and those towards the rear of the body are *posterior*; and in relation to the transverse plane, positions close to the centre of the body or trunk are referred to as *proximal* whilst those away from the centre as *distal*. For the foot, the terms *dorsal* and *plantar* are used to refer to its upper and lower surfaces, and for the hand the terms *dorsal* for the back and *palmar* or *volar* for the front are in common usage.

1.2.2 Movement of body segments

The movement of one body segment with respect to an adjacent body segment occurs about a joint at which the principal motions are rotational. The following terms are conventionally used to describe these motions.

In the sagittal plane, *flexion* refers to the 'bending' of a joint. At the hip this is a motion of the thigh anteriorly towards the pelvis, while at the knee, a posterior movement of the leg relative to the thigh is the movement of flexion. The opposite movement, which is termed *extension*, involves a straightening of the joint. The motions of flexion and extension give rise to joints which have positions described as *flexed* and *extended*. Special terminology is used for the foot and the hand. At the ankle, the term *dorsiflexion* describes a 'raising' of the foot, i.e. a movement of the dorsal aspect of the foot towards the leg, whilst *plantarflexion* is a 'pointing' of the foot, i.e. a movement of the dorsal aspect of the foot away from the leg. For the hand, *dorsiflexion* is a rotation which moves the back (dorsum) of the hand towards the forearm, and *palmar flexion* is the rotation which moves the front (palm) of the hand towards the forearm.

In the coronal plane, *abduction* is a movement of a distal segment away from the midline of the body, and *adduction* is the movement of the distal segment towards the midline. The motion of abduction leads to a distal segment which is *abducted* or in *valgus*, and the motion of adduction leads to a distal segment which is

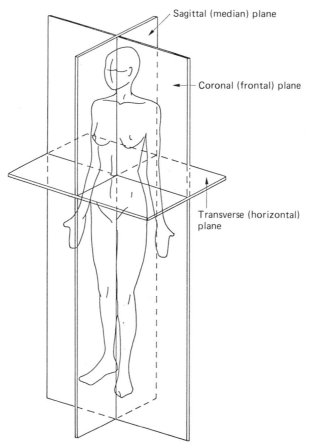

Figure 1.1 Body planes used to define body segment movements
(Reproduced with permission from Palastanga *et al.*, 1991)

adducted or in *varus*. Again special terminology is used for the foot and hand. For the foot, *inversion* is the motion of the foot in the coronal plane such that its plantar surface faces medially, and *eversion* is the motion of the foot in the coronal plane such that the plantar surface faces laterally. For the hand, *ulnar deviation* is rotation of the hand away from the midline and *radial deviation* is rotation towards the midline. In addition, coronal plane bending of the trunk is referred to as *lateral flexion*.

In the transverse plane, *internal rotation* is the motion causing the anterior surface of the distal segment to rotate medially relative to the proximal segment, and *external rotation* is the converse motion causing the anterior surface of the distal segment to rotate laterally relative to the proximal segment. These two motions lead to joint positions described as *internally rotated* and *externally rotated*, respectively. For the wrist, *supination* (with the arm in the ana-

tomical position) causes the palm to face anteriorly and *pronation* to face posteriorly.

1.2.3 Special motion of the foot

Although the three planar motions of the foot have been named individually, in practice, because of the nature of the subtalar joint complex, functional motion of the foot relative to the lower leg occurs in all three planes simultaneously and is termed either *supination* or *pronation*.

Supination is motion of the foot, relative to the leg, which involves simultaneous inversion, plantarflexion and internal rotation. Pronation is a motion of the foot, relative to the leg, which involves simultaneous eversion, dorsiflexion and external rotation. Note that in some older texts, the terms inversion and eversion are used instead of supination and pronation.

Some apparent ambiguity exists in the naming of positions and motions of the foot. This is because, although most other segments of the body tend to lie with their major axes in the sagittal and coronal planes, intersected by the transverse plane, the neutral position of the foot is such that its major axis lies in the transverse plane. Thus, some authors use the terms abduction and adduction instead of external rotation and internal rotation because, even though it is a transverse plane motion, it has historically been perceived as motion occurring in the 'foot coronal plane'. In this situation the reference axis passes through the centre of the hindfoot and along the second ray. This approach to terminology is still apparent in the names of many foot pathologies, for example, the common condition whereby the big toe lies across the adjacent second toe (resulting in a bunion) is termed hallux abducto-valgus.

Reference

Palastanga N., Field D. and Soames R. (1991) *Anatomy and Human Movement*. Butterworth-Heinemann, Oxford

2

An update in essential mechanics

Peter Bowker

2.1 Introduction

The aim of this chapter is to present a concise review of those aspects of mechanics which are relevant to orthotic function. *Mechanics* is about creating or preventing motion. It is therefore concerned with the description and analysis of motion itself and with the forces which either maintain an object in static equilibrium or cause it to move in some particular way. Finally, mechanics deals also with how forces are carried within components and how, as a result, these components may be deformed and ultimately damaged. *Biomechanics* is the application of the principles and techniques of mechanics to living things and to pieces of hardware, like orthoses, intimately attached to living things.

A fundamental difficulty in mechanics is that many of its most basic terms, for example force, work and energy, are words which are used every day but have a wide variety of meanings. In mechanics, these terms have very particular and precise definitions and a short glossary of these and other essential terms is included at the end of this chapter. A particular difficulty arises with the word *body*. Whereas in the biological sciences a 'body' refers specifically to the material frame of an animal, in mechanics it is the general term used to describe any physical object, animate or inanimate. The word has therefore been avoided and the term *object* used instead to refer to any physical entity, including the human body. However, lacking any alternat-

ive, the term *free-body*, which refers to an object or part of an object isolated from its surroundings, has been retained.

This chapter is presented in four sections. These deal firstly with the nature of forces themselves and their manipulation (Section 2.2), secondly with the analysis of objects which are at rest (Section 2.3; *statics*), then with objects which are in motion (Section 2.4; *dynamics*) and finally with the mechanics or deformation of materials (Section 2.5). Before moving onto those sections however it is necessary to briefly discuss the units of measurement which will be used.

2.1.1 SI units

The SI system of units, used throughout this book, is based on a series of core units. Those relevant to mechanics are shown in Table 2.1 together with their symbols. The SI system also provides a useful series of multiples to enable particularly large or small quantities to be conveniently described. These multiples, the most important of which are listed in Table 2.2,

Table 2.1 SI core units

Quantity	Name of unit	SI symbol
Length	metre	m
Mass	kilogram	kg
Time	second	s
Force	Newton	N
Plane angle	radian	rad

Table 2.2 Multiples used with SI units

Prefix name	SI symbol	Multiplying factor
micro-	μ	10^{-6}
milli-	m	10^{-3}
kilo-	k	10^3
mega-	M	10^6
giga-	G	10^9

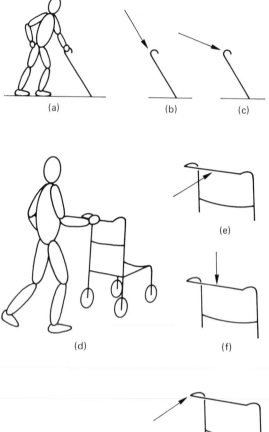

are attached as prefixes to the units, for example mm for millimetre (10^{-3}m). Similarly, 1234000 N may also be written as 1.234×10^6 N, 1.234 MN or 1234 kN.

When units are multiplied together as in newtons × metres, they are written Nm without punctuation. When units are divided, as in metres per second, the dividing quantity is shown with a −1 superscript, e.g. ms^{-1}.

2.2 Forces and their manipulation

Forces make things move, stop things moving, or make things change shape. They are, in common parlance, pushes or pulls. In the SI system of units, forces are measured in newtons (N).

Figure 2.1 shows two situations in which a force is being applied to an object. In each case, it is clear that the outcome of the application of that force will depend not only upon the *magnitude* (size) of the force applied but also on its *direction*.

Depending on the size and direction of the force applied to the walking stick, it may tend to bend (Figure 2.1(b)) or to slide along the ground (Figure 2.1(c)); depending on the size and direction of the force applied to the push-chair handle, the push-chair may travel forward, slowly or quickly (Figure 2.1(e)), or tip backwards (Figure 2.1(f)). All forces thus have two characteristics – magnitude and direction – and both need to be stated in order to describe the force fully. Force is a *vector* quantity, which simply means it has both direction and magnitude.

In addition, the precise effect of a force will depend upon the point on the object at which the force is applied, that is its *point of application*. A force identical to that in Figure 2.1(e), but applied to the push-chair handle at one end

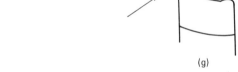

Figure 2.1 (a)–(g) The effect of a force depends upon its magnitude, its direction and its point of application

(Figure 2.1(g)), would tend to rotate the chair rather than to move it forward in a straight line.

2.2.1 Weight force and mass

All objects are made up of a certain amount of substance. The quantity of substance in an object is referred to as its *mass*. It is, in effect, a measure of the number of molecules or atoms which it contains. So long as no material is taken away from it, nor new material added, the mass of an object remains constant whatever new shape it is pressed or pulled into and wherever in the Universe it is taken. Mass is measured in kilograms (kg).

Any object having mass exerts a force of attraction on every other object. The strength of the pull is related to the masses of the two objects and the distance between them. For everyday objects, even when they are close together, this force is insignificant. However, the Earth itself is very large and all objects near or on the Earth experience an attractive force pulling them towards its centre. It is this force of attraction between the Earth and an object that we refer to as its *weight*.

Thus, whilst an object always has the same mass, its weight depends on how far it is from the centre of the Earth and therefore its weight changes with its height above the Earth's surface or its position on the Earth, because our planet is not truly spherical. However, for most practical purposes this variation is negligible, and it may be taken that the weight of an object is about 9.8 N for each kilogram of its mass. This factor is symbolized by g (for gravity). The relationship between mass and weight is thus given by the simple equation $W = mg$, where m is the mass in kg, g is the gravity value or weight per kilogram of mass in Nkg^{-1}, and W is the weight force. Thus the magnitude of the weight force is known as its direction, which is always vertically downwards.

However, in order to fully define the weight force, its effective point of application on an object must also be defined. That point, referred to as the *centre of gravity* of the object, is in effect identical to a point called the *centre of mass* which is the point at which the mass of the object is considered to be concentrated. For a symmetrical object such as a strip of metal or plastic (Figure 2.2(a)) the centre of mass will be situated at its geometric centre; for non-symmetrical objects, such as a foot or a shoe (Figure 2.2(b)) the centre of mass is situated at a point somewhere inside the object about which it will exactly balance. Note that in the case of the shoe, the centre of mass is located within the space enclosed by the shoe, rather than within the actual material of the shoe.

For an object of variable shape, such as the human body, the precise position of the centre of mass will clearly change with the positions of the limbs and body segments, and for any particular position may lie inside or outside the body (Figure 2.2(c) and (d)). In the standard anatomical position, the centre of mass of the adult lies within the pelvis in front of the upper part of the sacrum, its exact location depending on the build, sex and age of the individual.

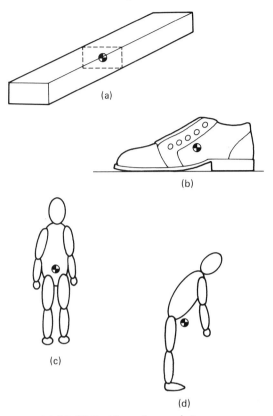

Figure 2.2 (a)–(d) Positions of centres of mass

2.2.2 Adding and resolving forces

In practical biomechanical problems, the limbs or orthoses which are analysed will usually be subjected to a number of forces acting in various directions. Often, we will wish to 'add' these forces together to determine their overall or resultant effect. However, as forces are vectors, that is, they have direction as well as magnitude, they cannot simply be added numerically. If all the forces involved act along the same line they can be added *algebraically* – that is forces acting in one direction are regarded as positive, whilst those acting in the opposite direction are regarded as negative. If, in Figure 2.3, forces acting to the right are positive, the resultant forces in the two cases are $50 + (-40) = 10$ N (positive, therefore to the right) in Figure 2.3(a), and $25 + (-100) = -75$ N (negative, therefore to be left) in Figure 2.3(b). Clearly, two equal and opposite forces give rise to a zero resultant as in Figure 2.3(c).

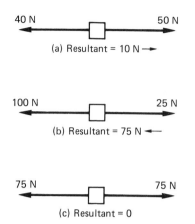

40 N   50 N

(a) Resultant = 10 N →

100 N   25 N

(b) Resultant = 75 N ←

75 N   75 N

(c) Resultant = 0

Figure 2.3 (a)–(c) Algebraic addition of forces acting along the same line

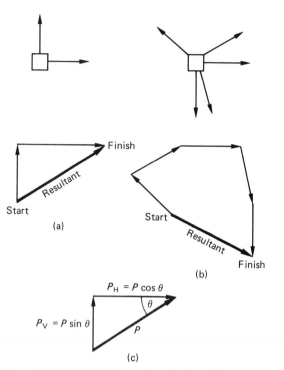

Finish

Resultant

Start

(a)

Start

Resultant

Finish

(b)

$P_H = P \cos \theta$

θ

$P_V = P \sin \theta$

P

(c)

Figure 2.4 (a)–(c) Addition and resolution of forces

If, however, the forces involved do not act along the same line, they need to be added using geometrical methods. Vectors are added graphically by drawing to scale the individual vectors nose to tail, in any order from some starting point to the finishing point. The total or *resultant* vector is then the single straight line connecting the starting point to the finishing point. If two vectors are added, the resulting figure is a triangle as shown in Figure 2.4(a). If five vectors are added, a six-sided polygon is the result as seen in Figure 2.4(b), and so on. In each case the effect of the single resultant force is identical to the effects of all the individual forces acting together.

However, as constructing scale drawings is time consuming and inaccurate, in practice the magnitude and direction of the resultant vector are nearly always obtained by calculation using a knowledge of the angles and side lengths of the geometrical figure. Such calculations can be complex if there are many forces acting but examination of Figure 2.4(a), which is a special case in which two perpendicular forces have been added to give a single resultant force, suggests a simple approach to calculating the sum of a number of vectors. Redrawing this arrangement as in Figure 2.4(c) reveals that any force F acting at an angle θ to the horizontal can be replaced by two forces (speaking formally: can be *resolved* into two *components*) P_H and P_V which act at right angles to each other; P_H in the horizontal direction and P_V in the vertical direction. Whilst it is usually easiest if the two perpendicular forces are

taken to be horizontal and vertical, this is not essential; they may be inclined at any angle so long as they remain at right angles to each other. The two components acting together have an identical effect to the single resultant, and are related to it by simple trigonometry:

$P_H = P\cos \theta$
$P_V = P\cos (90 - \theta) = P\sin \theta$

Thus, in order to add together any number of forces, acting in any direction, firstly it is necessary to calculate the vertical and horizontal components of each force. All the horizontal forces are then added together and then all the vertical forces (taking care to subtract those acting in the opposite direction). Finally the total horizontal and vertical forces can be combined to obtain the magnitude and direction of the resultant force using the relationships:

$$P = \sqrt{P_H^2 + P_V^2}: \tan \theta = \frac{P_V}{P_H}$$

The use of this procedure is illustrated in the worked example on page 13.

2.2.3 Forces and moments

Referring back to the wheelchair in Figure 2.1, it is clear that forces can cause objects to do two quite different things: to move in a straight line (*translate*) or to turn (*rotate*). Whether, in any particular situation, a body will tend to do the former, the latter, or indeed both, depends upon the way in which the object is able to move and on the direction and point of application of the force. Pushing forwards on the centre of the wheelchair handle causes it to move in a straight line; pushing the handle vertically downwards causes it to rotate about its rear wheels.

The turning effect of a force about a point is known as its *moment*. Its magnitude is proportional both to the magnitude of the force and to the perpendicular distance from the pivot to the line of action of the force. In Figure 2.5(a) the moment M of the force F about the knee joint centre is given by

$$M = Pl$$

where l is often referred to as the *moment arm*. Clearly then the force which must be applied to produce the turning effect necessary to raise the limb reduces as the moment arm is increased. It is thus always most efficient to apply a force as far away from the pivot or fulcrum as possible. Note that the units of moment are force × distance, that is Newtons × metres (Nm), and that is is usual to take clockwise moments as being positive, and anticlockwise moments as being negative.

Two possible situations in which the limb is pushed obliquely are shown in Figure 2.5(b) and (c). In these cases the moment arm is again the perpendicular distance, but this is now reduced to $l\cos\theta$ because the direction of the force is no longer perpendicular to the leg. Ideally then, to achieve maximum turning effect, the force would always be applied in the optimum direction with $\theta = 0°$ or perpendicularly. In the other extreme case in which $\theta = 90°$, as in Figure 2.5(d), the moment is zero; the line of action of the force passes through the pivot resulting in a moment arm of zero length.

Another way to calculate the moment of an inclined force is to break the force up into two perpendicular components. In Figure 2.5(b), the components along and perpendicular to the axis of the leg are $P\sin\theta$ and $P\cos\theta$ respect-

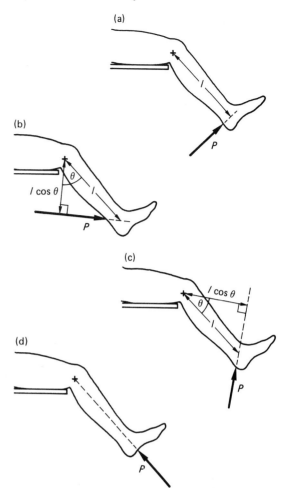

Figure 2.5 (a)–(d) Calculating the moment of a force

ively. The first of these acts through the pivot and has zero moment, the second has a moment arm l. The total moment is thus $P\cos\theta \times l$, which is exactly the same as the result found by the previous method. In practice, any pair of rectangular components has the same moment as the original force.

There are two further points about moments which are important. Firstly, a force can be considered to have a moment about any point, and that point may be inside or outside the object on which the force is acting. In Figure 2.6(a) a wheelchair is subjected to an upward angled push P on its handles. If the chair is standing against a low kerb, the moment tending to tip it forwards, about the pivot or fulcrum A, is $P \times d$ clockwise; if it rests against an obstruction at seat height, so that it

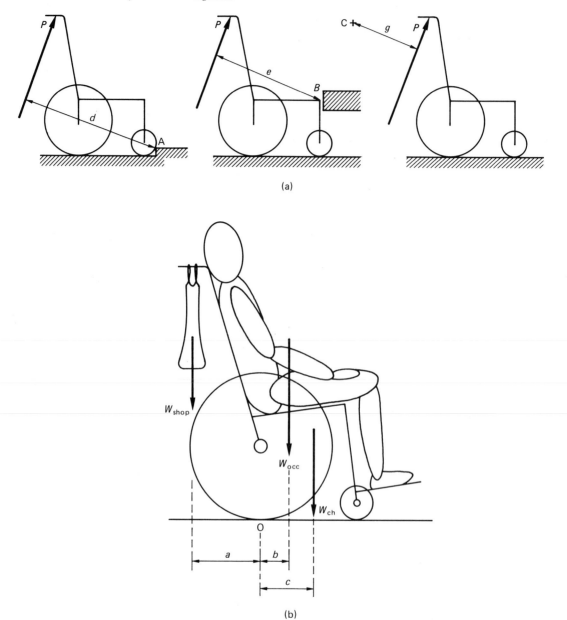

Figure 2.6 (a),(b) Moments on a wheelchair and occupant

rotates about B, the moment is $P \times e$ clockwise. The moment of the force P about some non-specific point C, which may allow a problem-solving equation to be developed, although the position of point C is of no practical significance, thus calculated is $P \times g$ anticlockwise.

Secondly, moments of individual forces about the same point can be added algebraically to obtain the total turning effect of the forces on an object. In Figure 2.6(b), the total moment on the wheelchair, its occupant and his shopping, about O, the point about which tipping would occur, is $W_{ch} \times c + W_{occ} \times b - W_{shop} \times a$ clockwise. The chair would tip over backwards if, following a visit to the supermarket, $W_{shop} \times a > W_{ch} \times c + W_{occ} \times b$.

A *couple* is a pair of equal and opposite forces acting on parallel lines. A couple has no translational effect because the vector sum of the two forces is zero, but it has a moment about any point of value F*l*, where *F* is the magnitude of the force and *l* is the perpendicular distance between the two forces.

Finally, whereas a moment is a rotational effect generated by a force applied at a distance, such as when using a spanner, a *torque* is a directly applied 'twisting force' such as in using a screwdriver. Rather than applying a particular force at a particular point, it is distributed around the pivot. Torque is measured in newton-metres (Nm) and can be treated as a 'ready made' moment.

2.3 Statics

In statics we apply the fundamental concepts of mechanics, force and moment, to the analysis of objects which are at rest. A good place to start is with the laws formulated by Newton.

2.3.1 Newton's laws

Sir Isaac Newton in 1687 published three simple laws which together enshrine the fundamental principles of mechanics. In looking at objects which are at rest, we need deal with only two of these laws, the first and the third, and it is helpful to deal with the third first.

Newton's third law

If one object exerts a force on a second object, then the second object exerts an equal and opposite reaction force on the first object. The person in Figure 2.7(a) is exerting a weight force on the floor. The floor must then be exerting an equal and opposite force on the person. Similarly, if the strap in Figure 2.7(b) is exerting a force on a limb, the limb must be exerting an equal and opposite force on the strap.

Newton's first law

If there is no resultant force acting upon it, a body will remain at rest [or will continue to move in a straight line with constant velocity]. As we are only dealing with objects which are

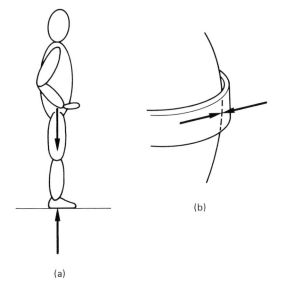

(b)

(a)

Figure 2.7 (a),(b) Newton's third law: to every action there is an equal and opposite reaction

stationary at present we need only concern ourselves with the first part of this first law: the final part, in square brackets, will be referred to in Section 2.4 which deals with moving objects. Thus the first law tells us that a stationary object will remain stationary if no resultant force acts upon it. This does not mean no force at all – in practice there must at least be a weight force – but rather that the forces are balanced so that there is no resultant, as shown in Figure 2.3(c). In addition, although the first law does not explicitly say so, the moments acting on the object must also be balanced so there is not only translational equilibrium but also rotational equilibrium.

2.3.2 Static equilibrium

The concept of static equilibrium is of the greatest importance in biomechanics because it enables us to calculate the values of forces which are unknown. Newton's first law tells us that if there is no resultant force or moment a stationary body will remain at rest. The reverse statement – that if a body is stationary there is no resultant force or moment acting upon it – is the *principle of static equilibrium*.

Thus we know that for any object at rest, the algebraic sum of the forces on the object, in any direction, is zero, and the algebraic sum of the moments acting on the object, about any point, is zero. This enables us to formulate a total of three equations of static equilibrium – two in which the algebraic sum of the forces in any two perpendicular directions is equated to zero ($\Sigma R_x = 0$, $\Sigma R_y = 0$), plus a third in which the algebraic sum of the moments about any point is equated to zero ($\Sigma M = 0$).

2.3.3 Free body analysis

Thus we have a framework for analysing the forces on any static object and thereby determining the size of unknown forces. There are, however, some difficulties in applying this procedure.

Let us suppose that for the climber negotiating an overhang shown in Figure 2.8, we wish to calculate the forces exerted on the rock by his hands and feet. First we draw onto the diagram all the forces acting – the weight force acting through the climber's centre of mass and the forces exerted on the rock by the climber, showing each of these as vertical and horizontal components. However, because New-

ton's third law states that every force has an equal and opposite reaction, the forces exerted on the rock by the climber must be opposed by equal and opposite forces exerted on the climber by the rock. Thus the complete picture is as shown in Figure 2.8(a).

The application of the principle of static equilibrium achieves little – the unknown forces do not appear in any of the equations which can be formulated because the actions and reactions cancel out. In order to solve this problem, some way has to be found to split up these equal and opposite pairs of forces.

In fact this is relatively easily done by, in effect, removing the climber from the rock face and thus isolating him from the environment around him. The drawing of the isolated climber (Figure 2.8(b)) will then show all the forces acting upon it, but *not*, of course, the forces exerted by it on its external environment. Thus application of the principles of static equilibrium to this diagram should now enable the values of the unknown forces to be calculated very easily. The item isolated from

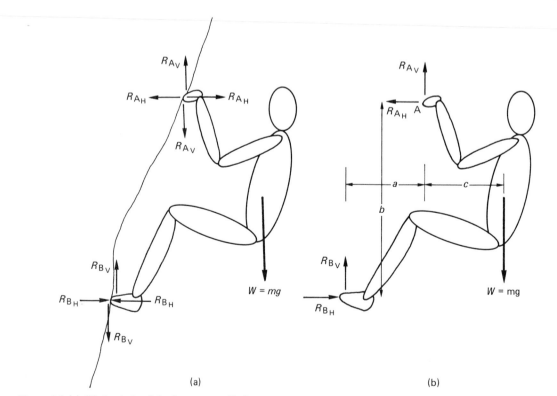

Figure 2.8 (a),(b) Analysis of the forces on a climber

its surroundings is known as a *free body*, and the drawing of its outline showing all the forces acting on it is a *free body diagram*.

Unfortunately, as frequently happens in biomechanical analysis, there are more unknown quantities than there are equations. In this case there are four unknowns (R_{A_H}, R_{A_V}, R_{B_H}, R_{B_V}) but only the three equations of equilibrium (sum of moments about any point is zero; sum of forces in two orthogonal directions is zero). In order to obtain a solution therefore, a fourth equation is required. To obtain this, let us assume that the climber's weight is shared between his hands and feet in the ratio ¼ : ¾. Thus:

$$R_{B_V} = 3R_{A_V}$$

Then considering the equilibrium of vertical forces ($\Sigma R_V = 0$)

$$R_{B_V} + R_{A_V} = W, \text{ so } R_{B_V} = \frac{3W}{4} : R_{A_V} = \frac{W}{4}$$

From the equilibrium of horizontal forces ($\Sigma R_H = 0$)

$$R_{A_H} = R_{B_H}$$

and from the equilibrium of moments about A ($\Sigma M_A = 0$)

$$R_{B_H} \times b = \frac{3W}{4} \times a + W \times c$$

$$\therefore R_{A_H} = R_{B_H} = \frac{W}{b}\left(\frac{3a}{4} + c\right)$$

Inserting realistic values $a = 0.25$ m, $b = 1.2$ m, $c = 0.25$ m, gives

$$R_{A_H} = R_{B_H} = 0.36W$$

Referring now to Figure 2.9, the resultant force exerted by the rock on the climber at A is

$$R_A = W\sqrt{0.36^2 + 0.25^2} = 0.44W$$

at an angle of $\theta = \tan^{-1}\dfrac{0.25}{0.36} = 34.8°$ to the horizontal

and at B

$$R_B = W\sqrt{0.36^2 + 0.75^2} = 0.83W$$

at an angle of $\theta = \tan^{-1}\dfrac{0.75}{0.36} = 64.4°$ to the horizontal.

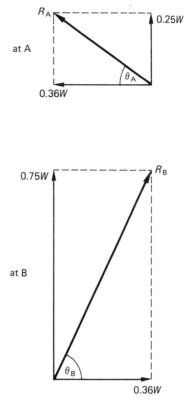

Figure 2.9 Calculation of magnitude and direction of resultant forces exerted by the rock on the climber

The forces exerted by the climber on the rock are equal and opposite to these.

Note what every climber knows – that the forces on the fingertips are reduced by keeping the body as close to the rock as possible (i.e. by reducing c) and by keeping the hands as high as possible (i.e. by increasing b).

As a further example, we may also wish to calculate the force in the climber's quadriceps muscle at the instant we are considering. However, this force does not even appear in our diagram, neither this nor any other muscle or joint force in the climber's body, because all internal forces, which have actions and reactions and therefore cancel out, have been ignored and only external forces shown. To determine such a muscle force, it is necessary to create a new free body by severing action and reaction so the unknown force becomes an external force. Such a free body with all external forces marked is shown in Figure 2.10.

The procedure for determining an unknown force either inside the body or on its surface can thus be described in three steps:

1. Isolate the free body by cutting around it so that the unknown force or forces required appear as external forces. The cut may be any shape and in any direction.
2. Onto the free body draw all the external forces acting. Clearly if one or more external forces are omitted from the free body diagram, erroneous results will be obtained so it is essential none are missed. In general, all free bodies will have a weight force acting through their centre of mass and will experience a surface force, with a normal and tangential component wherever material has been cut to create the free body. Some forces such as buoyancy or aerodynamic drag may be relevant in particular situations, whilst others such as electrostatic and magnetic forces will never normally need to be considered.

3. Formulate the three equations of equilibrium and manipulate these to yield the required values.

Applying these three steps to the calculation of the force in the climber's quadriceps:

1. The relevant free body of one lower leg, created by cutting through the knee, is shown in Figure 2.10.
2. The external forces acting on this free body are its weight force (assumed to equal $W/16$), the horizontal and vertical reactions at the rock (half the values for the two limbs found previously), the normal and tangential components of the joint force acting on the top of the tibia, and the force in the quadriceps tendon. This force must act along the line of action of the tendon – for the anatomical position considered at about 30° to the horizontal. The key dimensions from the point of contact of the force J with the tibia are also shown in Figure 2.10.

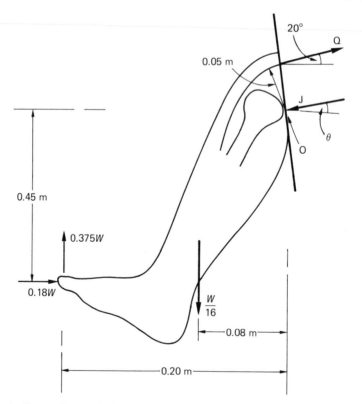

Figure 2.10 Free body diagram for calculation of force in climber's quadriceps

3. Equilibrium of moments about O ($\Sigma M_0 = 0$) then gives

$Q \times 0.05$ m $+ 0.375W \times 0.20$ m
$= 0.18W \times 0.45$ m $+ W/16 \times 0.08$ m

from which Q, the force in the quadriceps muscle, is obtained as:

$Q = 0.22W$

The horizontal and vertical components of the knee joint force and hence the magnitude and direction of the resultant may now, if required, be obtained by considering the equilibrium of horizontal and vertical forces. The solution is obtained as $J = 0.55W$ at 45° to the horizontal.

2.4 Dynamics

The previous section of this chapter dealt with the analysis of forces and moments acting on bodies in equilibrium. This section, *dynamics*, is concerned with the motion of bodies which are not in equilibrium, and the forces and moments which produce these motions. Dynamics, like statics, is based on Newton's laws of motion. However, before looking again at Newton's laws, three terms used to describe motion must be introduced: *displacement*, *velocity* and *acceleration*. The definitions of these terms, and the equations which interrelate them, depend upon whether the motion which is occurring is translational motion in a straight line or rotational motion along a circular path. We will briefly look at each of these in turn.

2.4.1 Translational motion

If a runner sets off from some point and runs along a straight path at increasing speed, three parameters are required to fully define his motion at any point; displacement, velocity and acceleration. *Displacement* measures the runner's change in position and is the straight-line distance between the starting point and the point being considered. For straight-line motion, displacement and distance are numerically the same, but displacement, like force, is a vector quantity and therefore requires both a magnitude and a direction to fully specify it. In Figure 2.11(a), the displacement of the runner

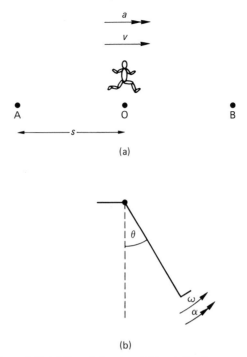

Figure 2.11 (a) Translational and (b) rotational displacement, velocity and acceleration

at O may be, for example, 15 m to the right. Linear displacement is usually denoted by s.

Velocity is the time rate of change of position, and again being a vector expresses both the magnitude and direction of motion at a particular instant of time. As the magnitude of velocity is called speed, velocity comprises speed and direction and thus a change in either or both of these is a change in velocity. The common units for velocity are metres per second (ms^{-1}), so the velocity of the runner at O may be 2.5 ms^{-1} to the right. Linear velocity is usually denoted by v. For the special case in which the runner is moving with constant velocity, his velocity from A to O could be obtained from $v = s/t$ where t is the time taken.

In the same way as velocity is the time rate of change of position, *acceleration* is the time rate of change of velocity: it is the rate of speeding up. Acceleration is also a vector quantity and is defined at a particular instant of time. Note that if either the magnitude or the direction of velocity, or both, change, then there is an acceleration. In biomechanical problems any accelerations will usually be assumed to be constant. Common units for acceleration are metres per second per second (ms^{-2}), so the acceleration of the runner at O may be 2 ms^{-2} to the right. (His acceleration would be to the left if he were slowing down.) Linear acceleration is usually denoted by a.

The following four equations describing the motion of an object undergoing constant acceleration are often useful in solving problems involving motion:

$$v = u + at$$
$$v^2 = u^2 + 2as$$
$$s = ut + \tfrac{1}{2}at^2$$
$$s = \tfrac{1}{2}(u+v)t$$

where u is initial velocity, v is final velocity, a is acceleration, s is distance travelled and t is time taken.

2.4.2 Rotational motion

For rotational motion the corresponding quantities and units are *angular displacement* θ in radians, *angular velocity* ω (in rad s^{-1}) and *angular acceleration* α (in rad s^{-1}) as shown in Figure 2.11(b).

Corresponding equations also interrelate the various quantities:

for constant angular velocity

$$\omega = \theta/t$$

for constant angular acceleration

$$\omega_2 = \omega_1 + \alpha t$$
$$\omega_2{}^2 = \omega_1{}^2 + 2\alpha\theta$$
$$\theta = \omega_1 t + \tfrac{1}{2}\alpha t^2$$
$$\theta = \tfrac{1}{2}(\omega_1+\omega_2)t$$

where ω_1 is the initial angular velocity, ω_2 is the final angular velocity, α is angular acceleration, θ is the angle moved through and t is the time taken.

When an object, such as a limb, has rotational motion, then any point on that limb, such as P in Figure 2.12(a), has translational motion. Thus, at any instant, P has a linear displacement. In Figure 2.12(b), the limb has rotated through an angle θ, so the point P has moved along a circumferential path of length $r\theta$ where θ is in radians. If the angle θ is small,

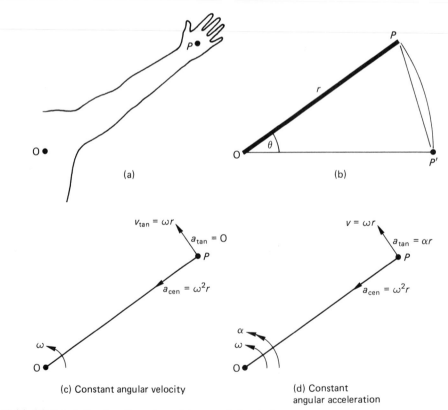

(a)

(b)

(c) Constant angular velocity

(d) Constant angular acceleration

Figure 2.12 (a)–(d) Translational motion of a point on a rotating body

this arc length will approximate to the chord length PP^1 which is the displacement of the point.

In addition, the point P has a linear velocity. As the displacement is instantaneously perpendicular to the radius line, the velocity is instantaneously tangential to the circular path and is hence called the tangential velocity. This linear velocity is given by the equation $v_{tan} = \omega r$, Figure 2.12(c).

If we assume for the moment that the limb is rotating with constant angular velocity, that is ω is constant, although the magnitude of v_{tan} is constant, as rotation proceeds, its direction constantly changes. P thus has an acceleration by virtue of its motion along a circular path, albeit at constant angular velocity. This acceleration is directed towards the centre of the circular path and is hence known as centripetal acceleration. Its value is given by the equation $a_{cen} = \omega^2 r = v^2/r$.

If now there is in addition an angular acceleration of the limb, α, ω and v will be instantaneous values and P will experience a tangential acceleration given by $a_{tan} = \alpha r$. The point P thus experiences two accelerations at right angles, a_{tan} and a_{cen}, as shown in Figure 2.12(d).

Having now dealt with the quantities describing motion, we can look at the relationship between the quantities and the force which causes the motion. For this, we need to return to Newton's Laws.

2.4.3 Newton's laws revisited

The first and third of Newton's Laws of Motion have already been stated and the third law and the first part of the first law have been used in solving problems concerned with objects at rest. For solving problems in dynamics the remainder of the first law and the second law are also required.

The first law says that if the forces acting on an object are balanced, that is in equilibrium, then the body remains at rest *or continues to move with constant velocity*. The first part of this law is straightforward enough – no resultant force, no motion. The second part however is less easy, for it says that once an object is moving, it will continue to move indefinitely in the same way without needing any force to be applied to it. In other words,

forces are only required to change motion, that is to cause accelerations.

This idea is a big problem in mechanics because it does not tie in with our everyday experience. We naturally make a fundamental distinction between rest and motion. We know that we must make an effort to keep moving and thus it appears that a force is necessary to maintain motion. The discrepancy between theory and experience is however easily explained. In practice there are always forces present which resist motion and which therefore must be balanced by some driving force in order to maintain steady motion. Objects sliding or rolling along have friction forces acting on them which always tend to decelerate them and bring them to rest. Air resistance has the same effect. For movement of the human body, forces are required to accelerate the limbs and bring them to rest again on each step; forces are also required to accelerate the body vertically because its centre of mass rises and falls with each stride. So an effort is needed to keep moving at a constant velocity – but only because the forces acting against motion must be balanced.

Thus, whilst under equilibrium conditions motion continues unchanged at constant velocity, unbalanced forces cause changes in motion, that is accelerations. The relationship between the magnitude of the unbalanced force which acts and the acceleration which results is given by Newton's second law.

Newton's second law

If there is an unbalanced force acting on an object, it experiences an acceleration in the direction of the force, proportional to the force and inversely proportional to its mass; mathematically this is written as:- $a = cF/m$, where a is acceleration, F is resultant force, m is mass and c is the constant of proportionality. In the SI system of units, c has been chosen to be unity, so $F = ma$, and the relationship effectively gives a definition of the unit of force. Thus if mass is expressed in kg and the acceleration in ms^{-2}, the force F is given in Newtons. That is $1\,N = 1\,kgms^{-2}$. Thus the relationship between the unbalanced force and the resulting straight-line motion of an object is established.

A similar relationship exists for rotating objects. In this case the equation is $M = I\alpha$ where

M is the moment of force, I the *second moment of mass* or the *moment of inertia* and α is the magnitude of the angular acceleration about some chosen axis. I (which has units of kgm^2 or Nms^2) is a measure of the mass distribution of the object about the axis of interest; its values about the centres of mass of a homogeneous solid cylinder, hollow cylinder and rectangular bar are shown in Figure 2.13. Values of I about any other point O are given by $I_o = I_G + mh^2$ where I_G is the value about the centre of mass, m is the mass of the object and h is the distance between G and O. Sometimes the second moment of mass is expressed in terms of the *radius of gyration* of the object, k. The relationship is then $I = mk^2$.

2.4.4 Solutions to dynamics problems

The key to solving dynamics problems is the same as that for statics problems – the free body diagram. However, instead of equating the resultant forces and moments to zero, the resultant forces will equal ma_x and ma_y, and the resultant moment $I\alpha$. It will also sometimes be necessary to use the equations relating linear and angular displacements, velocities and accelerations. In the following example, we examine the biomechanics of the lower leg during walking and look at the effects of adding an orthosis.

Figure 2.14(a) shows a tracing from a sagittal plane video recording of a subject walking barefoot taken at the instant at which the forward angular acceleration of the lower leg about the knee was a maximum. This peak value was 25 rad s^{-2} and occurred when the angle between the segment axis and the vertical was 40°. At the same instant, the angular velocity of the limb was 1.4 rad s^{-1}. Using the body weight of the subject and the overall segment length, standard anatomical data tables provided the following values:

mass of lower leg and foot = 4.5 kg

distance from knee centre to centre of mass = 0.25 m

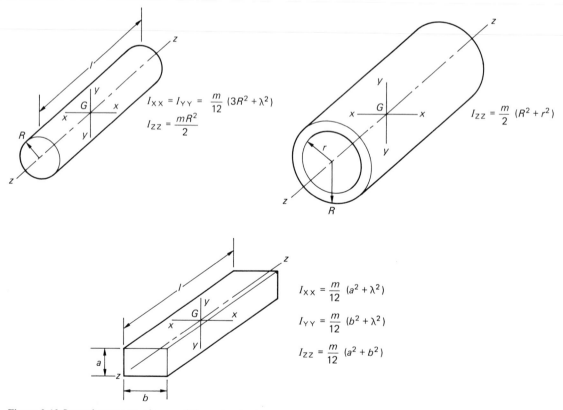

$$I_{XX} = I_{YY} = \frac{m}{12}(3R^2 + \lambda^2)$$

$$I_{ZZ} = \frac{mR^2}{2}$$

$$I_{ZZ} = \frac{m}{2}(R^2 + r^2)$$

$$I_{XX} = \frac{m}{12}(a^2 + \lambda^2)$$

$$I_{YY} = \frac{m}{12}(b^2 + \lambda^2)$$

$$I_{ZZ} = \frac{m}{12}(a^2 + b^2)$$

Figure 2.13 Second moments of mass of three simple shapes

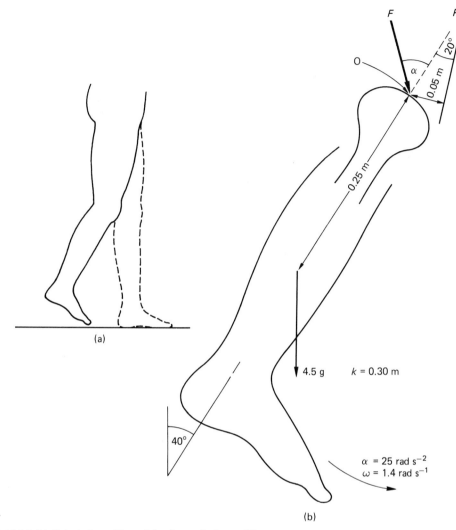

Figure 2.14 (a),(b) Calculation of knee joint forces during walking

radius of gyration about axis through knee = 0.30 m

The free body diagram of the lower leg (Figure 2.14(b)) shows the weight force (4.5 kg), the joint force, F, assumed to act through the centre of rotation, O, and significant muscle forces – in this instance, as the knee is extending, the force in the quadriceps, P. Examination of the video image indicated that at the instant of interest, the line of action of the quadriceps force (in the quadriceps tendon) was at 20° to the vertical as shown, and from anatomical measurement the moment arm of this force about the knee joint centre was estimated to be 0.05 m.

Analysis of the free body diagram then yields three equations which enable the calculation of the three unknowns – the muscle force and the magnitude and direction of the joint force. First, applying $\Sigma M = I\alpha$ about O gives the value of P:

$$4.5g \times 0.25 \sin 40 + P \times 0.05 = (4.5 \times 0.3^2) \times 25$$

$$7.08 + 0.05P = 10.13$$
$$P = 61 \text{ N}$$

Then consideration of forces along and perpendicular to the axis of the limb, and use of $\Sigma F = ma$ gives:

along limb axis: $P\cos20 - F\cos\alpha - 4.5\ g\cos40$
$= ma_{cen} = 4.5 \times 1.4^2 \times 0.25$
$57.32 - F\cos\alpha - 33.78 = 2.205$
$\qquad\qquad F\cos\alpha = 21.33$

perp. to limb: $-P\sin20 + F\sin\alpha + 4.5\ g\sin40$
$= ma_{tan} = 4.5 \times 25 \times 0.25$
$-20.8 + F\sin\alpha + 28.3 = 28.13$
$\qquad\qquad F\sin\alpha = 20.63$

from which $F = \sqrt{21.33^2 + 20.63^2} = 29.67$:
$F = 29.7N$

$$\tan\alpha = \frac{20.63}{21.33} : \alpha = 44°$$

Thus, during barefoot walking, at this instant in the gait cycle, the quadriceps tendon force is 61 N and the joint reaction force is 30 N; both, as would be expected, very low values.

If the subject is now fitted with a below-knee outside iron and a pair of 'sensible' shoes (total mass 1.5 kg), the resulting free body diagram is as shown in Figure 2.15. If the maximum

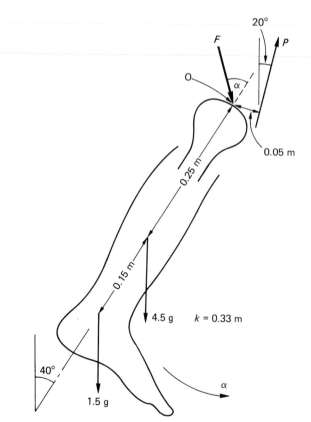

Figure 2.15 Free body diagram of lower leg with shoes and orthosis added

angulation acceleration remains 25 rad s^{-2}, applying $\Sigma M = I\alpha$ about the axis of rotation through the knee now gives:

$1.5\ g \times 0.4\sin40 + 4.5\ g \times 0.25\sin40 + 0.05P$
$\qquad\qquad\qquad = 6 \times 0.33^2 \times 25$
$3.78 + 7.09 + 0.05\ P = 16.13$
$\qquad\qquad\qquad P = 105.2\ N$

This would indicate that for the same gait speed and pattern as was achieved in walking barefoot, the quadriceps force has to be increased by 72% to 105 N. Conversely, the same equation can be used to show that if the muscle force remains unaltered from the barefoot case at 61 N, the maximum angular acceleration of the lower leg must be reduced to 21.6 rad s^{-2}. If then the assumption is made that during the swing phase of walking the lower leg accelerates uniformly from rest at toe off, when its angle to the vertical is 50°, to a maximum angular velocity when the lower leg is at an angle of 25° to the vertical, and decelerates similarly, the reduction in walking speed resulting from reducing the angular acceleration/deceleration from 25 rad s^{-2} to 21.6 rad s^{-2} can be estimated from $\theta = \omega_1 t + \frac12\alpha t^2$ to be 11%.

A summary of key items of anthropometric data which will be required in solving biomechanics problems is presented in Table 2.3, and a listing of typical joint and muscle forces generated during a range of everyday activities is in Table 2.4. These data and the techniques used for estimating joint and muscle forces have been discussed by Dowson *et al.* (1981).

2.4.5 Work and energy

A force does *work* when the object on which it acts moves through a distance. Mathematically, the quantity of work done is given by the product of the magnitude of the force and the distance moved in the direction of the force. The unit of work is thus Newtons × metres (Nm) which has the special name of Joules (J).

Imagine now a small object of mass m kg at rest on a frictionless table as seen in Figure 2.16(a). It is in static equilibrium under the action of its weight force and the normal reaction force. If a horizontal force of F N is applied to the object it will accelerate in the direction of the force according to the relationship $F = ma$. If, after the object has travelled a

Table 2.3 Anthropometric data for upper and lower extremities. Segment lengths from Drillis and Contini (1966), other data from Dempster (1955): as reported by Winter (1979)

| | *Length as % of total body height* | *Weight as % of body weight* | *Distance of centre of mass from proximal joint as % of segment length* | *Distance of radius of gyration, as % of segment length, for rotation about* | | | *Density (kg m^{-3})* |
				Centre of mass	*Proximal joint*	*Distal joint*	
Total leg	53.0	15.7	44.7	32.6	56.0	65.0	1060
Thigh	24.5	9.7	43.3	32.3	54.0	65.3	1050
Shank and foot	28.5	6.0	60.6	41.6	73.5	57.2	1090
Shank	24.6	4.5	43.3	30.2	52.8	64.3	1090
Foot	15.2	1.5	50.0	47.5	69.0	69.0	1100
Total arm	44.1	4.9	53.0	36.8	64.5	59.6	1110
Upper arm	18.6	2.7	43.6	32.2	54.2	64.5	1070
Forearm and hand	25.4	2.2	68.2	46.8	82.7	56.5	1140
Forearm	14.6	1.6	43.0	30.3	52.6	64.7	1130
Hand	10.8	0.6	50.6	29.7	58.7	57.7	1160

Table 2.4 Typical joint and muscle forces during various activities

JOINT FORCES (multiples of body weight)

Hip
One-legged stance	2.9	Rydell, 1965, 1966
	6.0	Williams and Svensson, 1968
	1.8–2.7	McLeish and Charnley, 1970
Quasi-static walking	5.4	Seireg and Arvikar, 1975
Level walking	3.3	Rydell, 1965, 1966
	2.3–5.8	Paul, 1967, 1971
Running	4.3	Rydell, 1965, 1966

Knee
Level walking	3.4	Morrison, 1969
	3.3–5.4	Winter, 1979
Walking up/down ramp	4.0	Morrison, 1969
Ascending stairs	4.3	Morrison, 1969
Descending stairs	3.8	Morrison, 1969
Rising from chair unaided by arms	2.8	Seedhom and Terayama, 1976
	4.0	Ellis *et al.*, 1979
Jumping	24	Smith, 1972

Ankle
Level walking	1.3–1.8	Sokoloff, 1969
	3–4	Weber, 1972
Jumping	8	Smith, 1972

MUSCLE FORCES (Newtons)

	Quads.	Hams.	Calf muscles	
Level walking	865	1400	1200	Morrison, 1969
Ascending stairs	2000	810	360	Morrison, 1969
Descending stairs	1720	400	702	Morrison, 1969
Rising from chair				
Using arms	950	870	500	Seedhom *et al.*, 1976
Unaided by arms	1800	1300	1600	Ellis *et al.*, 1979
Jumping	9600	—	3600	Smith, 1972

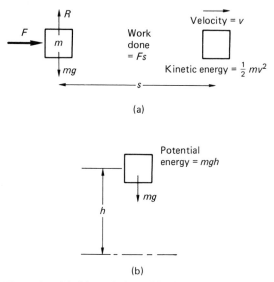

Figure 2.16 (a),(b) Work done, kinetic energy and potential energy

particular distance, s m, at which time it is travelling with a velocity v ms^{-1}, the force is removed, the object will continue to move with the same velocity. In acting upon it, the force has done work on the object (of magnitude Fs) and as a consequence the object has acquired *energy*.

If the object is now to be stopped, a force must be applied to it against its motion, that is negative work must be done on it – or, to look at it the other way around, the object does positive work on whatever is trying to stop it. In coming to rest, the work done by the object will be equal to the work done on the object to get it moving. Any moving object, because it has energy, is capable of doing work in being brought to rest. Energy is the ability to do work: work is the transfer of mechanical energy. The change in the energy of the object is equal to the work done on it or by it.

The energy associated with motion is called *kinetic energy* and is given by $\frac{1}{2}mv^2$ for linear motion and $\frac{1}{2}I\omega^2$ for rotation. (Both will be confirmed as having the same units as work, that is Joules, if it is remembered that $1 \text{ kg ms}^{-2} = 1 \text{ N}$). However, there is also another important form of mechanical energy. An object has *potential energy* by virtue of its height as shown in Figure 2.16(b). By applying a force $F = mg$ to an object it can be lifted through a height h. Work of mgh has been done on the object which, as a result, then has

a potential energy of mgh. This work can subsequently be recovered by allowing the object to fall to its original level: the weight force mg moves through a distance h. In falling, the potential energy is converted into kinetic energy.

A third form of mechanical energy, strain energy, which is stored in an object such as a spring or rubber band when it is deformed, is of lesser importance in biomechanics.

2.5 Mechanics of materials

This chapter so far has discussed forces in terms of their effects on stationary and moving objects. This section now looks briefly at the way forces change the shapes of objects. Depending upon the nature of the material concerned, its original shape and the way the force is applied to it, a piece of material may change shape in many different ways. However, only those forms of deformation which are of importance in the design and construction of an orthosis are considered here. These are compression, bending and buckling.

Figure 2.17(a) shows a piece of material in compression between two plates. There is no overall motion of the block of material because there is no resultant force; it is in equilibrium under the influence of an action and an equal and opposite reaction. There is, however, a squashing of the material – which is actually no more than a change in shape, because its total volume must remain the same. In an ideal situation in which there is no friction between material and compressing plates, the final shape would be a uniform cylinder of reduced height and increased cross-sectional area as seen in Figure 2.17(b). In practice, friction at the upper and lower surfaces will restrict the spread of the material and the cylinder will 'barrel' as it is compressed as seen in Figure 2.17(c).

The amount of compression which will be caused by a particular compressing load will depend upon three factors:

1. The original height of the material (a tall piece of material will compress more than a short piece).
2. Its cross-sectional area (a small piece will compress more than a big piece because in

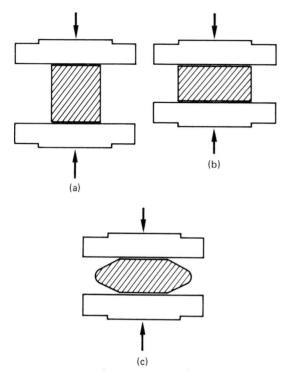

Figure 2.17 (a)–(c) Compression of a piece of material between two plates

the latter case the load is more spread out).
3. The compressibility of the material (a piece of spongy foam will compress very much more than a piece of wood, plastic or metal).

In general, a material which is compressed by a load will tend to spring back to its original shape when the force is removed. However, if the force is large, or if it is applied over an extended period of time, the structure of the material itself may be destroyed and it will become permanently compressed. This is particularly true for soft materials such as foams which we know often have a limited useful life in applications such as insoles.

Hard, structural materials, such as metals and plastics, compress very little when squashed; for normal levels of loading the changes in their dimensions can only be detected with very sensitive measuring equipment, and failure of these hard materials in compression is a problem only under the most extreme circumstances. However, such hard structural materials are often used in the form of long, thin pieces (referred to as beams), which will never fail by crushing but are at risk

of being damaged by distortion; the longer and thinner is the piece, the greater is this risk.

Distortion can occur in one of two ways, depending upon the way in which the beam is loaded. In Figure 2.18(a) loading is at right angles to the beam and as the load P is increased, the beam is distorted by *bending*. If the bending is slight, it will spring back to its initial straight shape when the load is removed. If the bending is greater, the beam may remain permanently distorted. The susceptibility of a beam to bending depends not only upon the stiffness of the material, the length of the unsupported beam and the size of its cross-sectional area, but also on the shape of its cross-section and its orientation with respect to the direction of bending. In essence, the deeper is the section, that is, the further away is the material from the central axis of bending, the stiffer is the beam. For a uniform rectangular cross-section, experience with a ruler confirms this to be true as highlighted in Figure 2.18(b). Alternatively, stiffness is increased by using flanged or hollow cross-sections to move material away from the axis of bending. In Figure 2.18(c) all the sections shown have the same area (that is all would produce beams of the same weight) but their stiffnesses vary by a factor of almost 40. This is why structures which must resist bending, such as structural beams, bicycle frames and long bones, use flanged or hollow sections.

The other way in which a beam may be distorted is by forces acting along rather than across its length. In this situation the beam is said to *buckle*, as seen in Figure 2.19. In contrast to bending, which gradually increases in magnitude as the load is increased from zero, buckling occurs suddenly once a critical value of load is reached. A buckled structure will usually recover its initial shape once the load is removed as can be demonstrated with a ruler or a woodsaw, but the structure is unlikely to continue to perform its function satisfactorily whilst deformed. The likelihood of buckling is minimized by the same factors which reduce bending, that is reducing the length of the unsupported span or increasing material stiffness or section thickness.

Finally torsional forces applied to a beam will cause it to twist as shown in Figure 2.20. Again susceptibility to twisting depends on the length of the unsupported beam, the size and shape of its cross-sectional area and the stiffness of the material used.

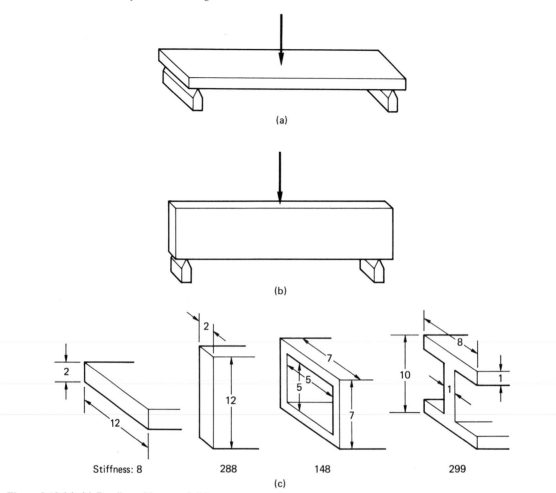

Stiffness: 8   288   148   299

(c)

Figure 2.18 (a)–(c) Bending of beams of different cross-sections

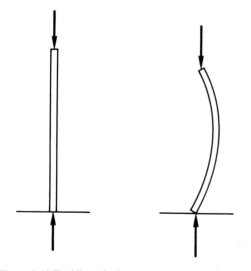

Figure 2.19 Buckling of a beam

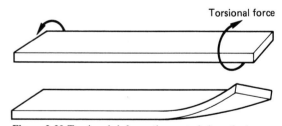

Figure 2.20 Torsional deformation or twisting of a beam

2.6 Glossary

acceleration: the rate of change of velocity

algebraic addition: addition of two or more quantities taking account of the sign of each

angular acceleration: the rate of change of angular velocity

angular displacement: the change in angular position of a rotating object

angular velocity: the rate of change of angular position

biomechanics: the application of the principles and techniques of mechanics to living things

body: any piece of matter or substance – animate or inanimate

buckling: failure of a long thin object through instability in compression

centre of gravity: point at which the weight force effectively acts; usually identical to the centre of mass

centre of mass: point about which all the mass of an object is evenly distributed, or at which the mass of the object may be considered to be concentrated

centripetal acceleration: the component of acceleration of a rotating body which is directed towards the centre of rotation

components: pair of vectors at right angles which add together to give a single resultant vector

compression: form of deformation in which an object is shortened

couple: pair of two equal and opposite parallel forces on different lines of action

deformation: change in shape of an object

displacement: change of position of an object

dynamics: the study of the motion of objects which are not in equilibrium and of the forces and moments which cause the motion

equilibrium: the condition in which the forces and moments acting upon an object are balanced

force: an influence which causes or prevents motion, or causes deformation

free body: object or part of object isolated from its surroundings for analysis

free body diagram: outline drawing of a free body showing the significant forces and moments acting on it

kinetic energy: mechanical energy arising from motion

mass: quantity of matter or substance in an object

mechanics: the study of the creation or prevention of motion

moment: the turning effect of a force

moment arm: the perpendicular distance from the line of action of a force to a particular axis of rotation

moment of inertia: second moment of mass

point of application: the point on or within an object at which a force may be considered to act

potential energy: mechanical energy arising from height above a given datum

principle of static equilibrium: if a body is stationary, there is no resultant force or moment acting upon it

radius of gyration: a measure k related to the second moment of mass of an object by the expression $I = mk^2$

reaction: equal and opposite force which arises in response to an applied force

resolve: determine the component of a vector acting in a particular direction

resultant: a single vector which is the sum of two or more vectors; the resultant has exactly the same effect as all the individual vectors acting together

rotation: angular displacement – motion in which an object turns about an axis

second moment of mass: a measure of the distribution of mass of an object about a particular axis

statics: the study of forces on stationary objects

tangential acceleration: the component of acceleration of a rotating body which is directed tangentially to the circle of motion

torque: turning effect about a point

torsional deformation: a twisting displacement in response to torsional forces on a beam

translation: linear displacement – motion in which an object moves without turning

vector: a quantity which has both magnitude and direction

velocity: the rate of change of position

weight/weight force: the force on an object caused by gravity

work: force multiplied by distance moved in the direction of the force

References

Dempster W.T. (1955) *Space Requirements of the Seated Operator, Wright Patterson Air Force Base.* WADC Technical Report, pp. 55–159

Dowson D., Seedhom B.B. and Johnson G.R. (1981) Biomechanics of the lower limb. In: Dowson D. and Wright V. (eds), *An Introduction to the Biomechanics of Joints and Joint Replacement.* Mechanical Engineering Publications, London, pp. 68–84

Drillis R. and Contini R. (1966) *Body Segment Parameters.* Report 1163-03. Office of Vocational Rehabilitation, Department of Health, Education and Welfare, New York.

Ellis H.I. Seedhom B.B., Amis A.A. *et al.* (1979) Forces in the knee joint whilst rising from normal and motorised chairs. *Eng. Med.* **8**, 278–282

Morrison J.B. (1969) Function of the knee joint in various activities. *Biomed. Eng.* **4**, 573

McLeish R.D. and Charnley J. (1970) Abduction forces in the one-legged stance. *J. Biomech.* **3**, 191–209

Paul J.P. (1967) Forces transmitted by joints in the human body. Proc. *Inst. Mech. Eng.* **181**, (3J), 8–15

Paul J.P. (1971) Load actions on the human femur in walking and some resultant stresses. *Exp. Mech.* **3**, 121

Rydell N. (1965) Forces in the hip joint: II Intravital studies. In: Kenedi R.M. (ed.), *Biomechanics and Related Bioengineering Topics.* Pergamon, Oxford

Rydell N. (1966) Forces acting on the femoral head prosthesis. *Acta Orthop. Scand. Suppl.* 88

Seedhom B.B. and Terayama K. (1976) Knee forces during the activity of getting out of a chair with and without the aid of arms. *Biomed. Eng.* **11**, 278–282

Seireg A. and Arvikar R.J. (1975) The prediction of muscular load sharing and joint forces in the lower extremities during walking. *J. Biomech.* **8**, 89–102

Smith A.J. (1972) A Study of Forces on the Body in Athletic Activities with Particular Reference to Jumping. PhD Thesis, University of Leeds, UK

Sokoloff L. (1969) *Biology of Degenerative Joint Disease.* University of Chicago Press

Weber B.G. (1972) *Die Verletzungen des Oberen Springgelenkes.* (Injuries of the Ankle Joint.) Hans Huber and Williams and Wilkins, Baltimore

Williams J.F. and Svensson N.L. (1968) A force analysis of the hip joint. *Biomed. Eng.* **3**, 365–370

Winter D.A. (1979) *Biomechanics of Human Movement.* John Wiley, New York

3

The biomechanics of orthoses

Peter Bowker

Having dealt with the basic principles of mechanics, that is, how forces create or prevent motion, the application of those principles to the function of orthoses will now be described. Whether the human body is stationary or moving, it is always subject to a system of external forces and moments. Except when the body is fully supported, these external forces and moments will tend to cause motion to occur at its joints.

Normally, the effects of the external forces and moments on the body are resisted or controlled by forces generated internally either in passive tissues, such as joint capsules, ligaments or articular cartilage, or in active tissues such as muscles. In this way a normal functional static posture or pattern of motion is generated. In a body segment in which injury or disease is present, one or more of these tissues is unable to produce the appropriate force. For example, a ligament may be stretched or torn, joint cartilage may have lost its structural integrity, or a muscle may have reduced tone (paralysis) or increased tone (spasticity). In all these cases a more normal function may be restored by modifying the system of external forces and moments acting across one or more of the joints of the body by using an orthosis.

There are four different ways in which an orthosis may modify the system of external forces and moments acting across a joint. The first three of these may be termed 'direct' in that the orthosis actually surrounds the joint being influenced. The fourth, by contrast, may

be termed 'indirect' as the orthosis modifies the external force system acting beyond its physical boundaries. These four patterns of action are summarized briefly below and then the biomechanics of each approach is analysed in some detail.

First, an orthosis may modify the moments acting about a joint. In doing so it may restrict, either partially or totally, the rotational motion at the joint. In partially restricting motion, the orthosis may limit the range of motion available about any particular axis, or may limit the number of axes about which motion may occur. For example, at the knee joint some rotation is available about all three of the perpendicular axes in the sagittal, coronal and transverse planes. A knee orthosis, which partially restricts motion, may be designed either to eliminate motion about the coronal and/or transverse plane axes whilst allowing functional motion in the sagittal plane, or it may restrict the range of motion in the sagittal plane. The restriction of rotational motion through the control of moments at a joint is the most common reason for prescribing an orthosis.

Secondly, an orthosis may modify the normal forces acting about a joint and thereby restrict translational motion at the joint. In theory, the restriction may be partial or total, but in practice, as functional joint motion is always rotational, the aim will always be to totally eliminate translational motion. An example of this form of intervention is the orthotic control of transverse plane motion of the knee resulting from damage to the passive supporting structures of the joint.

Thirdly, the orthosis may reduce the axial forces carried across a joint. This is achieved by sharing the loads between the anatomical structures and the orthotic exoskeleton. In the extreme case the orthosis is designed to completely 'by-pass' the limb and hence totally relieve load from it, the anatomical structures then becoming functionally redundant. This approach is useful in reducing joint pain arising from weight bearing in arthritic joints, or in reducing the deleterious effect of continued loading on such tissues.

Finally, the fourth indirect approach involves modifying the point of application and the line of action of the ground reaction force during either static or dynamic weight bearing. This approach can, in theory, result in a modification of both normal and axial forces and moments about a joint, but in practice is normally used to modify moments. This is a particularly useful strategy for reducing abnormally high moments about a joint, but can also be used to change the alignment of a joint, that is the 'neutral' position about which its functional motion occurs, during gait or other activity. In this way the function of a joint or joints, particularly those in the foot, can be returned to a more normal pattern of movement.

For each of these four patterns of action, the basic biomechanical function of the orthosis is the same whichever of the body's joints and whichever plane of motion is involved. The following analyses therefore are framed in terms of non-specific joints and segments. As will become apparent from the later chapters of this book, the principles derived may be applied, without modification, to the management of any functional deficit at any of the joints of the body, including those of the spine.

3.1 Control of moments across a joint

Figure 3.1(a) shows two load-carrying limb segments joined together in such a way that they are free to rotate relative to each other in the plane of the page. The same two segments, but drawn as two free bodies so that the force across the joint, now being an external force, appears on the diagrams, are shown in Figure 3.1(b).

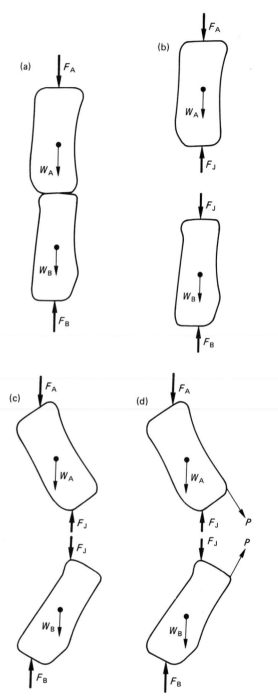

Figure 3.1

When the two segments are aligned, as in Figure 3.1(b), the structure is in equilibrium under the action of the external axial force system. However, if the joint moves out of this aligned position, even by the smallest amount, equilibrium is lost (Figure 3.1(c)) and, in the absence of other influences, the moment of the applied force about the joint centre leads to collapse in flexion. In the normal limb, control of the joint is maintained and collapse avoided through the action of muscles or passive soft tissue restraints such as capsular structures or ligaments acting across the joint. These are represented by the forces P in Figure 3.1(d), and produce an extending moment which balances the flexing moment of the external forces. In pathological cases however, in which these stabilizing influences have been lost, the resulting imbalance of moments needs to be controlled by fitting an orthosis.

The lower of the two free bodies in Figure 3.1(d) but without the muscular restraining force is reproduced in Figure 3.2(a). If we consider the rotational stability of this free body about its lower end (point O in Figure 3.2(a)), we see that it is necessary to apply an anticlockwise moment in order to restore equilibrium. This we will generate by applying some force R_1 acting at an arbitrary angle ϕ to the segment axis and with a point of application a distance b from O. However, whilst the addition of this force enables rotational equilibrium to be attained, it destroys translational equilibrium, and in order to restore this, a second force must be added, equal and opposite to R_1 and with a point of application nearer to point O so as to retain the required imposed net anticlockwise moment as in Figure 3.2(b). Then if the inclination of the segment axis to the vertical is θ, the segment length is L, and its centre of gravity is located at its midpoint, the equation expressing the equilibrium of moments about O is

$$R_1b\sin\phi = R_1a\sin\phi + W_B\tfrac{1}{2}\sin\theta + F_JL\sin\theta \tag{3.1}$$

which simplifies to

$$R_1\sin\phi(b-a) = \tfrac{1}{2}W_B\sin\theta + F_JL\sin\theta \tag{3.2}$$

As all the terms on the right-hand side of this equation are constant, it is apparent that the controlling force R_1 is minimized when the term $\sin\phi(b-a)$ is maximized, that is $\sin\phi=1$, $(b-a) = L$. Contact forces are therefore minimized when $\phi=90°$, $b=L$ and $a=0$, that is when the orthosis contacts the segment as near to and as far from the joint as possible, and when the controlling forces are applied to the

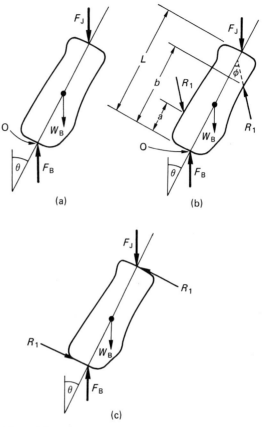

Figure 3.2

limb perpendicular to its longitudinal axis (Figure 3.2(c)).

For this ultimate case of $a=0$ and $b=L$, with $\phi=90°$, Equation (3.2) simplifies to the expression

$$R_1L = (\tfrac{1}{2}W_B + F_J)L\sin\theta \tag{3.3}$$

from which an estimate of the magnitude of the contact force between the orthosis and the limb may be made. It can be seen that as expected, the contact force is zero when the two segments are aligned, and increases with flexion according to the sine function to a maximum value at 90°.

Note that in the above analysis we have in effect controlled rotation of the limb segment by applying to it a couple – that is, two off-set equal and opposite forces. The magnitude or turning effect of the required couple (R_1L) is equal to the out-of-balance turning effect as shown in Equation (3.3). We have then sought to minimize the force required to produce the necessary turning effect by maximizing the moment arm, that is, positioning the two forces at the extremities of the segment.

It is important to note that the point on the limb segment about which moments are considered is immaterial. As the initial free body in Figure 3.2(a) is in translational equilibrium $(F_B = F_J + W_B)$, the same out-of-balance turning effect is obtained whichever point is chosen. Similarly, as established in Chapter 2, the turning effect of a couple is the same about any point.

An analysis on the free body of the upper segment yields a similar result, as demonstrated in Figure 3.3(a) (indeed, if the weights of the two segments are the same, an identical result), so that the final picture for the whole limb is as shown in Figure 3.3(b). The two forces acting at the joint centre, R_1 and R_2, have in effect become a single force, R.

In an orthosis the optimum positioning of R in line with the joint centre can be achieved, but practical considerations limit the maximum distance achievable between R_1 and R_2 and the joint centre. As the distances to R_1 and R_2 are increased, the orthosis becomes increasingly long and bulky, and its attachments to the limb

are more likely to interfere with the function of neighbouring joints. The situation represented in Figure 3.3(b) may represent the end point of a limited degree of flexion allowed by an orthosis. Much more commonly, however, the orthosis would fix the joint in the fully extended position.

Thus an orthosis which is effective in controlling the rotation of a joint will consist of a rigid framework incorporating pads or straps which apply three controlling forces to the limb: one placed over the joint centre, the other two, acting in the opposite direction to the first, placed proximal and distal to the joint. This is known as three-point fixation and is the arrangement which is needed, in every case, to control the moments acting at a joint. There is no exception to this rule. It is clear then that the positions of the controlling forces will be the same whether the objective of the orthosis is to totally prevent rotation in a particular plane, or to limit or resist rotation in that plane. It will in fact be the design of the orthotic joints which will determine the precise way in which the control of joint moments controls joint motion.

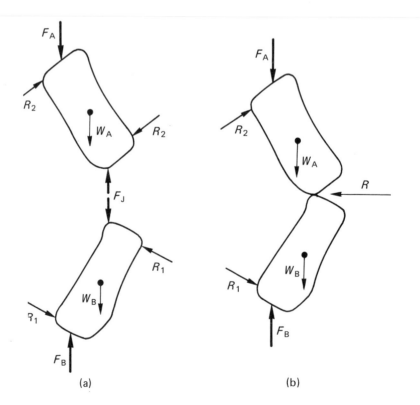

(a)   (b)

Figure 3.3

3.2 Control of normal forces across a joint

Whilst uncontrolled rotational motion can occur in the absence of normal stabilizers even under the effect of quasi-static weight-bearing forces, translational instability generally only arises in dynamic situations in which there are significant shear forces acting.

Figure 3.4(a) shows the free body diagrams of the two load-carrying body segments at an instant at which their long axes are vertical. The segments are subjected to a ground reaction force with vertical and horizontal components and are free to rotate in the plane of the page. The joints between the segments are maintained in extension by fixing moments generated by muscular forces. The shear forces F required to maintain the segments in equilibrium in the transverse plane are provided by the capsular and ligamentous structures of the joint.

Figure 3.4(b) presents the free bodies of the same segments under the same conditions but for a pathological joint which has lost the structures which restrain the transverse plane motion of the lower segment to the right. The lower segment is clearly no longer in equilibrium. In this case the main objective of orthotic management is to control this excessive translational motion. Application of the force R_1 as shown in Figure 3.4(c) restores translational equilibrium as required but, because it also introduces an additional clockwise moment about the joint, disturbs rotational equilibrium. This must then be restored by a balancing anticlockwise moment generated by the force R_2 acting in the opposite direction. The optimum points of application of the two orthotic controlling forces, R_1 and R_2, are then obtained as follows. If the shear force is F and the length of the lower segment is L, consideration of the equilibrium of moments about the joint centre for the healthy limb gives the value of the fixing moment at the knee as FL. The equations of rotational equilibrium about points A and B in Figure 3.4(c) then give $R_2 = Fa/b$ and $R_1 = -F(a+b)/b$,

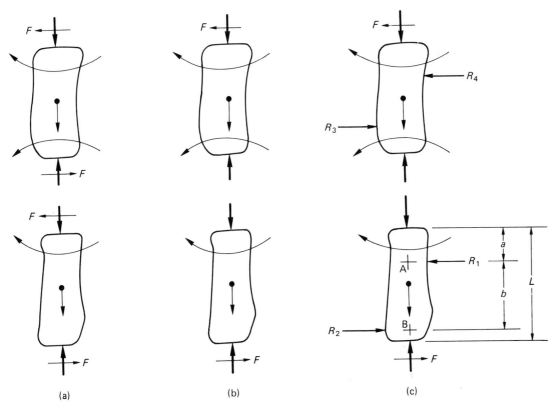

(a)   (b)   (c)

Figure 3.4

indicating that the applied forces are minimized when A is as close to the joint and B as far from the joint as practicable. A similar line of reasoning for the upper segment demonstrates that equilibrium is restored to this segment through the application of the two forces R_3 and R_4 in Figure 3.4(c), these forces again being minimized when R_3 is as close to the joint and R_4 as far from the joint as practicable. Thus, an orthosis which is effective in controlling the excessive translation within a joint with deficient ligamentous or capsular structures will consist of a rigid framework incorporating pads or straps which apply the four controlling forces R_1–R_4 to the limb. Such a device is often referred to as a 'four-point fixation' brace, and this is the arrangement needed, in every case, to control the normal forces acting across a joint. There is no exception to this rule.

However, the design of an orthosis such as that proposed, whilst being effective in preventing translation, because it encloses the joint in a rigid framework, also prevents normal functional rotation of the joint. To allow flexion to occur, this rigid brace must be hinged at the joint centre. We must therefore also examine the mechanics of the four-point fixation orthosis when the joint which it is controlling is

functioning in the flexed position. Looking initially at the mechanics of the normal limb with the joint partially flexed leads to the free body diagrams in Figure 3.5(a), in which the reaction forces at the joints are represented as components parallel and perpendicular to the longitudinal axis of the lower segment. Figure 3.5(b) shows the corresponding diagrams for the same segments of the pathological limb which has no restraint at the joint to translation of the lower segment to the right. The analysis is then similar to that for the previous case with the joint extended. Looking firstly at the lower segment, application of the external force R_5 in Figure 3.5(c) restores translational equilibrium to the lower segment and R_6 re-establishes rotational equilibrium, the optimum points of application of these forces being as before. Similarly for the upper segment, equilibrium is restored through the application of the two forces R_7 and R_8 as shown in Figure 3.5(c). It should be noted however that these latter two controlling forces have both normal and tangential components. As joint flexion increases, their tangential components progressively increase, until at 90° of flexion translation of the lower segment is prevented entirely by shear forces at the interface between the

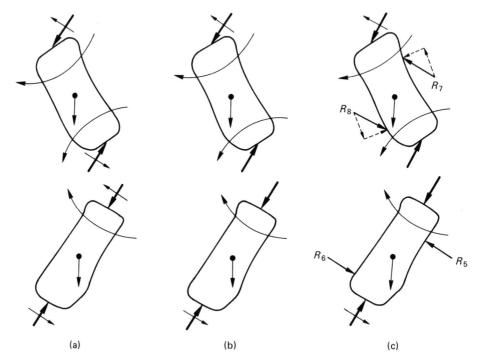

(a)   (b)   (c)

Figure 3.5

orthosis and upper segment. As these shear forces are generated through friction between the brace and the skin surface, a good grip between the orthotic pads or straps and the skin surface is required if the orthosis is to be maximally effective for all angles of joint flexion.

3.3 Control of axial forces across a joint

In a healthy limb, axial loading is carried across joints through bony structures and layers of articular cartilage which have sufficient strength and stiffness to enable them to continue to function without pain whilst load bearing. If however, as a result of some degenerative disease process, these load-carrying materials lose their structural integrity, the application of axial load will lead to excessive compressive deformation within the joint. This will disrupt the normal geometry of the articulation, often making movement painful and stiff.

For a joint of the lower limb, which must function whilst it is loaded for locomotion to take place, such a situation will potentially impair mobility. Alleviation of the problem will often depend on joint replacement surgery, but in some cases partial or total relief of load from a joint by means of an orthosis may be helpful.

Figure 3.6(a) again shows the free body diagrams of two load-carrying segments joined together with a simple hinge so that they are free to rotate relative to each other in the plane of the page. The objective in this case is to devise an orthosis which will effectively reduce the magnitude of the contact force F_J. Taking a rigid orthotic framework and strapping it at its ends to the two limb segments so that it spans across the joint (Figure 3.6(b)) provides an alternative pathway for the transmission of the applied loading which may relieve some of the load from the anatomical joint. Thus, in Figure 3.6(b), the total joint load F_J is divided into two parts, one part of magnitude F_{JA} passing across the anatomical joint, and the other part of magnitude F_{JO} passing down the orthosis, so that

$$F_{JA} + F_{JO} = F_J$$

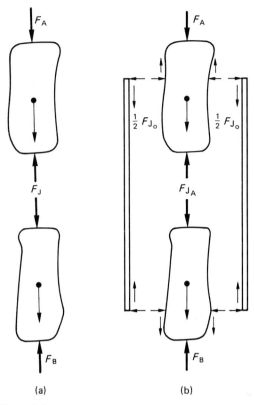

Figure 3.6

In the diagram it has been assumed that the load carried by the orthosis is equally divided between the two side members.

The extent to which load can be transferred from the joint to the orthosis clearly depends both on the fitting procedure adopted and also on the nature of the interface between the body segment and the orthosis and the contact pressure acting at the interface. Dealing with the fitting procedure first of all, imagine attempting to fit an orthosis of the general type depicted in Figure 3.6(b), so as to relieve as much load as possible from the anatomical joint. This will be most effectively done if the segments are firstly unloaded and distracted so that their adjacent ends are physically separated, precluding the possibility of direct load transfer between them, and the orthosis is then secured to the limb.

However, whilst in theory an ideal arrangement has been achieved, restoration of functional compressive loads to the segments changes the situation. Firstly, there is relative motion between the orthosis and the underlying skeletal bone as a result of shear deformation of the interposed soft tissues. Secondly, function results in the muscles within the soft tissue composite changing both in shape and volume so that the contact pressure between the orthosis and the limb is variable. And finally, gravity tends to displace the orthosis down the limb – a process aided by the fact that the majority of body segments tend to be tapered rather than cylindrical.

The net result of these three factors is that once functional weight bearing begins, contact within the joint between the bone ends is likely to occur thus re-establishing a direct load carriage pathway. Therefore, although the orthosis may have been fitted to the limb in the optimum way, the proportion of the applied load carried through the orthosis may in practice be quite small.

As previously mentioned, the success of the orthosis in off-loading the anatomical joint depends not only upon the care taken in applying the orthosis but also on the nature of the material interfacing to the skin and the value of the interface pressure. In theory, the higher the pressure, the higher F_{JO} may become. In the simplest case, transfer of load across the skin–orthosis interface will depend solely upon friction of the orthosis on the underlying skin as shown in Figure 3.7(a). In this case, the limiting value of F_{JO} is given by μF_N, and, in principle, as the value of μ may approach unity through the suitable choice of an interface material, quite large loads may be transferred in this way. However, shear forces in the soft tissues through which load is transferred will be correspondingly high and this may lead to tissue damage.

The above is a rather simplistic model. As the soft tissues overlying the skeletal structures are compressed by tightening the orthotic strap, they will deform so that the load transfer mechanism becomes much more complex. These load transfer mechanisms are discussed fully in Chapter 5. Load transfer now occurs partially via tangential friction and partially via normal contact forces as in Figure 3.7(b). The normal contact forces will be dramatically increased if the edge of the orthotic strap is tucked under a bony prominence as demonstrated in Figure 3.7(c). This is in fact the only practicable way of transferring significant loads across the interface and is utilized commonly in knee-ankle-foot orthoses (KAFOs) with an 'ischial seat' in which the top of the thigh cuff

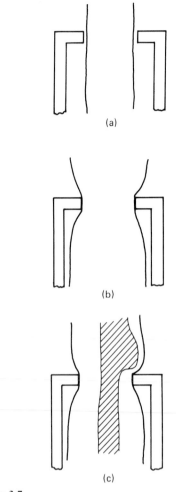

Figure 3.7

has a posterior ledge which fits under the ischial tuberosity (see Chapter 9). An alternative but relatively little used strategy is to relieve ankle loading by extending an ankle--foot orthosis (AFO) proximally and moulding it anteriorly over the flares of the tibial condyles and into the patellar tendon and posteriorly into the popliteal region (see Chapter 7).

Ultimately, all the difficulties can be overcome, and indeed a complete transfer of load from the anatomical joint to the orthosis achieved by a small redesign of the orthosis so that it extends beyond the distal segment (Figure 3.8). So long as some gap under the distal segment is maintained under functional load bearing conditions, the lower segment is mechanically redundant and the whole of the load will be carried through the orthosis.

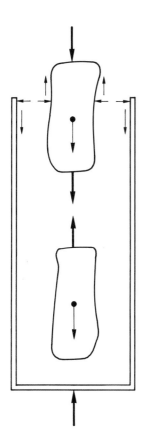

Figure 3.8

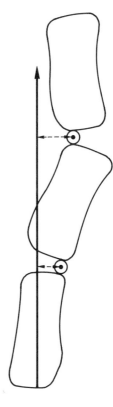

Figure 3.9

3.4 Control of line of action of ground reaction force

Use of the final type of orthotic mechanics is limited to the lower limb. As the foot contacts the floor during gait (described in detail in Chapter 4), it experiences a ground reaction force which has components in all three principal body planes. As the stance phase progresses from heel-strike to toe-off, the relative values of these three components change, so that the direction of the resultant ground reaction force also changes. In addition, as stance proceeds, its precise point of application on the underside of the foot moves progressively forwards from the heel at heel-strike to the area of the metatarsal heads at toe-off.

Thus, at any instant during the gait cycle, the ground reaction force has a particular line of action which, in general, will lie at some distance from the centre of rotation of each of the joints of the lower limb as seen in Figure 3.9. The ground reaction force will thus create a

moment about each of these joints, the sense of the moment being determined by whether the ground reaction force passes anteriorly or posteriorly (or medially or laterally) to the joint, and its magnitude being determined by the perpendicular distance between the joint centre and the line of action of the force. As the ground reaction force generated during gait is of considerable magnitude, being roughly equal to body weight for the majority of the period of contact between foot and floor, these moments exert a major influence on the motion and alignment of all the joints of the lower limb. Realignment of the ground reaction force using an orthosis thus offers considerable potential for changing the moments about the lower limb joints.

Perhaps the most obvious application of such an approach is in controlling the position of a joint which has an asymmetrical pattern of motion – that is one which can rotate from its neutral position to a significantly greater extent in one sense than in the other. The most obvious example of this situation is rotation of the knee joint from the extended position in the sagittal plane, but it may also be relevant to coronal

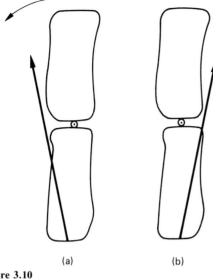

Figure 3.10

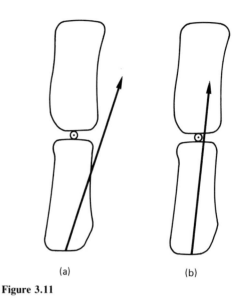

Figure 3.11

plane motion of the subtalar joint. If Figure 3.10 represents a joint of this type, in which rotation of the upper segment relative to the lower can occur only in an anticlockwise sense, a ground reaction force having a line of action lying to the left of the joint as in Figure 3.10(a) tends to cause rotation of the joint, whereas if the line of action is repositioned so it passes to the right of the joint centre as in Figure 3.10(b), there is no tendency to motion. Such a strategy may be useful if the muscles or passive structures controlling the joint and normally preventing excessive rotation cannot counter the collapsing moment either because the musculature itself is weakened, or because the passive structures are damaged, or because an abnormality of the load bearing pattern has caused a grossly abnormal force vector alignment, which the joint structures are unable to resist.

A rather more controlled approach to realigning the ground reaction force is illustrated in Figure 3.11. In this case the joint may rotate in either sense but a skeletal malalignment or an abnormality of gait has resulted in a substantial displacement of the line of the force away from the joint centre (Figure 3.11(a)). This gives rise to an abnormally large moment, which passive or active joint structures may be unable to resist, or to resist only at the cost of an energy expensive gait adaptation. In this case, the aim of orthotic management would be to reduce the moment by moving the line of

action of the force vector so that it passes through or close to the joint centre of rotation (Figure 3.11(b)).

An alternative objective of realigning the ground reaction force may be to subtly change the alignment of the lower limb during gait, so as to slightly change the position about which each of its joints functions. This approach is of particular value in realigning the joints of the foot so that they are operating from more normal positions and thereby facilitating more normal overall foot function.

The process of realigning the ground reaction force at any particular joint involves altering the angular relationship either between the plantar surface of the foot and the floor, or between the articulating segments at a more distal anatomical joint. A simple example of a case in which it is of value to modify the angular relationship between the foot and the floor is shown in Figure 3.12, in which the diagrams could represent the coronal plane view of the subtalar joint. In Figure 3.12(a), a skeletal malformation in the distal segment has led to an abnormal joint position. However, interposing an orthotic wedge between the distal segment and the floor, as in Figure 3.12(b), compensates for this malformation and realigns the joint into its correct neutral position. As an additional benefit, the repositioning of the joint has also reduced the joint moment. Orthotic management of this type is parti-

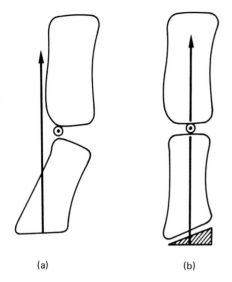

(a) (b)

Figure 3.12

cularly valuable in controlling the joints of the foot (see Chapter 6) and has the significant benefit that joint realignment is achieved without placing any restriction on its functional motion.

Similarly, in instances in which the alignment of the ground reaction force at one joint is controlled by changing the position of a more distal joint, the desired result is achieved not through the direct action of the orthosis itself but as a compensation for its effect at the distal joint. For example, fixing the position of the ankle joint using an AFO will require a subject to fundamentally modify his gait pattern to compensate for the lack of ankle dorsiflexion and plantarflexion. This altered gait pattern will involve a change in the whole pattern of lower limb motion and thus in the alignment of the ground reaction force relative to the knee and hip. This strategy, which can be beneficial in controlling the moments at the more proximal joints, is discussed further in Chapter 7.

4

A description of gait

Brendan McHugh

4.1 Introduction

This chapter describes normal gait and considers the effects of pathological conditions on the normal patterns of walking. The purpose of describing gait in this context is to aid patient assessment and orthotic prescription, and to monitor changes in walking ability leading up to and following orthotic treatment.

From a casual observation of people walking, normal gait might appear to involve walking beside another person, looking regularly towards that person, occasionally speaking and gesturing, constantly changing direction and carrying a bag or similar object. It is not realistic to examine gait scientifically in these circumstances. Thus it is customary in the clinic or the laboratory, for gait to be observed when the subject walks alone in a straight line unencumbered by luggage. The ability of subjects to walk and turn under these circumstances, and to negotiate slopes and steps, is generally considered to give a reliable indication of their gait capabilities in everyday living. Abnormal gait patterns are often discernible, even to the untrained observer, but the rehabilitation professional seeks to understand the underlying causes and the potential for improvement in gait, and needs to be able to monitor changes which occur during treatment.

Normal and abnormal gait will be described in the following stages:

1. A description of the features of normal gait in Section 4.2

2. An outline of the scientific techniques used to study gait in Section 4.3
3. A detailed consideration of normal gait in terms of movements, forces and energy consumption in Section 4.4.
4. Finally a discussion of gait abnormalities which result from specific functional disabilities in Section 4.6.

4.2 Observable features of normal gait

The rhythmic reciprocal motion of the legs, arms and trunk, which constitute gait, occur in a repetitive gait cycle. This gait cycle may be conveniently described by subdividing it into a sequence of events as shown in Figure 4.1.

The right leg will be considered and the gait cycle will be deemed to commence at the instant the right foot makes contact with the ground. Since, in normal gait, initial contact is made by the heel, this instant is referred to as heel-strike. The gait cycle is completed at the next heel-strike by the right leg. The period during which the foot remains in contact with the ground is the 'stance phase', which constitutes some 60% of the gait cycle. The remainder of the cycle, when the foot progresses forward, is the 'swing phase'. In walking, the stance phase exceeds the swing phase in duration because there are periods when both feet are in contact with the ground simultaneously. This distinguishes walking from

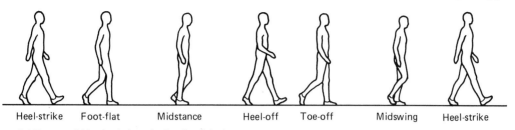

| Heel-strike | Foot-flat | Midstance | Heel-off | Toe-off | Midswing | Heel-strike |

Figure 4.1 Events within the gait cycle for the right leg

running, in which the swing phase is of longer duration than stance phase.

Observation of the gait cycle during walking reveals the following approximate time sequence of events:

1. *Sagittal plane:*
   (i) *0–10% of cycle.* At heel-strike the right leg is in a forward position with the right hip at its most flexed. The knee is extended and the ankle is in the neutral position. The ankle gradually plantar-flexes until the foot is flat on the ground. Meanwhile knee flexion is seen to occur while there is no appreciable change in hip attitude. This sequence is referred to as the shock absorption phase.
   (ii) *10–45% of cycle.* During this 'midstance phase' the foot remains flat on the ground while the remainder of the body continues to progress forward. It commences with 'foot-flat' and ends with 'heel-off'. Between these two identifiable events is the point where the left foot, swinging forward, passes the stationary right foot. This instant is often referred to as 'midstance'. During the midstance phase the hip gradually extends and the ankle dorsiflexes as the body progresses forward over the stationary foot. The knee initially continues to flex, but before the instant of midstance it begins to extend and continues to do so for the remainder of this phase. At the instant of midstance the knee is noticeably flexed.
   (iii) *45–60% of cycle.* This is the so-called 'push-off phase' which commences with 'heel-off' and ends with 'toe-off'. This phase is characterized by rapid plantarflexion of the ankle accompanied by flexion at both the knee and the hip.
   (iv) *60–100% of cycle.* During this 'swing phase' the right foot has no contact with the ground. This phase begins with acceleration of the thigh, which produces forward motion of the leg, and ends with a corresponding deceleration in readiness for heel-strike. The hip flexes throughout this phase while the knee initially continues to flex but later extends so that by heel-strike it is again fully extended. Initially the ankle dorsiflexes to the neutral position and remains so for the remainder of the swing phase. One definable event in swing phase is 'midswing' when the right foot is passing the left foot (which is itself, by definition, at midstance). At midswing the hip is flexed while the knee is at its maximum flexion and the ankle is in the neutral position (relative to the lower leg).

2. *Frontal plane:*
   A slight lowering of the non-supporting hip, due to a tilting motion of the pelvis about the supporting hip, is normally observed during midstance. There is also a barely noticeable motion of the trunk towards the supporting side during early stance and in the opposite direction in late stance phase. Throughout the normal gait cycle the knee and ankle do not conspicuously deviate towards either side. On uneven terrain, the foot supinates and pronates in response to the changing contour of the ground. A striking feature of frontal plane observation during normal gait is how little side to side movement is seen.

This has been a description of the movements of the legs as might be observed visually or with the aid of simple photographic equipment. However, it is by no means a complete description of the leg movements which occur during gait since it lacks precise quantification of joint motion. Furthermore, normal gait involves more than merely leg movements. In unhindered gait, it is normal for each arm to move in harmony with the contralateral leg such that, as the right hip flexes, the left arm moves forward. Such arm movements are not always present in slow ambling but as gait becomes more purposeful, and walking speed increases, they are seen more consistently.

The aforementioned leg and arm movements are often exhibited by cartoon characters, as they walk; yet their gait appears unreal. This is probably due to the absence of the trunk movements characteristic of normal gait. As a direct consequence of the leg movements which occur during walking, the body undergoes vertical displacement; it reaches its maximum height at midstance and is at its lowest point during the double support period. Thus the body is seen to rise and fall twice in each gait cycle. This vertical oscillation, coupled with the forward motion of the body, produces a waveform trajectory (sinusoidal in appearance) of the centre of gravity of the body during walking (Figure 4.2).

The vertical displacement of the centre of gravity of the body would be even greater were it not for certain joint movements during gait which either lower the body at midstance or raise it during double support. First, due to the plantarflexed attitude of the foot, the ankle joint rises towards the end of the stance phase. This helps to limit the descent of the body during double support. Secondly, the flexed attitude of the knee during midstance reduces the maximum height of the body. Thirdly, the

slight adduction of the supporting hip joint at midstance, and the consequent dipping of the pelvis, lowers the body at midstance. Fourthly the pelvis rotates, about a vertical axis, such that during double support, with the right leg leading, the right hip is displaced forward of the left hip. For a given stride length this causes the legs to adopt a more vertical attitude thus increasing the height of the centre of gravity of the body during double support. It is interesting to note that, even at midstance, the subject is not as tall as when standing erect, since the maximum height has been reduced by knee flexion and pelvic dipping.

Simple measurements of gait provide other information. One of the easiest parameters to measure is the cadence (number of steps per minute). Finley and Cody (1970) in a study of 1106 pedestrians walking in an urban environment found that the natural cadences for men and women were 110.5 (standard deviation 10.0) and 116.5 (standard deviation 11.7) respectively. The stride length (the distance travelled in one gait cycle), which is related to body height, is about 1.5 m for males and 1.3 m for females. The gait velocity can be determined (in metres per minute) as stride length × one half of the cadence. The average walking velocity for normal healthy adults is approximately 80 m min^{-1}. Waters *et al.* (1988) determined the normal walking speed related to age group and sex, for each of 260 subjects (Table 4.1).

Table 4.1 Walking speed (metres per minute) by age and sex, expressed as mean (standard deviation) after Waters *et al.* (1988)

Age range (yr)	Male	Female	Total
6–12	70.72 (8.02)	68.29 (9.19)	69.64 (8.57)
13–19	73.41 (11.58)	73.16 (8.96)	73.28 (10.17)
20–59	81.58 (9.41)	77.67 (10.71)	79.76 (10.16)
60–80	76.64 (9.01)	71.83 (10.04)	73.55 (9.93)

4.3 Scientific techniques used to study gait

4.3.1 Kinematic (motion) analysis

Gait has been discussed in terms of observable movements and simple measurements. It is possible to study such movements in a more

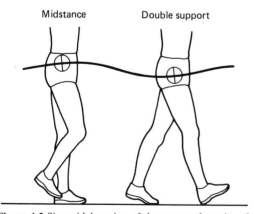

Midstance   Double support

Figure 4.2 Sinusoidal motion of the centre of gravity of the body during walking

detailed manner and to record data for subsequent analysis. Gait analysis techniques will now be briefly described.

Early studies involved the use of still photography using techniques such as multiple exposure or single exposure with stroboscopic illumination. Subsequently, much use was made of cine photography in the pioneering studies of the late 1940s (University of California, 1947). In order to track the motion of identifiable points on the anatomy, researchers used markers which would be visible on film. It was recognized that markers attached to the skin would not necessarily reflect the motion of the underlying skeleton. Where skeletal motion was to be investigated, efforts were made to achieve a more intimate relationship between marker and bone. However, this is not always possible as it requires either surgical fixation of the marker to the bone or the application of a rigid clamp anchored to a suitably shaped bone. Most investigators rely on surface markers attached to the skin surface by adhesive.

In the past, analysis required many hours of painstaking measurements on film to produce the kinematic data in a useful form. It was necessary to build into the calculations corrections for parallax and perspective effects (as the camera was normally stationary). Analysis in any given plane was often complicated by rotation of the limb segments. For example, a marker attached to the lateral malleolus would, if viewed in the sagittal plane, move anteriorly if the leg were internally rotated. Thus if the leg were swinging forward and rotating, a correction for such rotational effects would be necessary in the calculation of flexion-extension angles. For this reason, it is necessary to record a full three-dimensional trajectory for each marker, even if only a sagittal plane analysis is being undertaken. This can be achieved by employing two cameras – usually one viewing the sagittal plane, and the other capturing frontal plane data.

Much of the drudgery of kinematic analysis has disappeared due to the development of opto-electronic gait analysis systems. Typically, reflective markers are attached to predetermined anatomical landmarks. As the subject walks, the successive positions of the markers are detected using television cameras and then fed into a computer for rapid processing. The emergence of these systems makes

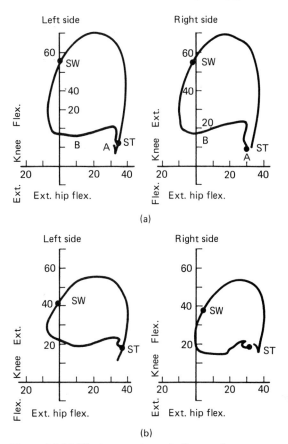

Figure 4.3 (a) Hip–knee angle–angle diagram for a normal 11-year-old girl walking at her natural cadence. ST = initiation and SW = termination of stance phase. (b) Hip–knee angle–angle diagram of a 9-year-old girl with spastic diplegia. She was ranked first for most mildly affected in the degree of clinically assessed dysfunction. (Reproduced with permission from DeBruin *et al.*, 1982)

routine clinical gait analysis a more practical proposition, although the equipment can be prohibitively expensive.

Another tool used widely in kinematic gait analysis is the electrogoniometer. One of its uses has been to monitor hip and knee joint motion. The data can be presented as an 'angle–angle' diagram – a graph on which hip angle is plotted against knee angle for a full gait cycle as shown in Figure 4.3. Such plots can be used to characterize various gait abnormalities. Although it iisss possible to indicate specific events in the gait cycle, some may find the absence of a continuous timebase to be a drawback. There remain significant difficulties in the accurate location of a goniometer and in measuring the three-dimensional motion of universal joints such as the hip.

A recently introduced flexible electro-goniometer, the end block of which are attached to the limb on opposite sides of the joint axis was designed to overcome these difficulties. It functions in close contact with the skin and does not need to be precisely aligned with the anatomical joint axis of rotation, although it must be located in the appropriate plane.

4.3.2 Kinetic (force and motion) analysis

Kinetic analysis gives a more complete description of gait and it becomes possible to explain observed movements in terms of the interplay of the various force actions which cause them. It is also possible to use the data to estimate muscle and joint forces. This has been of great value in the design of internal and external prostheses and for developing orthotic devices.

The forces acting between the feet and the ground may be measured by a force plate. This is a plate which is supported on a force transducer assembly such that it is level with the surrounding floor. As its rigidity is not perceptibly different from that of the surrounding floor, the plate is undetectable to the test subject. The transducer assembly measures the forces along three orthogonal axes (vertical, fore-aft and side-side) and produces corresponding electrical outputs which can then be processed by computer. It is relatively simple to derive the moment about each of the orthogonal axes, and to calculate the centre of force application (or centre of pressure). Figure 4.4 shows the three orthogonal components of the ground reaction force plotted against time. For any instant in the gait cycle, the magnitude and direction of the resultant ground reaction force, exerted on the foot by the ground, can be derived from these components. Consider a typical result at say 50% of the gait cycle. The vertical component of force (F_z) is 800 N while the fore and aft shear (F_x) is 120 N. These can be combined to give the magnitude and direction of the resultant ground reaction (R) in the sagittal plane (Figure 4.5). A similar procedure involving the vertical force and lateral shear force yields the resultant ground reaction as it affects the frontal plane. As will be seen later, these projections of the ground reaction onto the sagittal and frontal planes are useful for visualizing its effect on joint motion. If required, the total ground reaction force R can be calculated using the relationship

$$R = \sqrt{(F_x^2 + F_y^2 + F_z^2)}$$

One method of presenting force plate data in a readily usable form is to display successive ground reaction vectors on a single graph. The typical butterfly shape of this plot of sagittal plane data may be recognizably distorted if pathological gait abnormalities are present as seen in Figure 4.6.

Kinetic data can give the magnitude and direction of the ground reaction vector and its line of action in relation to the various joints and segments of the body. When an individual is stationary the total ground reaction force (both legs) is equal and opposite to body weight. During walking the ground reaction force on each leg is mostly inclined to the vertical. Viewed in the plane of progression, the horizontal component acts posteriorly during early stance and anteriorly during push-off. These horizontal components, acting simultaneously in opposite directions during double support, almost cancel one another with only a small net forward effect, to overcome external resistance to progression such as that due to air resistance.

Fluctuations in the total vertical component of the ground reaction will occur because bipedal gait involves vertical accelerations of the body mass. As discussed earlier, the trajectory of the centre of gravity of the body during walking is similar to a sine wave in form. The relationship between this motion and the measured forces is demonstrated in Figure 4.7. The vertical force required to produce the described sinusoidal motion is in phase with the vertical acceleration of the body due to the relationship between force and acceleration $(F = ma)$. It is therefore reasonable to anticipate such a force waveform during the gait cycle. When the vertical component of the ground reaction force for each leg is drawn on the same baseline and the total vertical reaction (the sum of the reactions for the right and left legs) is also drawn, the result is an approximately sinusoidal waveform as expected. In general, the total ground reaction force exceeds body weight if the body accelerates

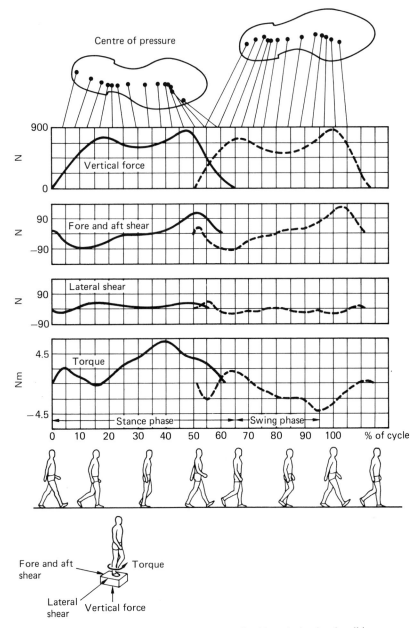

Figure 4.4 Typical force-plate results for a normal subject during level walking. (Reproduced with permission from Eberhart *et al.*, 1954)

upwards and is less than body weight when the acceleration is downward.

The force plate can provide information about the successive 'instantaneous' ground reaction forces, but it cannot determine how that force is distributed under the foot. More detail of foot pressure distribution can be obtained with the use of multiple discrete transducers either floor mounted or embedded in an insole. These transducers normally measure the force applied to them, and from this the mean pressure over the area of the transducer can be recorded. This may be quite different from the peak value if there is a large variation in pressure over the measuring surface. Errors due to bending of the transducer and difficulty in separating direct and shearing forces may affect the reliability of measurements. In recent

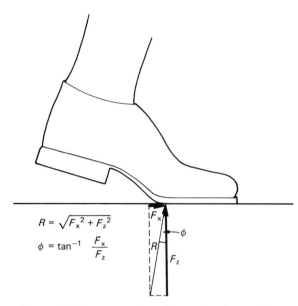

$$R = \sqrt{F_x^2 + F_z^2}$$

$$\phi = \tan^{-1} \frac{F_x}{F_z}$$

Figure 4.5 Vector summation of force-plate data to give magnitude and direction of the ground reaction force in the sagittal plane

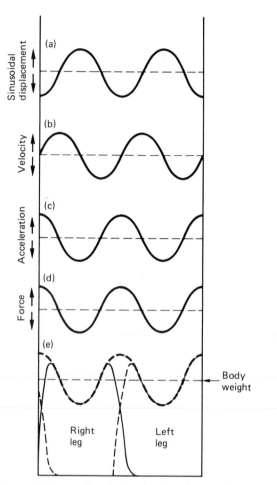

Figure 4.7 The total vertical ground reaction waveform (e) is similar to that of the force (d) associated with a sinusoidal displacement versus time curve (a)

Direction of progression

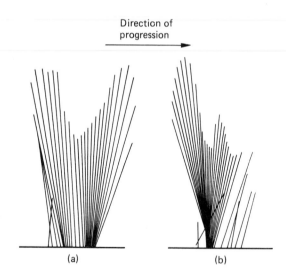

Figure 4.6 Example of 'butterfly' plots of the ground reaction vector in the sagittal plane. (a) Normal, (b) dorsiflexor insufficiency (note the sudden forward displacement of the centre of pressure in early stance)

years it has become possible using a pedobaro-graph to investigate pressure under the foot during walking. This device provides a video display, in the form of a contour map, of the pressure variations over the contact area between the foot and an instrumented glass plate. If shoes are worn, the contact area is the interface between the shoe and the glass plate and thus the true pressure distribution under the foot cannot be recorded. An overview of foot pressure measurement methodology and clinical findings, including examples of graphically displayed data, has been presented by Lord, Reynolds and Hughes (1986).

Kinetic data may also be used to identify the forces, moments and torques to which skeletal structures are subjected. In addition, it is possible to deduce the required muscle force if the line of action of a muscle relative to a joint which it controls is known. This deduction is dependent on the assumption that a single muscle group is active about the given joint. Where this is not the case it may still be possible to estimate joint loading. To establish precisely which muscle groups are active at any given phase of the gait cycle, electromyographic (emg) studies can be carried out. The size of the electrical impulses, which are detected by the emg electrodes, can be integrated and analysed to give a percentage figure for the mechanical activity of that muscle. Inman et al. (1981) have reported that the onset of electrical activity coincides reasonably well with the start of muscular contraction but that there can be a delay between the cessation of the e.m.g. signal and end of muscle contraction, thus requiring some caution in interpretation. Nevertheless, emg analysis has contributed greatly to the investigation of the phasic activity of muscles during walking.

Much of the muscle activity during the stance phase of walking is necessary to oppose the moments exerted about the hip, knee and ankle by the ground reaction force. For example, when the line of action of the ground reaction force is posterior to the knee this will create a knee flexion moment which must be opposed by the action of the knee extensors (Figure 4.8). In this static situation where the joint is neither flexing nor extending, the extension and flexion moments are equal. In a dynamic situation, such as gait, joint control is more complex. Stability of the knee joint is of paramount importance for safe gait but this does not always require knee extensor activity. For example, a contraction of the hip extensors, producing a hip extension moment, causes a posterior thrust at the knee and thus has a stabilizing effect on the knee (Figure 4.9). This

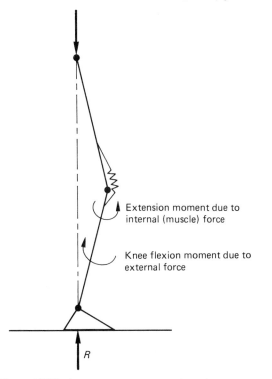

Extension moment due to internal (muscle) force

Knee flexion moment due to external force

R

Figure 4.8 The knee extensors are exerting a knee moment which counteracts the flexion moment imposed by external loads

action is reflected in an induced anterior tilting of the ground reaction vector such that its flexion moment about the knee is eliminated. Whether it is the hip muscle activity, or its resulting effect on the ground reaction force which is considered to be the important factor,

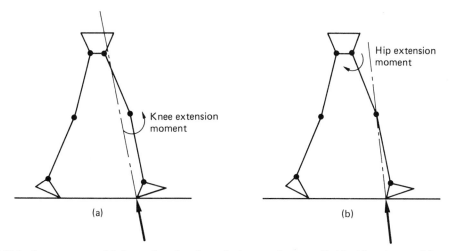

Knee extension moment

Hip extension moment

(a)   (b)

Figure 4.9 If the knee extensors (a) do not function, knee flexion may be controlled by hip extensors (b)

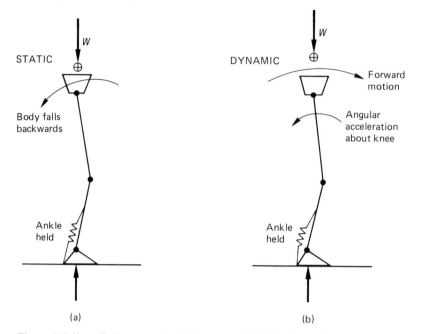

Figure 4.10 Knee flexion occurs in (a) but not in (b) if the forward velocity of the body is sufficient and the ankle is controlled

the outcome is the same – increased knee stability. Secondly (Figure 4.10), in static single support, an unopposed knee flexion moment induces an angular acceleration of the joint towards flexion. If the ankle were held stable the portion of the body above the supporting knee would collapse posteriorly. On the other hand, if the body is in a state of forward motion then the knee flexion moment will cause it to decelerate and will only lead to collapse if this deceleration is sufficiently great to arrest forward motion completely. These effects are relevant in both normal and pathological gait.

In order to explain the interrelationship between external force, muscle action and motion during the entire gait cycle it is helpful to refer to graphical displays such as those of Peizer *et al.* (1969). Using their style of presentation, three graphs are plotted on the same time-base (Figures 4.11–4.13) showing the joint angle, the externally applied moment and relevant muscle activity about that joint for the hip, knee and ankle respectively. Thus, at a given instant in the gait cycle, the relationship between these parameters may be readily seen. For example, at 50% of the cycle the ankle is in approximately 10° of dorsiflexion and is rapidly plantarflexing. This implies a net plantarflex-

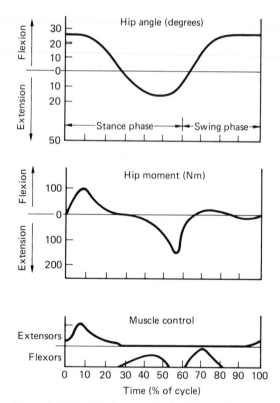

Figure 4.11 Hip joint in normal gait: joint motion, externally applied moment and relevant muscle activity. (Reproduced with permission from Peizer *et al.*, 1969)

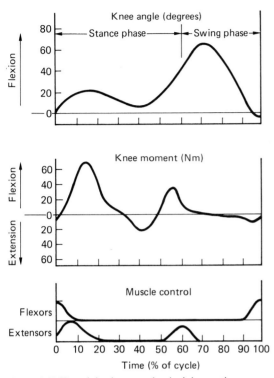

Figure 4.12 Knee joint in normal gait: joint motion, externally applied moment and relevant muscle activity. (Reproduced with permission from Peizer *et al.*, 1969)

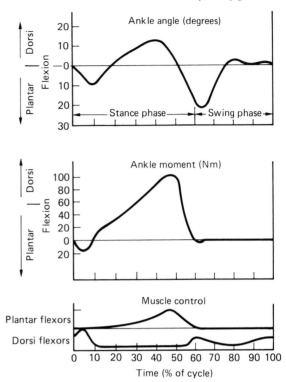

Figure 4.13 Ankle joint in normal gait: joint motion, externally applied moment and relevant muscle activity. (Reproduced with permission from Peizer *et al.*, 1969)

ion moment. There is, in fact, a large external dorsiflexion moment of around 100 Nm acting (Figure 4.13). It is possible to estimate the force which must be exerted by the plantar-flexors, to overcome this dorsiflexion moment (Figure 4.14). The muscle force P, acting at a perpendicular distance d from the joint, counteracts an external dorsiflexion moment of 100 Nm (due to the ground reaction acting anterior to the ankle joint). Thus $P \times d = 100$ and if d is equal to say 4 cm (0.04 m) then P is equal to 2500 N or approximately a quarter of a ton. The ankle joint is subjected to a force (J) which is the vector sum of the muscle force (P) and external ground reaction force (R). In this particular case the joint force will be around 3300 N (assuming a ground reaction force of 800 N).

Such calculations, although only approximate, indicate the considerable magnitude of the forces which muscles must be able to generate and joints must withstand during walking. Using gait analysis data Paul (1965) was able to estimate maximum hip joint loading during

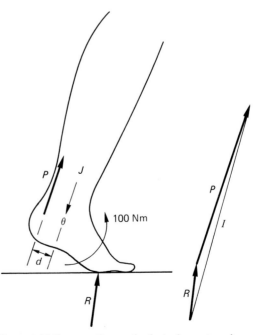

Figure 4.14 Forces acting on the foot when external dorsiflexion moment is 100 Nm in late stance phase

walking as almost six times body weight. Other activities such as running and jumping have been shown to involve substantially greater forces. Thus the large internal forces associated with walking are well within the capacities of a normal healthy individual. For this reason, normal walking is possible with less than full muscle power. Perry (1985) has stated that the hip abductors require only 40% of their full strength for an individual to walk without a limp. Similarly, the necessary strength of the hip flexors and extensors was 15% of full strength and the quadriceps could be sufficiently strong at less than 5% of full strength as long as the hip extensors and plantarflexors of the foot were normal. It is also worth noting that, with the exception of the hip extension and ankle dorsiflexion, normal ranges of joint motion far exceed those required for normal gait.

The use of instrumented gait analysis techniques permits a detailed description of the process of walking. It is theoretically possible to obtain simultaneous readings of all body movements, external forces, muscle activity and, as will be discussed in the following section, the energy consumption throughout several consecutive gait cycles. In practice not all of these parameters are routinely studied by any single gait laboratory. If ground reaction forces are measured these are usually for only one or two strides as variability of stride length makes it difficult to achieve clean foot-strikes on a larger number of plates arranged in series. However, even in this limited configuration the force place has contributed enormously to our understanding of gait.

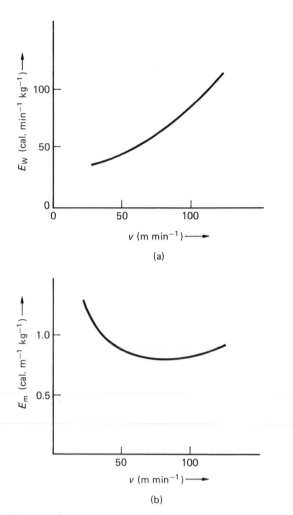

Figure 4.15 A plot, versus walking speed, of energy consumption (a) per minute and (b) per metre walked

4.3.3 The energy required for gait

The energy cost may significantly limit both walking speed and potential range and is clearly an important factor when discussing gait. The physiological cost of walking can be investigated by studying oxygen consumption, and carbon dioxide production using lightweight systems, carried by the patient, for the collection of expired air. Using this technique, Ralston (1958) concluded that the average rate of energy consumption in calories per minute per kilogram of body weight (E_w) was directly proportional to the square of walking speed (v) and could be represented by the formula $E_w = b + m\,v^2$ where b and m are constants (Figure 4.15(a)). The values of b and m were initially determined by Ralston to be 29 and 0.0053 respectively but were later updated by Inman *et al.* (1981) to 32 and 0.0050 respectively based on further data which had accrued since the original study. Zarrugh *et al.* (1974) noted that this equation loses accuracy towards the upper limit of walking speed but is adequate for walking speeds up to 100 m min^{-1}. If the above equation is divided throughout by v, it becomes $E_m = E_w/v = b/v + mv$ where E_m represents the energy consumed per metre walked. This may be expressed graphically (Figure 4.15(b)). By differentiating this expression with respect to *v*, and equating the result to zero, it is found that the minimum rate of energy consumption per metre is $2\sqrt{bm}$ at a walking speed of $\sqrt{b/m}$. Using the more recent values of *b* and *m* this yields, on average, a minimum energy consumption of 0.8 cal m^{-1} kg^{-1} at a normal walking speed of 80 m min^{-1}.

Bard and Ralston (1959) observed that the walking speed which minimizes the energy consumption per metre walked is approximately the same as the 'comfortable' speed which is naturally adopted by the subject.

Even lightweight gas collection systems may, in themselves, affect the energy consumption they are intended to measure. In an attempt to develop a less intrusive technique, MacGregor (1981) experimented with heart rate. Due to the physiological differences between individuals, the heart rate alone cannot reflect energy consumption but it was found that the so-called physiological cost index (PCI) was a useful parameter. This was defined as:

$$\text{PCI} = \frac{\text{heart rate (walking)} - \text{heart rate (resting)}}{\text{walking speed (metres/min)}}$$

This section has given an overview of instrumented gait analysis techniques. A more com-prehensive account is given by Gage and Oun-puu (1989), and a detailed coverage of the subject, including theoretical aspects, is presented by Winter (1979).

4.4 Analysis of gait

At the beginning of this chapter a description of the observable features of gait was given. It is now possible to complete this description by including kinetic data derived from instrumented gait analysis systems. The sagittal and frontal planes will be considered separately. In each of the following figures, the lower limb is shown as a stick diagram and the ground reaction force is represented by a vector. The length of this vector indicates its magnitude and its line of action is represented by an extended dotted line.

4.4.1 Sagittal plane

(a) Heel-strike to foot-flat (Figure 4.16)

At heel-strike, the hip is flexed by some 25–30° and remains so throughout this phase. It is controlled by the hip extensors (gluteus maximus and hamstrings) which counteract the

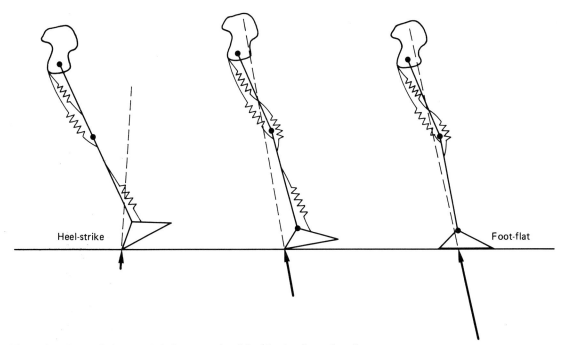

Figure 4.16 Lower limb control during normal walking; heel-strike to foot-flat

flexion moment produced by the ground reaction passing anterior to the hip joint.

The knee flexes gradually from full extension to about 15° of flexion. This flexion is induced by the ground reaction passing behind the joint aided by the hamstrings which are controlling the hip but, as biarticular muscles, also affect the knee. Knee flexion is opposed and thereby controlled by the knee extensors (quadriceps).

The ankle undergoes plantarflexion from the neutral position to some 10° of plantarflexion due to the plantarflexion moment created by the ground reaction passing posterior to the ankle. The rate of plantarflexion is controlled by the action of the dorsiflexors (anterior tibial muscles).

(b) Foot-flat to heel-off (Figure 4.17)

During this phase, the hip extends to about 15° of extension, initially under the action of the hip extensors which overcome the flexion moment due to the ground reaction passing anterior to the hip joint. This flexion moment gradually reduces and is replaced by an exten-

sion moment as the body progresses forward over the supporting foot. As this occurs, hip extensor action is replaced by hip flexor (iliopsoas) activity.

The knee may flex a little further but the predominant motion during this phase is extension.

The foot is firmly located on the ground and as the lower leg moves forward the ankle joint attitude changes from 10° of plantarflexion to about 10° of dorsiflexion. Dorsiflexion occurs because the ground reaction force moves anterior to the ankle joint. It is controlled by the plantarflexors (calf muscles). The fact that the ankle and hip are controlled and the body has forward impetus, removes the need for knee extensor control as described in section 4.3.2.

(c) Heel-off to toe-off (Figure 4.18)

During this phase the hip initially continues to extend by a few degrees then flexes reaching about 10° of extension by toe-off. The hip flexors (iliopsoas) control the initial extension and induce the subsequent flexion in opposi-

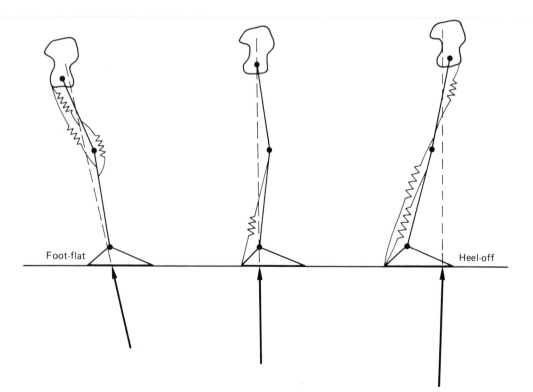

Figure 4.17 Lower limb control during normal walking; foot-flat to heel-off

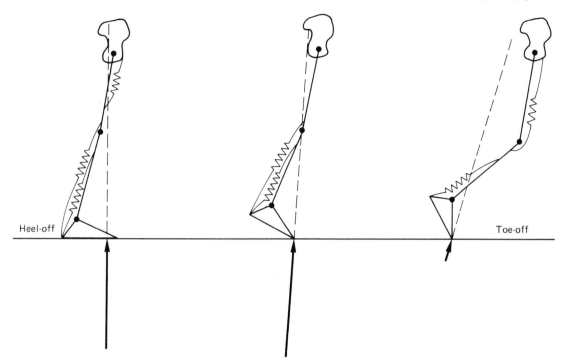

Heel-off

Toe-off

Figure 4.18 Lower limb control during normal walking; heel-off to toe-off

tion to the extension moment of the ground reaction force.

The knee joint is close to full extension at heel-off but begins to flex, in harmony with the hip, possibly influenced by the gastrocnemius muscle which is both an ankle plantarflexor and a knee flexor. The ground reaction force rapidly passes behind the knee and the resulting flexion moment is then controlled by the quadriceps.

The characteristic feature of this phase is the rapid plantarflexion of the ankle from 10° of dorsiflexion to 20° of plantarflexion. This occurs, due to the plantarflexor (gastrocnemius and soleus) activity, in spite of the large dorsiflexion moment induced by the ground reaction force. During this phase extension of the toes occurs progressively, as the heel rises, to a maximum just before toe-off. Using simple geometry, it can be calculated that the required toe extension at any instant during this phase is approximately equal to the sum of the angles of hip extension, knee flexion and ankle plantarflexion. This assumes that the toe is horizontal and that midtarsal flexion/extension is relatively small during push-off.

(d) Swing phase (Figure 4.19)

During this phase the hip flexes from around 10° of extension to 25–30° of flexion. The hip flexors initiate motion and the hip extensors act later to decelerate the leg prior to heel-strike. As the leg accelerates the knee continues to flex due to inertial effects. This flexion is restrained by the knee extensors. Towards the end of the swing phase the deceleration of the thigh reverses the inertial effect on the lower leg; the resulting tendency towards knee extension is opposed by the action of the knee flexors. The maximum knee flexion achieved during the swing phase is about 65°. Throughout the swing phase the anterior tibial muscles maintain the foot in a neutral attitude to aid toe clearance.

4.4.2 Frontal plane

One aspect of gait which is not observed in the sagittal plane, but is of great importance, is the control of hip adduction in stance phase (Figure 4.20). During midstance the pelvis dips on the non-supported side; this involves adduction

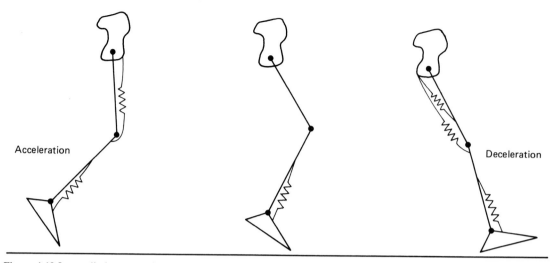

Figure 4.19 Lower limb control during normal walking; swing phase

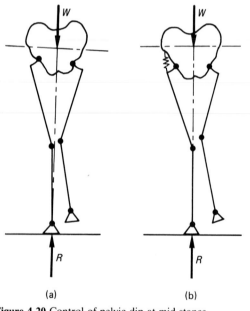

(a)   (b)

Figure 4.20 Control of pelvic dip at mid-stance

lines would normally be about 5–10 cm apart (Figure 4.21). This 'walking base' is somewhat wider than the side to side translation of the body centre of gravity, as might be expected in the dynamic situation where a small degree of medially directed instability at midstance initiates the return oscillation towards the contralateral side in anticipation of the next step. The side to side movement of the body and axial rotation of the leg during midstance phase, while the foot remains flat on the ground, are possible because of the mobility of the joints within the foot itself, particularly the subtalar joint. This will be discussed in more detail in Chapter 6 which deals with foot orthotics.

of the supporting hip and is due to the line of action of the ground reaction force relative to the hip. To control this effect, the hip abductors contract producing a countermoment which restricts pelvic dip to around 5° from the horizontal.

Also observed in the frontal plane is a side to side oscillation of the pelvis with a total excursion of some 5 cm. If the positions of the midpoints of successive footprints for each foot were connected by lines then the two resulting

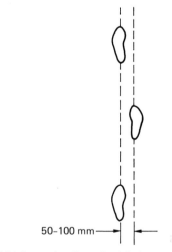

50–100 mm

Figure 4.21 Successive 'footprints' during normal walking

4.5 The range of normality

The analysis of normal gait provides a description of movement and a rationale for muscle activity which are both useful in the discussion of the effects of pathological and congenital abnormalities. However, it must be recognized that the gait patterns described may vary from one individual to another. Repeatability studies, involving three tests on each of three separate days, were carried out by Kadaba *et al.* (1989) on 40 normal subjects walking at their natural speed. They found that, for a given subject, both single-day and between-day repeatability of sagittal plane data was excellent. Poor between-day repeatability was found for the frontal and transverse planes but this was partly attributed to the difficulty in accurately repositioning skin markers. Winter (1987) reported low variability in repeated testing of a given subject and noted that there were identifiable differences between two different normal subjects. For example, the minimum knee flexion angle in stance phase was approximately 5° for one subject and 15° in the other.

Larger differences are found in the gait of children. Grieve and Gear (1966) found the gait of young children to be more variable and apparently experimental up to about 4–5 years of age. In terms of stride length, step frequency, time of swing and walking speed, children aged over 5 exhibited adult gait. In a study of 186 normal children aged from 1 to 7 years, which included joint motion analysis, Sutherland *et al.* (1980) observed that adult joint rotation patterns were approximated by the age of 2 years. The gait of young children exhibited greater knee flexion and dorsiflexion during the stance phase and pronounced external rotation of the hips, although reciprocal arm swing and heel strike were well established by 18 months. According to their criteria (duration of single limb stance, walking velocity, cadence, step length, and ratio of pelvic span to ankle spread), they concluded that mature gait was well established by 3 years. An investigation into the development of gait in 230 normal children between 3 and 16 years was carried out by Norlin *et al.* (1981). They studied velocity, stride length, cadence and the temporal phases of walking and concluded that there were discernible age-related changes up

to 8 years; thereafter leg length became the dominating factor.

Variations from the normal patterns might be expected in later life. In a study of 64 normal men, aged between 20 and 87 years, Murray *et al.* (1969) found that age-related gait changes occurred. For example, walking speed and stride length were significantly reduced beyond about 65 years, stride width appeared to increase beyond 74 years and out-toeing increased after 80 years.

The measurement and analysis of kinetic parameters has provided an explanation of how human beings walk. There will be variations in these parameters within the limits of normal gait but the underlying logic of the relationship between external forces (body weight, ground reaction force and inertial effects) and internal forces (muscle and joint forces) remains and greatly facilitates the analysis of pathological gait resulting from neuromuscular and musculoskeletal causes.

4.6 Pathological gait

In discussing normal gait it has been helpful to define a number of identifiable 'landmarks' in the gait cycle such as foot-flat and heel-off. Such definitions can become meaningless in the presence of gross gait abnormalities. Nevertheless, for convenience, the effects of abnormal conditions will be identified herein by examining their effects in relation to the normal gait cycle. In some cases the full impact of an abnormality such as muscular weakness can be predicted by considering the consequences in purely mechanical terms. However, in other cases, where sensory and proprioceptive feedbacks are intact, there will be the possibility of compensatory abnormal motion at unaffected joints.

Some illustrative examples will now be considered.

4.6.1 Reduced or absent dorsiflexion power

The dorsiflexors contribute significantly to ankle joint control in early stance phase and swing phase. Between heel-strike and foot-flat they control the plantarflexion of the foot induced by the ground reaction force. Weakness of this muscle group would be manifested, in early stance, by rapid plantarflexion often ending with a characteristic audible foot slap. During swing phase they exert the small dorsiflexion moment required to support the weight of the foot. If there is marked weakness, there may be insufficient power even to support the foot in swing phase. This will often lead to toe contact with the ground (drop-foot, toe-drag) at mid-swing and the consequent danger of tripping. If proprioceptive feedback is unimpaired, the danger can be averted by increased knee and hip flexion during swing phase. Toe clearance could also be achieved by circumduction (swing phase abduction of the non-supporting hip), hip hiking (elevation of the pelvis and non-supporting leg during midstance) or vaulting (midstance plantarflexion of the supporting foot). In more severe cases heel-strike will be replaced by flat footed or even toe contact.

4.6.2 Reduced or absent plantarflexion power

One consequence of severe plantarflexor weakness is an inability to oppose the external dorsiflexion moment, induced by the ground reaction acting anterior to the ankle joint, between the instants of midstance and toe-off. This reduces stability and eliminates the contribution of the ankle, at this stage, in preventing excessive lowering of the body centre of gravity. During the midstance phase, the role of ankle control by the plantarflexors in stabilizing the knee may be replaced by knee extensor activity. Where there is bilateral absence of plantarflexion power, even simple standing can be quite precarious since anterior foot support is lost.

Weakness of the plantarflexors will also result in the absence or impairment of the active plantarflexion which contributes significantly to the forward propulsion of the body during the normal push-off. In its absence some compensation by increased hip extensor activity is possible.

4.6.3 Loss of ankle motion

Consider first the consequences of ankle fixation in the neutral position. A normal heel-strike occurs but foot-flat can only be achieved by excessive knee flexion which may be controlled by the knee extensors. Forward progression can continue; the knee extends as the forward momentum of the body carries it over the fixed ankle. Once the knee reaches full extension, with the foot flat, further forward motion will require the heel to rise. This transfers the ground reaction force to the forefoot prematurely and moves its line of action anteriorly relative to the knee joint. Thus the knee joint will be subjected to an abnormally high extension moment after the midstance point. A normal push-off cannot occur but at least collapse into dorsiflexion is also impossible. An increase in hip extensor activity can, as already stated, compensate for the absence of push-off.

Consider now the differences introduced if the ankle is fixed in dorsiflexion or plantarflexion. The dorsiflexed ankle will experience heel-strike but a greater degree of knee flexion will be necessary for the achievement of foot-flat. Again the knee extensors can control this process; this will result in a prolonged period of heel loading. Knee flexion of about twice the angle of fixed dorsiflexion (as measured between the lower leg and the sole of the shoe) will be present at the midstance point and thereafter there will be an absence of push-off as before.

On the other hand, if the ankle is relatively plantarflexed, foot-flat is reached more readily. The knee will reach full extension early, possibly before the instant of midstance and, for the remainder of the stance phase, will experience an extension moment due to the anterior location, on the foot, of the ground reaction force. There may also be the danger of the plantarflexed foot contacting the ground during swing phase.

4.6.4 Abnormal supination/pronation

This can result from weakness or hyperactivity of the pronators or supinators of the foot. Whether the cause is weakness or hyperactivity, the resulting gait abnormality can be readily observed from behind during the swing phase and foot contact will be made by the medial or lateral margin. Where the cause is muscle weakness, the external moment will cause the foot to assume a normal alignment during stance phase. Where spasticity is present, the deviation will persist during weight bearing as long as the internal supinating or pronating moment exceeds the external correcting moment.

4.6.5 Knee extensor weakness

The knee extensors are active in early stance phase and early swing phase. Their role in early stance is to control the rate of knee flexion induced by the ground reaction force. In the absence of knee extensor power, uncontrolled knee flexion may be avoided if the ground reaction is prevented from passing behind the knee joint. This may be achieved by increased hip extensor activity and anterior trunk bending (which displaces the centre of gravity of the body anteriorly). A reduced range of plantarflexion, such as is experienced when high heels are worn, would add potential danger because early knee flexion would be induced without the extensor power to control it. Normal stair climbing is impossible in the absence of knee extensor power. If one leg is sound it must lead upstairs and follow downstairs so that the potentially unstable knee remains fully extended. A possible long-term consequence of this condition is hyperextension of the knee due to the continued thrusting of the joint into full extension for security. If hyperextension develops, the knee will become more inherently stable due to its posterior displacement relative to the line of the ground reaction force during stance phase. However, the increased extension moment will induce a further hyperextension deformity such that this secondary problem may assume major clinical importance.

4.6.6 Hip abductor weakness

The role of the hip abductors is to control the attitude of the pelvis, as viewed from the front, in stance phase. If they do not have adequate power, the trunk will dip excessively giving the so-called 'positive Trendelenburg sign'. The individual may attempt to counteract this by lateral bending of the trunk towards the supporting side. This displaces the ground reaction/weight line towards the supporting hip joint, thus reducing the hip adduction moment and the countermoment which has to be supplied by the abductors to control it.

4.6.7 Pain

In the presence of otherwise normal structure and function, the gait may still be significantly affected by the presence of pain. For example, pain occurring in the foot during ground contact may lead to the development of a compensatory gait deviation which will reduce the force at the site of the pain. Thus pain associated with hindfoot contact might result in lack of heel-strike since forefoot contact would avoid the application of force to the painful zone of the foot.

On the other hand, pain related to forefoot contact will become troublesome in late stance phase when the ground reaction force is concentrated at the metatarsal heads and toes. The pain may be alleviated by permitting the affected foot to dorsiflex, instead of actively plantarflexing, and transferring weight to the sound leg as quickly as possible. If the pain is occurring in one or more joints of the foot during forefoot loading, internal or external rotation of the leg may give relief by reducing the external moment which is causing the pain.

The foregoing discussion is intended as a series of examples of the logic which links gait abnormalities to particular impairments. It should be noted, however, that some pathological conditions such as muscular dystrophy (Sutherland *et al.*, 1981) and cerebral palsy (Meadows, 1984) produce complex patterns of gait which combine several abnormalities, of the types discussed above, in the one condition.

It is clear that, for pathological gait, the terminology employed in describing normal walking is inadequate. An alternative terminology was suggested by Perry (1985) to facilitate the description of pathological gait (Table 4.2).

There are various reasons to be concerned about abnormal gait patterns. Gait abnormalities may increase the energy needed for walking. Fisher and Gullickson (1978) generalized that disabled persons decrease their speed of walking so that their energy consumption per minute decreases towards the normal range.

Table 4.2 Adapted terminology proposed by Perry (1985)

Adapted terminology	Equivalent normal gait terminology
Initial contact	Heel-strike
Loading response	Shock absorption
Midstance	Midstance
Terminal stance	Early push-off
Pre-swing	Double support push-off
Initial swing	Acceleration
Midswing	Midswing
Terminal swing	Deceleration

Thus, on the one hand, the disabled person expends more energy in completing a given journey and, on the other, that journey requires more time than it would for an able-bodied individual. An abnormal gait pattern may also involve dangerous instability, it may cause tissue damage and pain due to abnormal loading, or promote the development of skeletal deformity as a result of abnormal joint moments. As will be seen in later chapters, orthotic treatment based on a sound understanding of the principles described in this chapter has an important contribution to make in overcoming these problems and improving gait.

4.7 Glossary

cadence: the number of steps taken per unit time during gait

force transducer: a device which produces an electrical signal related to the magnitude of the applied force (and therefore used to give a measurement of that force)

gait cycle: the repeating cycle of walking usually taken from heel-strike of a given foot to the next heel-strike of the same foot

ground reaction (force): the force (usually expressed in Newtons) exerted by the ground on the foot at any time during stance phase

kinematics: the branch of mechanics concerned with only the motion of a body

kinetics: the branch of mechanics concerned with the forces acting on a body and the effects of those forces on its motion

moment of force about a point: the product of the force and the perpendicular distance of its line of action from the point in question

stance phase: the part of the gait cycle during which the limb under consideration is in contact with the ground

step length: the distance between a given point on the left foot and the same point on the right foot at an instant at which they are both on the ground during walking

stride length: the distance between two successive stance phase positions of a given foot during walking (on average, stride length is twice step length)

swing phase: the part of the gait cycle during which the limb under consideration is not in contact with the ground

walking base: if a line were drawn connecting successive stance phase positions of the centre of the right foot, and a similar line were drawn for the left foot, then the distance between these two lines would be the walking base

walking velocity: the rate of linear motion of the body in the direction of progression (normally expressed in metres per minute)

References

Bard G. and Ralston H.J. (1959) Measurement of energy expenditure during ambulation, with special reference to evaluation of assistive devices. *Arch. Phys. Med. Rehabil.* **40**, 415–420

DeBruin H., Russell D.J., Latter J.E. *et al.* (1982) Angle-angle diagrams in monitoring and qualification of gait patterns for children with cerebral palsy. *Am. J. Phys. Med.* **61**, 176–192

Eberhart H.D., Inman V.T. and Bresler B. (1954) The principal elements in human locomotion. In: Klopskey P.E. and Wilson P.D. (eds), *Human Limbs and their Substitutes.* Reprinted 1968 by Hafner, New York

Finley, F.R. and Cody K.A. (1970) Locomotive characteristics of urban pedestrians. *Arch. Phys. Med. Rehabil.* **51**, 423–426

Fisher S.V. and Gullickson G. (1978) Energy cost of ambulation in health and disability: a literature review. *Arch. Phys. Med. Rehabil.* **59**, 124–133

Gage J.R. and Ounpuu S. (1989) Gait analysis in clinical practice. *Semin. Orthop.* **4**, (2), 72–87

Grieve, D.W. and Gear R.J. (1987) The relationship between length of stride, step frequency, time of swing and speed of walking for children and adults. *Ergonomics* **9**, 379–399

Inman V.T., Ralston H.J. and Todd F. (1981) *Human Walking.* Williams and Wilkins, Baltimore.

Kadaba M.P., Ramakrishnan M.E., Wootten J. *et al.* (1989) Repeatability of kinematic, kinetic, and electromyographical data in normal adult gait. *J. Orthop. Res.* **7**, 849–860

Lord M., Reynolds D. P. and Hughes J. R. (1986) Foot pressure measurement: a review of clinical findings. *J. Biomed. Eng.* **8**, 283–294

MacGregor J. (1981) The evaluation of patient performance using long-term ambulatory monitoring technique in the domiciliary environment. *Physiotherapy* **67**, 30–33

Meadows C.B. (1984) The Influence of Polypropylene Ankle-foot Orthoses on the Gait of Cerebral Palsied Children. PhD Thesis, University of Strathclyde, Glasgow, UK

Murray M.P., Kory R.C. and Clarkson B.H. (1969) Walking patterns in healthy old men. *J. Gerontol.* **24**, 169–178

Norlin R., Odenrick P. and Sandlund B. (1981) Development of gait in the normal child. *J. Paediatr. Orthop.* **1**, 261–266

Paul J.P. (1965) Bioengineering studies of the forces transmitted by joints. In: Kenedi R. M. (ed), *Biomechanics and Related Bioengineering Topics*. Pergamon, Oxford

Peizer E., Wright D.W. and Mason C. (1969) Human locomotion. *Bull. Prosthet. Res.* **10**, (12), 48–105

Perry J. (1985) *Atlas of Orthotics*, 2nd edn. CV Mosby, St Louis

Ralston H.J. (1958) Energy–speed relation and optional speed during level walking. *Int. Z. Agnew. Physiol.* **17**, 277–283

Sutherland D.H., Olshen R., Cooper L. *et al.* (1980) The development of mature gait. *J. Bone Joint Surg.* **62A**, 336–353

Sutherland D.H., Olshen R., Cooper L. *et al.* (1981) The pathomechanics of gait in Duchenne muscular dystrophy. *Dev. Med. Child Neurol.* **23**, 3–22

University of California, Berkeley (1947) *Fundamental Studies of Human Locomotion*. Serial No. CAL 5 (2 vols)

Waters R.L., Lunsford R., Perry J. *et al.* (1988) Energy–speed relationship of walking: standard tables. *J. Orthop. Res.* **6**, 215–222

Winter D.A. (1979) *Biomechanics of Human Movement*. John Wiley, New York

Winter D.A. (1987) *The Biomechanics and Motor Control of Human Gait*. University of Waterloo Press, Canada

Zarrugh M.Y., Todd F.N. and Ralston H.J. (1974) Optimisation of energy expenditure during level walking. *Eur. J. Appl. Physiol.* **33**, 293–306

5

The patient–orthosis interface

Dan Bader and Andrew Chase

5.1 Introduction

The patient–orthosis interface may be defined as the junction between the body tissues and the orthosis and/or support surface through which forces are transmitted. These forces may arise in one of two ways. First, they may result directly from the transmission of partial or total body weight to a supporting surface, such as the seating interface (Figure 5.1). At this interface, in accordance with Newton's third law, the weight force of the body acting on the supporting area of the seat is balanced by an equal and opposite reaction force imposed on the body by the support surface. A similar situation arises at the junction between the

plantar surface of the foot and the insock or insole of a shoe.

Alternatively, the interface forces may be generated because an orthosis has been designed specifically to hold one or more joints in particular positions; the orthosis therefore restrains motion which would otherwise have occurred either as a result of body weight or of an unbalanced muscle force having a moment about the joint centre of rotation. This process is illustrated schematically in Figure 5.2 in which an orthosis is preventing forward flexion of the intervertebral joints under the influence of the weight force of the trunk. The figure indicates the components of the orthosis through which forces may be applied.

Ultimately, the sustained application of pressure to an area of soft tissue will lead to the progressive breakdown of that tissue and the formation of a pressure sore. These sores are described in the following section.

5.2 Pressure sores

5.2.1 Classification

Four grades of pressure sores can be identified on the basis of the pathophysiology of soft tissue breakdown overlying bony prominencies (Shea, 1975). The most apparent superficial clinical presentation of a Grade I pressure sore is an irregular, ill-defined area of soft tissue swelling and induration, with associated heat and redness or erythema, overlying a bony prominence. It is always limited to the epi-

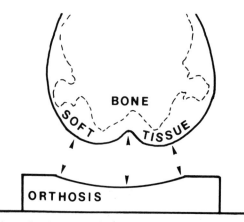

Figure 5.1 A cross-section through the seating–support interface

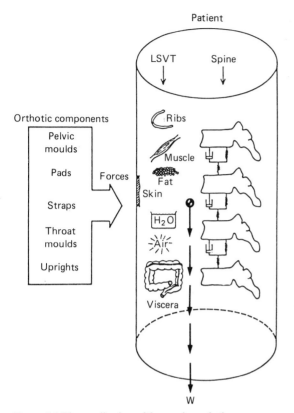

Patient

LSVT   Spine

Orthotic components

Pelvic moulds

Pads   Forces

Straps

Throat moulds

Uprights

Ribs

Muscle

Fat

Skin

H_2O

Air

Viscera

W

Figure 5.2 The application of forces through the interface between spinal orthosis and the body (based on White and Panjabi, 1990)

dermal layer but may expose the underlying dermis. The Grade II pressure sore presents clinically as a shallow full-thickness skin ulcer whose edges are more distinct, and with early fibrosis and pigmentation changes merging into a broad indistinct area of heat, erythema and induration. Clinically, the Grade III pressure sore involves an irregular full-thickness defect extending into the subcutaneous fat and exposing a draining, foul-smelling, infected, necrotic base which has undermined the skin for a variable distance. This type of sore also commonly involves adjacent muscles and joints. Grade IV sores resemble those of Grade III except that in the base of the ulceration bone can be identified which is more extensively undermined with necrosis of tissues and often profuse drainage. Clearly management is correlated with the extent of the lesion, and ranges from local wound care, relief of pressure and irritation and systematic support for Grades I and II, to major surgical intervention

for the more extensive Grades III and IV sores (Crow and Clark, 1990).

5.2.2 Incidence

The reported incidence of pressure sores in the UK is 30 000 per annum, but this figure is likely to be erroneously low due to a significant number of undocumented lesions, particularly those occurring in the community. This represents a large burden on the finances and the manpower of the Health Service. In fact, present estimates of the total cost of pressure sores to the Health Service exceed £250 million per annum. These figures can only increase in an ageing population unless a preventative care programme is rigorously introduced for subjects at particular risk of tissue breakdown. The individual cost of treating one Grade IV sore in an elderly patient in a London teaching hospital (Hibbs, 1990) has been estimated to be equivalent, in terms of both finances and manpower, to 16 hip or knee replacement operations. This takes no account of medico-legal costs, which are likely to become an increasingly important factor. In a recent English court settlement a patient was awarded over £100 000 for a pressure sore which arose during hospitalization.

However, the response of a particular area of the skin of a particular individual to the application of external forces depends on many factors. These include both *extrinsic factors*, that is the external physical parameters at the interface which place demands on the tissue, and *intrinsic factors*, physiological and pathological in nature, which through systemic or localized effects influence the response of the tissues to those environmental demands, and thus affect tissue viability. The effects of extrinsic and intrinsic factors will be considered separately.

5.3 Factors affecting tissue response to its environment

5.3.1 Extrinsic factors

(a) Pressure

A knowledge of the stresses occurring at the interface is essential in the evaluation of the potential damage to soft tissues of the body. It is well known that body tissues can support high levels of hydrostatic pressure which has equal components in all directions, with no resulting tissue distortion. This is well illustrated by deep sea divers, who are regularly exposed to hydrostatic pressures in excess of 750 mmHg (100 kPa) for prolonged periods with no ill-effects to their soft tissues. However, if the pressures are non-uniform, tissue distortion may lead to localized tissue damage. This occurs in many situations in which the body interfaces externally with load-carrying devices. For example, it is relevant in the provision of support surfaces for wheelchair-bound individuals as well as in the design of orthoses and prosthetic sockets.

The interface pressures are supported by the intervening soft tissues, and stress and strain fields will be established within the interstitium. This mechanical environment may be sufficient to impair the local blood supply and lymphatic circulation. Impairment of the former will limit the availability of the vital nutrient, oxygen, to the localized tissues, while lymphatic impairment will result in an accumulation of toxic intracellular materials in the tissues. If such interface conditions are applied over a prolonged period, cell necrosis may occur, leading to possible tissue breakdown and the development of pressure sores. As the soft tissues exhibit viscoelastic behaviour, the extent of tissue deformation will depend upon the rate and duration of loading as well as its magnitude. In general, short-term loading produces only elastic deformation, whilst long-term loading results in creep deformation as well, which leads to increasingly high tissue strains. Indeed it has been well established that tissue damage is often apparent following prolonged loading even at relatively low level pressure intensities (Reswick and Rogers, 1976).

Any significant period of loading may result in vascular occlusion. However, if the pressure is relieved intermittently higher pressures can be tolerated for a longer overall time period than if that pressure is applied continuously. This forms the basis of pressure relief regimens, which involve regular turning or lift-off from the support surface and which are recommended for all individuals who are 'at risk' and particularly those who are insensitive. The nature of the tissue recovery on load removal is determined by the resilience and structure of the specific tissues, including the blood and

lymph vessels. Commonly there is a reactive hyperaemia, which is a period of increased blood flow through the tissues which had been ischaemic. This phenomenon is a consequence of a local regulatory mechanism whereby the arterioles are dilated and the resistance to blood flow is reduced. The identity of the vasodilator agents remains unclear but histamine- and prostaglandin-like substances have been implicated in this response in the past.

(b) Shear

Shear stresses arise from any external contact surfaces causing distortion; for example, those which induce localized pressure, non-uniform pressure distribution, and surface shear or tangential forces developed particularly on weight-bearing surfaces. These shear forces can be a particular clinical problem when a patient is transferred from one support surface to another or for a patient who has been propped up and tends to slide on an inflexible bed support, as illustrated in Figure 5.3. Clearly the fabrics for sheets and cushion covers will also influence the possibility of skin damage due to friction. Shear forces are also established within any ill-fitting orthosis where there is relative movement between the orthosis and body tissues or where the forces transmitted through an orthotic component, such as a cuff, are not normal to the limb surface, as indicated in Chapter 8.

Shear forces also develop within the soft tissues where there is relative movement between the soft tissues and the underlying bone. Reichel (1958) discussed the presence of shear forces and increased compressive forces within the posterior sacral tissues and concentrated in the deeper portion of the superficial fascia. Such forces affect the structural integrity of the blood vessels which pierce the deep fascia and supply nutrients to the surrounding tissues and skin. Lymph flow is similarly restricted (Reddy *et al.*, 1981). An experimental study has shown that a tangential force of 1.33 N mm^{-1} and strain of 10% are sufficient to produce virtual obliteration of capillary blood flow (Bader *et al.*, 1986). In a separate study, Bennett *et al.* (1979) has shown that the pressure level required to disrupt blood flow can be reduced by half in the presence of shear forces.

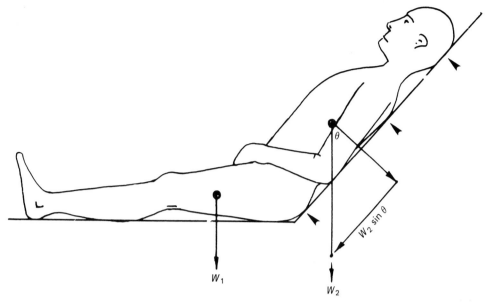

Figure 5.3 Support forces acting on the sacrum when a subject is supported on an inclined surface. The shear forces in the scaral region are indicated

(c) Interface microenvironment

The microenvironment of the patient–orthosis interface greatly influences the likelihood of tissue breakdown. High moisture levels at the interface can be produced by incontinence or perspiration adjacent to an impermeable close-fitting orthosis or within closed shoes. This excess moisture can lead to maceration of the epidermis, a precursor of tissue breakdown, which is accelerated by an alkali environment. In addition, wet skin is more likely to adhere to clothing or to the orthosis itself, thus increasing substantially the shearing forces.

Microorganisms may also thrive at the patient–orthosis interface, for example in the environment of the foot, resulting in a deterioration in the overall wear of the shoe uppers and a poor cosmetic appearance. A further important aspect of the presence of organisms in footwear is their likely direct effect on the foot. The best known example of fungal attack is athletes' foot, which is a degradation of skin between the toes by *Trichophyton interdigitalis*.

The need to provide dry and hygienic conditions at all patient–orthosis interfaces is thus clearly essential for the well-being of the soft tissues. In this context, the use of cotton is superior to man-made fibres in that it promotes a wick effect at the interface to remove excess moisture. This should always be considered at the time of an orthotic fitting.

Soft tissues are also sensitive to slight changes in temperature. For example, temperature increases at the patient–orthosis interface produce significant effects by increasing the rate of cell metabolism in the local tissues (Tortora and Anagnostakos, 1981). In fact it has been reported that a 1°C temperature rise increases the metabolic rate by about 13%. This is particularly important in patients with reduced peripheral circulation, in whom an inability to meet the increased tissue demands may lead to local tissue necrosis. The temperature at the interface should be considered particularly in warm ambient conditions, or when a patient is required to wear a close-fitting orthosis, such as a spinal brace made of thermoplastic materials, for long periods of the day. Conversely some subjects, particularly the elderly, benefit from the warming effects of orthoses, as discussed in Chapters 12 and 13.

5.3.2 Intrinsic factors

(a) Tissue viability

Whilst all the external physical factors discussed above are important in determining the prognosis of the tissues at the patient–orthosis interface, the monitoring and control of these is, alone, insufficient to alert the clinician to potential areas of tissue breakdown. For this some measure of the viability of the tissues themselves is also required.

The normal viability of the body's superficial tissues may be compromised by very many factors. Probably the most important requirement for the maintenance of viability is an adequate supply of nutrients via the blood stream. The measurement of blood flow is thus an essential part of determining the viability of the soft tissues. However, many other factors potentially compromise tissue viability and should be taken into account by the clinician who is prescribing an orthosis for a particular individual. The more significant of these are listed in Table 5.1.

In addition to these major factors, other variables such as local tissue integrity, the age of the patient, the presence of oedema, repeated application of pressure, infection within the body, altered sensation, neurotrophic and psychosocial factors may also influence the eventual success of the prescribed orthosis. Poor nutrition, resulting in loss of weight and reduced fatty 'padding' over the bony prominences, is another important factor. The body's normal tissue integrity is dependent upon a correct nitrogen balance and vitamin intake. Hypoproteinaemia leading to mild generalized oedema causes the skin to become less elastic and more susceptible to inflammation as the rate of oxygen transfer from the capillaries to the tissues is reduced, thus compromising tissue viability. Several rating scalings, for example the Norton and the Waterlow Scales (Crow and Clark, 1990), have been developed to assess whether a subject is at particular risk of tissue breakdown. These can be used at the time of prescription of the orthosis or at any time thereafter, particularly if there is a change in the medical condition of the subject.

Table 5.1 Intrinsic risk factors associated with the development of pressure sores

Reduced sensation (some failure of pain sensation)
Diminished attention (sedation, coma, depression)
Paralysis
Diminished tissue turgor (dehydration, hypotension)
Failed vasomotor reflexes (recent cord injury)
Peripheral vascular disease
Malnutrition
Systemic disease

The individual's attitude towards skin care and good outlook on life also correlate with the risk of skin breakdown. These factors are particularly relevant for the long-term wearing of orthoses.

5.4 The mechanics of the patient–orthosis interface

5.4.1 Tissue mechanics

The compression characteristics of the soft tissues influence their susceptibility to the breakdown process: the more compressible the tissues the more likely it is that blood vessels will be occluded. Areas at particular risk include the sacrum and the greater trochanter, which have minimal soft tissue covering over bony prominences. These present areas of high compressive stiffness to deforming loads. The overall properties of the skin and soft tissue as a composite in compression have received relatively little attention. Bader and Bowker (1983) used a counterbalanced beam to load the skin and soft tissue composite. They determined the estimated values of compressive stiffness derived from tissue recovery and found them to be on average 25% higher than those derived from tissue indentation tests. This was evident for subjects of different ages and from differing tissue sites.

An alternative approach to establishing stiffness values is to characterize changes in the shape of soft tissues when loaded compared to their unloaded shape using ultrasound techniques (Kadaba *et al.*, 1984) or magnetic resonance imaging (MRI; Reger *et al.*, 1990). The MRI technique in particular permitted the visualization of tissues and, from these images, measurements of tissue deformation were recorded at various applied compressive loads. A clear distinction was demonstrated between the mechanical response of healthy tissues adjacent to the ischial tuberosities from a normal subject compared to the atrophied tissues of an age-matched paraplegic. For the paraplegic subject, a compressive stiffness of 3.4 N mm^{-1} was estimated for muscle and 6.8 N mm^{-1} for skin and the tissues were observed to be more distorted under load, suggesting an increased risk of tissue trauma.

5.4.2 Load transmission across the interface

The transmission of forces across the patient interface and the resulting stress and strain distributions in the soft tissues are complex in nature. This is reflected in the relatively few attempts to produce mathematical (Murphy and Bennett, 1971; Bennett, 1972; Chow and Odell, 1978) and empirical (Reddy *et al.*, 1982) solutions to the problem. A description of the mathematical approach is beyond the scope of this chapter, but it is worth noting that all models must be inaccurate as they assume that the soft tissues exhibit linearly elastic and isotropic properties, which is not the case *in vivo*. The physical factors which principally determine the stress distributions in both the materials and at the patient–orthosis interface are important. When force is applied through the interface there will be some deformation of both surfaces, the strains in each of the two contacting materials depending on their relative moduli and thicknesses, the relative shapes of the underlying rigid structures and the level of the applied force.

Factors which affect the pressure distribution under the ischium when sitting include: subject weight and body build (Garber and Krouskop, 1982), the geometry of both the soft and bony tissues, the composition of the soft tissues, the mechanical properties of the various soft-tissue components (Bader and Bowker, 1983) and the geometry and the mechanical properties of the support surface. Further variations are also introduced both by postural changes and the fact that the mechanical properties of support surfaces change with time.

The sum of the incremental pressures multiplied by the area over which they act equals the total force exerted across the interface. In most cases a maximum conforming support area will provide a uniform distribution of pressures, with absolute pressure levels at a minimum. Thus, by contrast, if the number of support points is reduced, the interface pressure will increase with disastrous consequences, as illustrated in Figure 5.4. A maximum support area can be achieved in two distinct ways, as illustrated in Figure 5.5. In the first case the support surface, made of relatively high modulus material, can be matched in shape to that of the area of the body with which it interfaces.

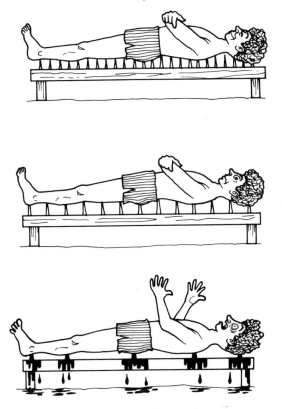

Figure 5.4 A person supported on a bed of nails

There is high congruity between body and support surface. This situation occurs for many body support systems such as in spinal bracing (see Chapter 13) and seating for the severely physically disabled (see Chapter 14). It is obvious that a relatively rigid support will only provide a maximum surface area provided that the body shape remains constant. In cases where this does not apply, for example in the case of a young subject with progessive muscular atrophy, the support surface must be regularly modified.

In the other case, illustrated in Figure 5.5(b), the support surface can be flat but made of relatively soft material, which can deform under load. This situation is common in many seating applications and when support is required over delicate and sensitive skin. It is important to recognize that tension will be established in a deforming surface and this may be transferred to the soft tissues. The use of a two-way stretch cover as part of the support surface will minimize this effect.

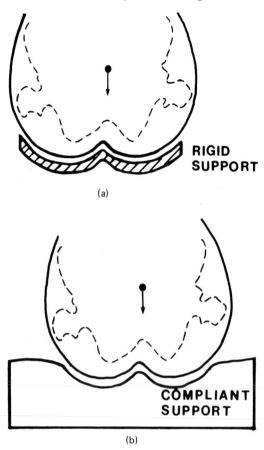

(a)

RIGID SUPPORT

(b)

COMPLIANT SUPPORT

Figure 5.5 Load transmission at the patient–orthosis interface: (a) with rigid support, matched to body shape; (b) with compliant support and a flat surface

The radius of curvature of the body contour to be supported is also a critical factor in determining the load transfer characteristics. Large body contours provide a large surface area for support, as is the case for a knee orthosis positioned over the anterior aspect of the thigh. Conversely, small body contours, particularly over bony prominences with minimal tissue covering, may be difficult to support. High contact pressures are common in these instances and the resulting high stress distribution in the soft tissues may cause tissue damage.

Consideration must also be given to the conditions at the edges of the support area, as discussed by Bennett (1972). Many orthoses contain straps, rivets and fasteners, etc., which are very stiff compared with the contacting soft tissues. These produce both sharp stiffness gradients and very high shear stresses at the edges of these structures, and typically produce erythema of the skin observable after the orthosis has been removed, with the possible generation of cysts. Various practical solutions to this problem include the bevelling or rounding off of edges or making the orthosis of variable stiffness. In such a case the orthosis would contain stiff sections in the centres of the supporting area, through which the forces creating the appropriate bending moments are applied, whilst it would contain less stiff flexible sections near to the edge of the supported area and over the areas of the skin which are not loaded.

In many orthotic applications, such as a knee-ankle-foot orthosis (KAFO) correcting a valgus knee or a moulded ankle-foot orthosis (AFO) holding a subtalar joint in neutral using three-point fixation, uniform pressure is clearly not possible. Asymmetry of loading is also inevitable in many physically disabled subjects with pelvic obliquity, spinal deformity or limb amputations. In these cases a compromise solution is often sought with the need to take into account postural and functional requirements in addition to optimum pressure distribution at the patient–orthosis interface.

5.5 Design solutions at the patient–orthosis interface

Support materials at the patient–orthosis interface should provide a safe, stable and comfortable means of transmitting loads to the body. This may be achieved in most cases by designing a support surface which provides a fairly uniform pressure distribution over a maximal support area. However, even if a totally uniform pressure distribution can be achieved, the physics of the support problem, i.e. the weight of the body divided by the projected area available to support the body, precludes the possibility of having all pressures less than 10 mmHg (1.3 kPa) even in the supine position. Normal tissue care programmes must therefore always be followed.

Additionally, it may be necessary to reduce, relieve or avoid pressure in particularly sensitive areas or over areas of existing tissue damage, and it must therefore be possible to shape the support material or introduce appropriate 'cut-outs' in the support surface. Also, to achieve clinically acceptable interface conditions, the choice of support material should take into account other physical, functional and aesthetic factors (Ferguson-Pell *et al.*, 1986; Krouskop *et al.*, 1986). These include stability, durability, permeability to water vapour and heat dissipation. The materials should also be biocompatible with the host tissues and they should not elicit any skin irritations or allergic reactions.

Compliant, viscoelastic materials form the basis of most of the common support surfaces. The inner linings over load bearing areas are generally made of foam, for example the polyethylene foam which makes up the compression pads within many orthotic systems for the spine. In the case of seating materials, a combination of foam, gel and air supports are regularly used. Viscoelastic materials, such as Temper foam, will accommodate changes in body position, thus maximizing the surface area of support. Contoured support surfaces, as described in Chapter 14, provide maximum support for those subjects with severe physical disability, who have limited functional capacity. Compliant support surfaces must also be thick enough to accommodate the large deformations produced by high levels of force across the interface and should still retain some compliance. In extreme cases, the stresses may be sufficient to 'bottom-out' the compliant material and the body tissues may then be supported locally on a rigid support with an associated increase in interface pressures. Most of the compliant materials used at the patient–orthosis interface demonstrate non-linear stress–strain curves, as illustrated in Figure 5.6. Characteristics such as these preclude the use of a single stiffness modulus value or Poisson's ratio in design calculations. Indeed urethane foams exhibit three-phase characteristic curves due to the bending, buckling and collapse of the cellular structure (Ferguson-Pell *et al.*, 1986). During phase 1 the material is highly compressible, producing large compression for small applied loads, and is relatively linear. The phase 2 region, however, is highly non-linear and is followed by phase 3, in which most foam cells have collapsed and the material becomes increasingly compacted. It is during this last phase of progressively increased stiffness, when the foams are commonly observed to 'bottom-out'. A study of the mechanical properties of common support materials in seating has indicated a large variation

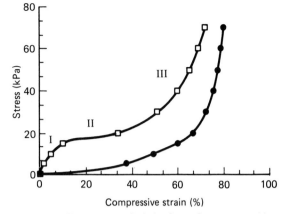

Figure 5.6 The stress–strain behaviour of two support foams tested in uniaxial compression (based on Ferguson-Pell *et al.*, 1986)

in compression moduli (Ferguson-Pell *et al.*, 1986). Values for the initial modulus of compression ranged from 14 kPa to 122 kPa, whilst values in phase 3, measured at a stress level of 50 kPa, had increased to a range from 447 kPa to 740 kPa. As these levels of stress are commonly experienced on the plantar aspect of the foot, foam insoles should be regularly inspected for permanent change of shape. It should also be noted that due to the viscoelastic nature of some materials, such as Temper foam, the values of compression moduli will depend on the strain rate during testing.

5.6 Measurement techniques

5.6.1 Pressure

Different types of patient–orthosis interface will experience different physical conditions. Physical measurement systems, such as interface pressure transducers, will therefore need to be related to the particular interface at which they are to be used. This is illustrated in Table 5.2.

There have been several excellent review articles describing pressure transducers designed for use at the patient–orthosis interface (e.g. Ferguson-Pell, 1980; Wych *et al.*, 1989). These discuss the strict requirements necessary to achieve acceptable performance. In summary, any device which accurately measures pressure at an interface between two conforming surfaces must itself be conforming if it is

Table 5.2 Transducer specifications

Interface system	Pressure range	Frequency response	Monitoring period
Seating/mattress Spinal bracing	0–300 mmHg (0–40 KPa)	up to 5 Hz	30 min
Foot/lower leg prosthesis	0–300 mmHg (0–400 KPa)	minimum 50 Hz	10 s

not to be disruptive. Therefore the device should be thin, with an optimum thickness to diameter ratio of less than 0.1. In addition, it should be flexible to accommodate body contours while being sufficiently robust to be used in different clinical situations. It must also have good spatial and temporal resolution.

Pneumatic sacs, small enough to evaluate localized pressure, meet these specifications. Many such devices, for example the single Skin Pressure Evaluator (Talley Group Ltd, Romsey, Hampshire, UK), which has a diameter of 28 mm and is thin enough to be flexible, incorporate a pair of internal electrical contacts. The pressure in the sac is increased using a pressure measuring sphygmomanometer, until the sac inflates, thus breaking the contacts. The pressure at this instant can then be recorded. However, using a single cell, it is not possible to map a non-uniform pressure distribution at the patient–orthosis interface. For this an array of multiple sensors, such as the Texas Pressure Evaluation Pad (Krouskop *et al.*, 1986), is required. This device incorporates an array of sacs, each of which contains a pair of electrical contacts made from resistive paints. However, our experience with this device has highlighted that the internal contacts are not sufficiently robust and tend to fail, thus limiting the life of each device. An alternative multiple cell system, the Oxford Pressure Monitor (Talley Group Ltd, Romsey, Hampshire, UK) based on pneumatic techniques has been described by Bader and Hawken (1986). A constant mass of flow of air is pumped into the cell and a pressure/time trace is electronically monitored. At the point at which the air pressure inside the cell becomes equal to the applied pressure, a change in the gradient of the pressure–time relationship is sensed due to changing volume caused by the opening of the cell. At this instant the system pressure is recorded and the air flow is reversed exhausting the system. The system

sampling rate, although dependent on the applied pressure and the pump characteristics, is typically only 2–3 Hz. The device measures pressures in the range of 0–300 mmHg (40 kPa) with an accuracy of ±3%. Thus it is able to measure interface pressures at many of the patient–orthosis interfaces including seating, spinal orthoses and lower limb orthoses.

These systems are, however, unable to measure the high pressure under the foot or at the base of the stump socket interface which are very much higher (Table 5.2). In addition, to assess changes in interface pressure during the gait cycle the transducer should have a high resolution exceeding 50 Hz. For this, either reactive electrical transducers or transducers made of piezoelectric films, based on polymer vinylidene fluoride (PVDF), may be more appropriate (Wych *at al.*, 1989). These can be manufactured as an instrumented insole which registers foot loading during normal activity in shoe-wearing subjects.

5.6.2 Other environmental parameters

The mapping of the temperature at the patient–orthosis interface can be simply performed using an array of miniature thermistors. Separate studies on shear measurements have been reported at the patient–seat interface (Bennett *et al.*, 1979) and the foot–shoe interface (Tappin and Robertson, 1991), although the physical bulk of the transducers may affect the measurement. To date, there has been no successful transducer to measure the moisture content directly at the patient–orthosis interface.

The time during which load is transmitted across the patient–orthosis interface, which is equivalent to the compliance time of an orthosis, is an important physical property. By using miniature switches, set at a threshold load, the compliance time of an orthosis can be estimated. This principle has been used to study the duration of load bearing under different areas of the foot. Small cylindrical footswitches composed of a rubber matrix loaded with silver-plated copper spheres were embedded into a polymeric insole (Miller and Stokes, 1979). This information may provide the clinician with supportive evidence of how often the orthosis is worn in an effective manner.

5.6.3 Tissue viability

In many cases the measurement of interface pressures alone will not alert the clinician to potential areas of tissue breakdown. Some measure of tissue viability, which is primarily dependent on an adequate supply of nutrients supplied by the blood, is required. This is illustrated in the following case study:-

A 27-year-old man with motor neurone disease presented to the seating clinic at the Mary Marlborough Lodge in Oxford with persistent tissue breakdown in an area marginally distal to the left ischial tuberosity. The Oxford Pressure Monitor was used to assess the pressure distribution under both ischia while the subject was seated on his normal support cushion (a 75-mm variegated foam cushion). The results are illustrated in Figure 5.7. Close examination reveals some asymmetry in the pressure distribution but no obvious high peak pressures or high pressure gradients under the left ischium

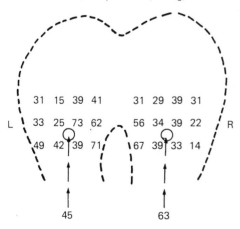

Figure 5.7 Mapping of the interface pressure distribution under the ischia of a patient with recurrent tissue breakdown at the left ischium

compared with the right. The question remained: Why was the left ischium more prone to tissue breakdown? A measure of transcutaneous oxygen tension was performed over identical areas on each unloaded ischium. Although there were no baseline levels for transcutaneous oxygen tension (T_cPo_2), the difference in values between the two sides appeared significant. Thus it appeared that the measured interface pressures of up to 9.7 kPa (73 mmHg) were sufficient to reduce the tissue oxygen from an inherently compromised level to a non-viable level under the left ischium, but did not produce the same effect on the tissue under the right ischium with normal unloaded oxygen levels.

A series of reports have described the effects of external loading on skin blood flow using various techniques, including radioisotope clearance, photoplethysmography and transcutaneous gas monitoring. The latter technique has proved an accurate and repeatable method for investigating the effects of loads on tissue viability (Newson and Rolfe, 1982). Further work has examined the effects of prolonged loading at the sacrum on tissue viability for a mixed group of debilitated subjects who were considered to be particularly prone to the development of pressure sores (Bader and Gant, 1988). The results have indicated a wide range of values of integrated pressure and time which the soft tissues would tolerate. This has emphasized the individual nature of the tissue response, which should be determined before clinical guidelines of safe pressure levels can be established.

This work was extended to investigate the effects of cyclic loading on the viability of the soft tissues of debilitated subjects (Bader, 1990). Two distinct responses were observed, as illustrated in diagrammatic form in Figure 5.8. The normal response produced a rapid and complete tissue recovery to unloaded levels of T_cPo_2 and the apparent effect of the applied load diminished with successive cycles. In contrast, however, in some cases recovery was not fully achieved within a 5-minute period and subsequent loading had a cumulative effect on the diminution of T_cPo_2 levels. It is this latter group who require surveillance during orthotic wear if they are to avoid the development of pressure sores.

Bader (1990) has also discussed the effectiveness of a dynamic support cushion, which

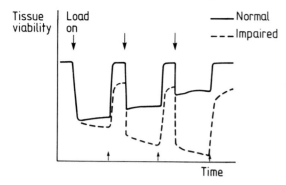

Figure 5.8 A diagrammatic representation of the two distinct effects observed on the viability of soft tissues subjected to repeated loading

produced repeated loading in the region of the ischial tuberosity. The cushion incorporated 48 individual, cylindrical-shaped, soft inflatable bellows arranged in eight rows (BASE, Talley Medical Equipment Ltd, UK). Each row of six bellows could be inflated or deflated as dictated by a control unit. A combined transcutaneous electrode was attached over one ischial tuberosity for each subject. The subject was positioned carefully upon the instrumented cushion, with a pressure measuring cell attached to the top of each bellow. The pressure distribution across the cushion and the transcutaneous gas tension levels were recorded throughout the test. The response of one subject with syringomyelia is illustrated in Figure 5.9. Initially as the subject sat on the cushion, there was a significant reduction in the $T_cP_{O_2}$

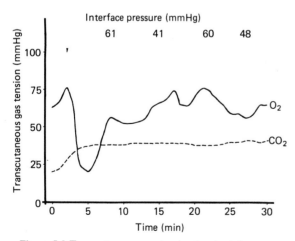

Figure 5.9 Transcutaneous gas tension levels at the ischium of a female subject with syringomyelia, during a period of sitting on the dynamic support cushion

levels, which was followed by recovery on successive deflation phases of the cushion cycle. The transcutaneous carbon dioxide tension ($T_cP_{CO_2}$) stabilized at about 5.3 kPa (40 mmHg) throughout the sitting period. A similar overall response was obtained with young healthy subjects indicating an active vasomotor control mechanism alerted by the change in mechanical stress. Other debilitated subjects demonstrated a tissue response suggestive of an impaired physiological control mechanism. Subjects demonstrating this response would appear to be at particular risk of developing pressure sores and require particular skin care and adequate pressure relief when they are prescribed an orthosis.

5.7 Conclusions

The success, or otherwise, of an orthosis is dependent on its biomechanical performance as it interfaces with the soft tissues of the body. Conditions at the patient–orthosis interface are important for both the functional requirements of the orthosis and the overall comfort of the user. In designing for the best conditions at the patient–orthosis interface, including a minimization of interface pressures, the orthotist must consider the following:

— Maximizing the pad size.
— Contouring the pad to the body shape.
— Positioning the pad to maximize the moment arm.
— Minimizing the level of the applied force by good orthosis design.
— Ensuring a good fit between the orthosis and body contour.

The orthotist should also consider the benefits of measuring extrinsic factors, such as interface pressure and, in patients who are at particular risk of tissue breakdown, of making some measure of tissue viability.

References

Bader D.L. (1990) The recovery characteristics of soft tissues following repeated loading. *J. Rehabil. Res. Dev.* **27**, 141–150

Bader D.L. and Bowker P. (1983) Mechanical characteristics of skin and underlying tissues *in vivo*. *Biomaterials* **4**, 305–308

Bader D.L. and Gant C.A. (1988) Changes in transcutaneous oxygen tension as a result of prolonged pressures at the sacrum. *Clin. Phys. Physiol. Meas.* **9**, 33–40

Bader D.L. and Hawken M.B. (1986) Pressure distribution under the ischium of normal subjects. *J. Biomed. Eng.* **8**, 353–357.

Bader D.L., Barnhill, R.L. and Ryan T.J. (1986) Effect of externally applied skin surface forces on tissue vasculature. *Arch. Phys. Med. Rehabil.* **67**, 807–811

Bennett L. (1972) Transferring load to flesh Parts 3 and 4. *Bull. Prosthet. Res.* **10–16**, 38–63

Bennett L., Kavner D., Lee B.Y. *et al.* (1979) Shear vs pressure as causative factors in skin blood flow occlusion. *Arch. Phys. Med. Rehabil.* **60**, 309–314

Chow W.W. and Odell E.I. (1978) Deformations and stresses in soft body tissues of a sitting person. *J. Biomech. Eng.* **100**, 79–87

Crow R.A. and Clark M. (1990) Current management for the prevention of pressure sores. In: Bader D.L. (ed.), *Pressure Sores – Clinical Practice and Scientific Approach.* Macmillan, Basingstoke pp. 43–52

Ferguson-Pell M.W. (1980) Design criteria for the measurement of pressure at the body/support interfaces. *Eng. Med.* **9**, 209–214

Ferguson-Pell M.W., Cochran G.V.B., Palmieri V.R. *et al.* (1986) Development of a modular wheelchair cushion for spinal cord injury persons. *J. Rehabil. Res. Dev.* **23**, 63–76

Garber S.L. and Krouskop T.A. (1982) Body build and its relationship to pressure distribution in the seated wheelchair patient. *Arch. Phys. Med. Rehabil.* **63**, 17–20

Hibbs P. (1990) The economics of pressure sore prevention. In: Bader D.L. (ed.), *Pressure Sores – Clinical Practice and Scientific Approach.* Macmillan, Basingstoke, pp.35–42

Kadaba M.P., Ferguson-Pell M.W., Palmieri V. *et al.* (1984) Ultrasound mapping of the buttock–cushion interface contour. *Arch. Phys. Med. Rehabil.* **65**, 467–479

Krouskop T.A., Noble P.C., Brown J. *et al.* (1986) Factors affecting the pressure-distributing properties of foam overlays. *J. Rehabil. Res. Dev.* **23**, 33–39

Miller G.F. and Stokes I.A.F. (1979) A study of the duration of load-bearing under different areas of the foot. *Eng. Med.* **8**, 128–132

Murphy E.F. and Bennett L. (1971) Transferring load to flesh Parts 1 and 2. *Bull. Prosthet. Res.* 10–16, 38–63

Newson T.P. and Rolfe P. (1982) Skin surface PO_2 and blood flow measurement over the ischial tuberosity. *Arch. Phys. Med. Rehabil.* **63**, 553–556

Reddy N.P., Cochran G.V.B. and Krouskop T.A. (1981) Interstitial fluid flow as a factor in decubitus ulcer formation. *J. Biomech.* **14**, 879–881

Reddy N.P., Patel H., Cochran G.V.B. *et al.* (1982) Model experiments to study the stress distribution in a sitting buttock. *J. Biomech.* **15**, 493–504

Reger S.I., McGovern T.F. and Chung K.C. (1990) Biomechanics of tissue distortion and stiffness by magnetic resonance imaging. In: Bader D.L. (ed.), *Pressure Sores – Clinical Practice and Scientific Approach.* Macmillan, Basingstoke, pp. 177–190

Reichel S. (1958) Shearing force as a factor in decubitus ulcers in paraplegics. *JAMA* **166**, 762–763

Reswick J.B. and Rogers J.E. (1976) Experience at Rancho Los Amigos Hospital with devices and techniques to prevent pressure sores. In: Kenedi R.M., Cowden J.M. and Scales J.T. (eds), *Bedsore Biomechanics.* London: Macmillan, Basingstoke, pp. 301–310

Shea J.D. (1975) Pressure sores – classification and management. *Clin. Orthop. Rel. Res.* **112**, 89–100.

Tappin J.W. and Robertson K.P. (1991) Study of the relative timing of shear forces on the sole of the forefoot during walking. *J. Biomed. Eng.* **13**, 39–42.

Tortora G.J. and Anagnostakos N.P. (1981) Metabolism. In: Tortora G.J. and Anagnostakos N.P. (eds), *Principles of Anatomy and Physiology.* Harper and Row, New York, pp.645–666

White A.A. and Panjabi M.M. (1990) In: White A.A. and Panjabi M.M. (eds), *Clinical Biomechanics of the Spine*, Lippincott, Philadelphia, pp. 479

Wych R., Neil G. and Kalisse C. (1989) Skin–orthosis interface pressure transducers – a review. *Care-Sci. Pract.* **7**, 100–104

6

Foot orthoses

David Pratt, David Tollafield, Garth Johnson and Colin Peacock

6.1 Introduction

Effective orthotic management of the pathological foot can have dramatic effects not only within the foot itself but also more proximally on the rest of the lower limb. Unfortunately, often the assessment for and the production of 'insoles' or the adaptation of footwear, has been poorly carried out because of a lack of understanding of the function of the foot.

Unlike most other orthotic devices, foot orthoses invariably work by realigning the ground reaction force rather than by applying forces or moments directly to joints. For a mobile foot, in which the deformity or malalignment is correctable, the aim of the realignment is to place the foot in its optimum functional position. This essentially involves placing the subtalar and midtarsal joints in their neutral positions. For a rigid foot with fixed deformities, the aims may be to accommodate deformity, to redistribute plantar pressure, to relieve dorsal pressure, or to realign the plantar surface of the shoe in order to obtain more normal contact forces.

6.2 Anatomy of the foot

6.2.1 Bony architecture

The bony skeleton of the foot consists of a total of 20 bones (Figure 6.1). These can be usefully considered as three groups: the rearfoot, midfoot and forefoot. The rearfoot consists of the calcaneus and the talus. The body of the talus is inclined at about 25° medially to the sagittal plane and articulates proximally with the leg through the talocrural joint, commonly called the ankle joint. The neck of the talus extends anteriorly, medially and dorsally from the body and then forms the head. The head articulates with the navicular, the anterior facet of the calcaneus and the calcaneonavicular ligament. Distally the body of the talus articulates with the calcaneus via its posterior, medial and anterior surfaces. Between the posterior and medial surfaces lies a groove, the sulcus calcanei, which in conjunction with the sulcus tali forms the sinus tarsi. In addition, the calcaneus articulates with the sustentaculum tali and with the cuboid.

The midfoot consists of the cuboid, medial, intermediate and lateral cuneiforms and the navicular. The cuboid articulates with the calcaneus, the navicular and the fourth and fifth metatarsals. The cuneiforms are wedge shaped, with their apices pointing dorsally, and they articulate with the first, second and third metatarsals distally. The navicular lies at the top of the medial arch articulating on its proximal surface with the talus. On its distal surface it articulates with the three cuneiforms and a small facet on the lateral surface articulates with the cuboid.

The forefoot consists of the metatarsals and phalanges. There are five metatarsals each of which has a broad base, a distally tapering shaft and dome-shaped heads, with the first being the shortest and widest. This metatarsal articulates proximally with the medial cunei-

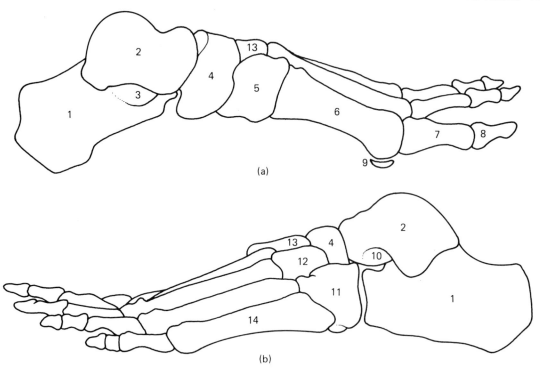

Figure 6.1 Skeleton of the foot: (a) medial view; (b) lateral view. 1=calcaneus, 2=talus, 3=sustentaculum tali, 4=navicular, 5=medial cuneiform, 6=first metatarsal shaft, 7=proximal phalanx, 8=distal phalanx, 9=sesamoid bone, 10=tarsal sinus, 11=cuboid, 12=lateral cuneiform, 13=intermediate cuneiform, 14=fifth metatarsal shaft

form and distally with two sesamoids on the plantar surface and the proximal phalanx of the hallux. The second metatarsal is longer than the others and at its proximal end articulates with all three cuneiforms to form a stable 'key' type of configuration. The other metatarsals are similar to each other with the exception of the fifth whose base possesses a large styloid process laterally.

The phalanges of the toes, numbering two for the first (the hallux) and three for each of the other toes, are all concave on their plantar surfaces. The trochlear-shaped heads of the proximal and middle phalanges provide enhanced stability, with the middle phalanges being shorter and broader than the proximal. The distal phalanges are the smallest with distal expansions to aid weight distribution during the latter stages of the stance phase of gait.

The sesamoid bones of the hallux are ovoid, lying within the flexor hallucis brevis tendon and articulating with the plantar surface of the first metatarsal head. Accessory bones may also be present elsewhere in the foot associated with, for example, the lateral metatarsals, and the tibialis anterior, posterior and peroneus longus tendons.

6.2.2 Joints of the foot

The joint axes of orthotic interest in the foot are shown in Figure 6.2. The ankle joint is a modified synovial hinge, the articular surfaces of which involve the distal ends of the tibia and fibula proximally and the talus distally. The articular surface of the tibia is concave antero-posteriorly, slightly convex transversely and has a sagittal ridge which fits into a corresponding groove on the dome of the talus. The articular surface of the fibula is almost triangular with the apex directed distally. The body of the talus forms all of the distal ankle joint and is convex anteroposteriorly with a central groove. This joint achieves its stability because of its saddle shape and its two malleoli. Additional stability is provided by the collateral ligaments and the joint capsule. The medial collateral ligament, or deltoid ligament, is fan shaped and interconnects the tibia, talus, calcaneus

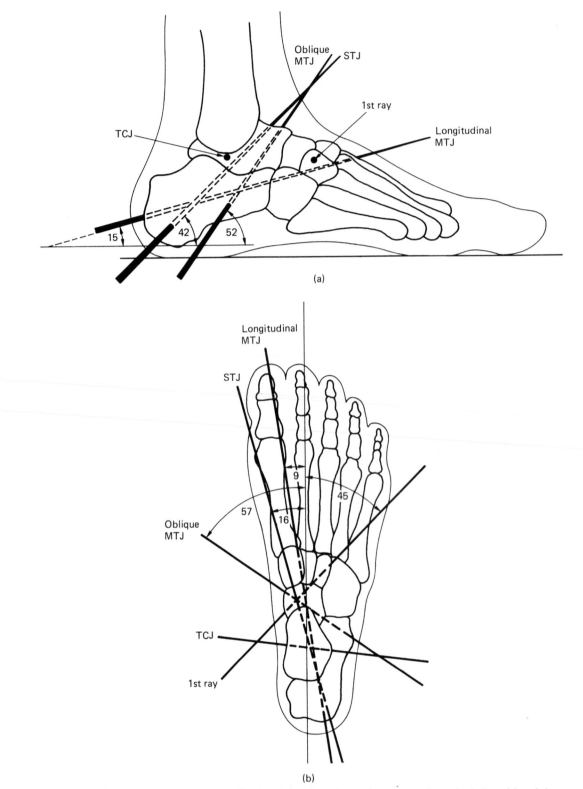

Figure 6.2 Details of joint axes in the foot indicating their orientation projected onto the sagittal plane (a) and the transverse plane (b). TCJ=talocrural joint.

and navicular. The lateral ligament consists of three parts, the anterior and posterior talofibular ligaments and the calcaneofibular ligament. Damage to these ligaments produces ankle instability.

The subtalar joint (STJ) consists of three articulations and, for easier comprehension, needs to be considered as having two aspects. The posterior aspect consists of the talocalcaneal joint, and the anterior aspect, the talocalcaneonavicular joint. The talocalcaneal joint is synovial and relies upon the medial and lateral talocalcaneal ligaments for its stability together with the interosseus talocalcaneal ligament which controls pronation, and the cervical ligament which controls supination. The talocalcaneonavicular joint comprises two articulations, the larger of the two being with the sustentaculum tali. Significant ligaments include the medial bifurcated calcaneonavicular ligament, the more dorsally sited talonavicular ligament and the 'spring' ligament medially. The STJ surface can be considered to be cylindrical with its axis running obliquely from anterior, medial and superior to posterior, lateral and inferior. In addition to ligamentous and capsular stabilization, the STJ relies upon muscular activity to provide the necessary stability for walking, particularly from the peroneal muscles and flexor hallucis longus.

The midtarsal joint (MTJ), sometimes called Chopart's joint, consists of two joints, the calcaneocuboid laterally and the talonavicular medially. These function about two common axes of motion, known as the longitudinal and oblique axes. The talonavicular joint is synovial and of the ball and socket variety, the ball being the head and part of the neck of the talus and the socket being formed by the surrounding bone and ligaments. Ligaments around the joint include the long and short plantar ligaments, which connect the calcaneus to the cuboid and to the lesser metatarsals in the case of the long plantar ligament. The bifurcate calcaneonavicular ligament supports the joint complex laterally.

The calcaneocuboid joint is the articulation between the anterior surface of the calcaneus and the posterior aspect of the cuboid. It is approximately quadrilateral in shape and comprises both concave and convex features. A simple capsule completely surrounds the joint and is thickened both above and below by the dorsal and plantar calcaneocuboid ligaments respectively.

The first ray is a functional unit consisting of the first metatarsal which has articulations (i) between the first metatarsal and both the second metatarsal and medial cuneiform, and (ii) between the medial cuneiform and the navicular, intermediate cuneiform and the second metatarsal. This results in a complex motion described by Ebisui (1968), primarily involving the cuneonavicular and first metatarsocuneiform joints. The interosseous ligament supports the cuneiform bones together with the medial and lateral dorsal ligaments. The medial dorsal ligament runs from the lateral aspect of the medial cuneiform to the medial aspect of the base of the second metatarsal. The lateral dorsal ligament is a series of fibres connecting the intermediate cuneiforms with the second and third metatarsals.

The first metatarsophalangeal joint (MTPJ) consists of the articular surfaces of the first metatarsal head and the base of the proximal phalanx of the hallux. In addition, the two sesamoid grooves under the first metatarsal head articulate with the sesamoid bones.

6.2.3 Joint musculature

Movements about the various joints of the foot are controlled by muscular activity. The primary functions of the important muscles and the timing and sequence of their activity are well documented (Table 6.1, Figure 6.3). The actions of the principal muscles controlling the foot are summarized below.

(a) Tibialis anterior

The tendon of this muscle passes nearly perpendicular to the axes of the ankle joint and the first ray and produces a large moment about both, hence its dorsiflexion function. It also passes medial to the STJ and longitudinal MTJ axes with a larger moment arm about the latter, hence its supinatory function. The moment arm of the tendon about the oblique MTJ is negligible.

(b) Triceps surae (gastrocnemius and soleus)

The gastrocnemius passes posteriorly and almost perpendicularly to the ankle joint axis with a large moment arm and, when the knee

Table 6.1 Primary specific functions of some foot muscles

Muscle	Primary function
Tibialis anterior	1. Dorsiflexion of toe at toe-off 2. Dorsiflexion of foot in swing 3. Assist supination of foot prior to heel-strike 4. Prevent excessive pronation during swing and stance phases 5. To resist plantarflexion of foot after heel-strike
Gastrocnemius	1. Plantarflexion of foot during late stance phase 2. Assistance with STJ supination during middle and late stance 3. Externally rotates the leg 4. Prevents excessive internal rotation of the leg towards the end of stance
Soleus	1. To assist the gastrocnemius 2. Stabilization of the lateral forefoot during late stance
Extensor hallucis longus	1. To stabilize the first MTPJ for propulsion 2. To dorsiflex the foot during early swing phase 3. Maintains the hallux dorsiflexed in early swing
Tibialis posterior	1. To supinate the STJ during midstance 2. To assist the soleus 3. To decelerate STJ pronation during early stance 4. To stabilize the MTJ 5. Assist with heel-lift
Peroneus longus and brevis	1. Stabilize the first ray 2. Assist with medial weight transfer in late stance 3. To assist, weakly, ankle joint plantarflexion 4. Pronation of the STJ

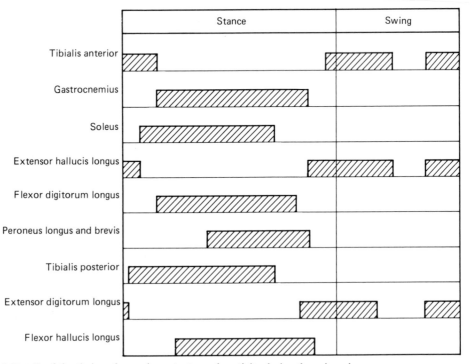

Figure 6.3 Details of the timing of some important muscle activity during the gait cycle

is extended, produces strong plantarflexion about this axis. It also has a reasonably large moment arm about the STJ, but because it crosses this axis at about 48° (Root *et al.*, 1977) its supinatory effect is reduced. When the knee is flexed all of these actions are reduced in strength because of the origin of the muscle on the femoral condyles. The soleus muscle can be considered as the same in function as the gastrocnemius having much the same position and direction. Due to its different origin from the tibia, it is not affected by knee flexion.

(c) Extensor hallucis longus

The tendon of this muscle passes anteriorly and almost perpendicularly to the ankle joint axis and is a strong dorsiflexor about this axis. It does this without pronating or supinating the foot about the STJ because it runs nearly parallel to and very close to the STJ axis. In addition this tendon passes dorsally and perpendicular to the first MTPJ axis, which enables it to function as a stabilizer of this joint during the final stages of stance.

(d) Flexor hallucis longus

The tendon of this muscle passes posteriorly to the ankle joint, around the talus and under the sustentaculum tali, attaching distally on the foot. The long moment arm created by the talus results in a strong plantarflexion action of the foot about the ankle or, conversely, a strong deceleration of the forward motion of the tibia. It also has a large moment arm about the STJ axis which, being at an acute angle, reduces its supinatory action. This muscle also plantarflexes the hallux at the first MTPJ axis, as well as flexing the IP joint of the hallux.

(e) Tibialis posterior

The tendon of this muscle passes posterior to the ankle joint axis around the medial malleolus. As this gives the muscle only a small moment arm, it is thus a weak plantarflexor of the foot. It has, however, a large moment arm about the STJ axis and is thus a strong supinator about this axis. In addition it passes almost perpendicularly to the oblique MTJ axis with a large moment arm and also produces strong supination about this axis. It has little or no action about the longitudinal MTJ axis.

(f) Peroneus longus and brevis

Both peronei pass posterior to the lateral malleolus with a small moment arm about the ankle joint axis and are thus weak ankle plantarflexors. Peroneus longus has a large moment arm about the STJ axis producing pronation, but passes through the oblique MTJ axis and has no effect here. Peroneus brevis acts similarly about the STJ axis but has a small moment arm about the oblique MTJ axis and acts perpendicularly to this axis to produce pronation.

(g) Soft tissue

In addition to these muscles, the plantar aponeurosis fulfils an important role in relation to the function of the foot. It has three parts, medial, lateral and central, the latter being the major one and having the role of maintaining the longitudinal arch of the foot. It is triangular in shape and extends from the calcaneus proximally to a divided structure distally. The medial and lateral sections are thinner and may be incomplete. When the toes are dorsiflexed in terminal stance, the aponeurosis is in tension and draws the two ends of the foot together. This results in the bones of the foot being held tightly and functioning as a single unit rather than separate bones. The truss-like structure thus created has been likened to a Spanish windlass (Figure 6.4).

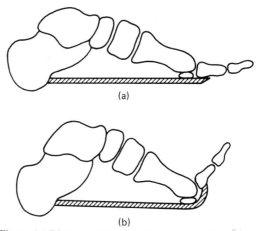

Figure 6.4 Diagram of the combined truss and Spanish windlass representation of the plantar fascia with the toes in neutral (a) and with the toes extended (b), locking the joints and making a single functional unit with a raised longitudinal arch

Table 6.2 Nerve supply to the foot

Location on the foot	Nerve
Medial ankle, medial foot to first metatarsal head	Saphenous (L3,L4)
Anterior and lateral shin/ankle across all toes dorsally except 1–2 toe space and lateral fifth metatarsal	Superficial peroneal (L4,L5,S1)
1–2 toe space	Deep peroneal (L4,L5)
Posterior-lateral malleolus to fifth toe and lateral plantar heel	Sural (L5,S1,S2)
Posterior heel	Medial calcaneal branch of tibial (S1,S2)
Plantar heel	Tibial (S1,S2)
Lateral plantar foot from anterior heel to lateral fourth and fifth toes	Lateral plantar branch of tibial (S1,S2)
Medial plantar from anterior heel to all toes except lateral fourth and fifth toes	Medial plantar branch of tibial (L4,L5)

6.2.4 Innervation

The principal nerves of the foot are associated with L4, L5 and S1 spinal segments (Table 6.2). An impairment in this innervation can lead to a number of problems such as muscle weakness, paralysis, numbness, pain and paraesthesia.

6.3 Biomechanics of the foot

6.3.1 Kinematics

The joints of the foot are all triplanar in nature, that is their motion gives rise to rotations in all three principal body planes. An appreciation of this is important when assessing the foot and describing its function. The motions of the joints during walking have been determined experimentally (Figure 6.5). The ankle joint provides mainly dorsiflexion and plantarflexion, although a small degree of transverse or horizontal plane motion is also present. Estimating the position of the ankle joint axis by palpating the distal tips of the two malleoli and pointing the two palpating fingers at each other, indicates that the ankle joint axis is inclined in the coronal plane. It is this inclination which produces abduction during dorsiflexion and adduction during plantarflexion. The effect of this is to modify the requirements for horizontal plane motion in the STJ. Little

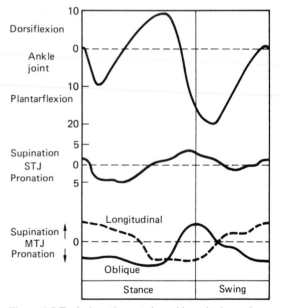

Figure 6.5 Typical motions at the ankle, subtalar and both midtarsal joints during the gait cycle

or no significant coronal plane motion takes place at the ankle joint (Close, 1956).

The STJ provides most of the horizontal plane motion in the foot to allow for the normal internal and external rotation of the leg during stance; pronating in response to internal rotation and supinating in response to external rotation. At heel strike the STJ is slightly supinated and, because the leg is internally rotating, starts to pronate as the foot is loaded. Some slight adduction of the foot may also take place but this is usually only a few degrees (Close, 1956; Isman and Inman, 1969). Pronation continues as weight is transferred to the front of the foot, such that by about 25% of the stance phase maximum pronation occurs with a resulting calcaneal eversion of about 6°.

During midstance the leg is externally rotating and the STJ supinates such that just before heel-lift the STJ is in neutral, at about 60% of the stance phase. After this the STJ is supinated and continues supinating, with further external rotation of the leg, so that the calcaneus inverts. Just before toe-off, the STJ, which is still supinated, starts to re-pronate (Wright *et al.*, 1964).

During the swing phase, the STJ continues to pronate until at midswing it is slightly pronated. It then moves into STJ neutral and just prior to heel strike, supinates to prepare for weight bearing.

This motion of the STJ has been likened to that of a spiral of Archimedes (Manter, 1941). The right foot exhibits motion about a right-handed thread and the left foot about a left-handed thread.

Because motion at the STJ is triplanar (because of its axis orientation), the effect of STJ motion on the rest of the foot is determined by whether the foot is weight bearing or not (Jones, 1945; Root *et al.*, 1966). When non weight bearing, motion of the STJ causes either pronation or supination to occur with little talar motion. The calcaneal motion thus produced takes the rest of the foot with it. When weight bearing, STJ motion is the same but the foot is unable to abduct or adduct because of friction with the ground so the calcaneus cannot move in these directions either. Thus the talus takes on a new action, abducting during STJ supination and adducting during STJ pronation. Similarly, the non-weight-bearing plantarflexion and dorsiflexion components of pronation and supination of the foot do not occur during weight bearing and again the talus moves to compensate, this time in the sagittal plane. On STJ pronation the talus plantarflexes and on supination it dorsiflexes. This illustrates the way in which foot function can affect the proximal limb, as any

dysfunction in these interrelated motions can lead to changes in leg rotation and possible problems in proximal joints, particularly the knee (Inman, 1969; Bates *et al.*, 1979; D'Amico, 1986). It also illustrates how leg rotation leads to pronation/supination of the foot as part of the natural torque converter mechanism.

Both axes of the MTJ are triplanar but to different degrees. The longitudinal axis produces a significant amount of inversion/eversion during supination/pronation with little other motion. The oblique axis allows significant amounts of motion in both the sagittal and horizontal planes and is important for horizontal plane motion (Sanner, 1987). The inclination of these two axes makes it possible for forefoot motion to be tailored to the requirements of the foot, e.g. large amounts of inversion or eversion to compensate for rearfoot eversion or inversion or or adapt to irregular surfaces such as a side-sloping terrain.

During the inital part of the stance phase, the position of the MTJ is influenced by muscle activity. Following forefoot contact it is principally controlled by ground reaction forces.

At heel-strike the forefoot is inverted about the longitudinal MTJ axis and pronated about the oblique MTJ axis, which locks the joint so that the forefoot is ready to weight bear. As the fifth metatarsal head makes ground contact, a combination of an everting ground reaction force and controlled relaxation of tibialis anterior allows the forefoot to load smoothly from lateral to medial and the joint to pronate about the longitudinal MTJ axis. There is no motion about the oblique MTJ axis, about which the foot remains pronated. This position is maintained during midstance by ground reaction force. Additionally, pronation occurs about the longitudinal MTJ axis until the MTJ is fully pronated. This coincides with the STJ reaching its neutral position. This flexibility of the foot during early contact with the ground is an important element of the shock attenuation process in the foot.

The concept of the subtalar neutral position is important to understand. Root *et al.* (1971b) have emphasized that the ST neutral position is that position where the range of inversion is equal to double the range of eversion. It is established by clinically examining the heel and STJ. Much orthotic practice in the foot focuses on positioning the heel in a ST neutral position.

During propulsion, no further motion takes place about the longitudinal MTJ axis but the peronei lift the lateral side of the foot to shift the forefoot load medially. This causes the MTJ to supinate about its oblique axis. This is further assisted by external leg rotation and the action of the plantar intrinsic muscles. This position increases joint stability in the foot and creates the rigid lever necessary to provide effective propulsion. Finally, during the swing phase, motion at both joints reverses, passing through neutral at about midswing; the forefoot then becoming supinated about the longitudinal MTJ axis and pronated about the oblique MTJ axis in preparation for heel strike (Root *et al.*, 1977).

It has been suggested (Sanner, 1987), and clinical evidence supports this view, that MTJ pronation occurs in two phases. Phase I follows the description presented so far and ends when STJ pronation reaches a maximum. In Phase II, further medial midfoot motion occurs without further calcaneal eversion. This causes leg rotation without talar motion because the calcaneus rotates on its tubercles to allow midfoot adduction. This allows the cuboid and the navicular to abduct. This would explain the often observed continued leg rotation beyond the point of maximum STJ pronation.

The axis of motion of the first ray is almost parallel to the horizontal plane. Thus, although its motion is strictly triplanar, the amount of horizontal plane motion is small. Principally as the first ray dorsiflexes it inverts and vice versa. The motion at this joint is particularly important as it is required to allow forefoot compensatory mechanisms to operate. Any restriction in its motion will thus lead to plantar callosities or excessive motions elsewhere, causing discomfort.

The first MTPJ has two axes of motion, transverse and vertical. The observed function of this joint is dependent upon three factors: heel-lift, STJ supination (the first metatarsal being shorter than the second), and finally sesamoid function (Root *et al.*, 1977). These factors combine to create the following sequence of motions. As heel-lift occurs, the metatarsal heads need to remain in contact with the ground and, because the first metatarsal shaft is shorter than the second, it needs to plantarflex more. As this happens the metatarsal head moves posteriorly upon the sesamoids until the distal plantar aspect of the first metatarsal head comes to rest on the sesamoids. This motion causes the transverse axis of the first MTPJ to move dorsally and posteriorly. This in turn stabilizes the hallux for propulsion (Shereff *et al.*, 1986).

The motion of the foot is affected by the use of footwear. Nicol and Paul (1988) have examined this and found that the range of motion at the ankle joint is increased from typically 15° of plantarflexion and 10° of dorsiflexion when walking barefoot, to over 20° of plantarflexion and 12° of dorsiflexion when wearing shoes. Forefoot motion is reduced from over 45° of extension to under 40°.

6.3.2 Kinetics

During the stance phase of walking the ankle joint force varies as shown in Figure 6.6. There are generally two peaks in the vertical joint force curve, with the second being higher and of about four to five times body weight in magnitude. This higher peak occurs during the acceleration phase of the gait cycle with the posteriorly directed shear force peaking at the same instant (Stauffer *et al.*, 1977). Variations in this force pattern are generally indicative of dysfunction in the locomotor system.

The centre of force between the foot and the floor during walking follows a well-established

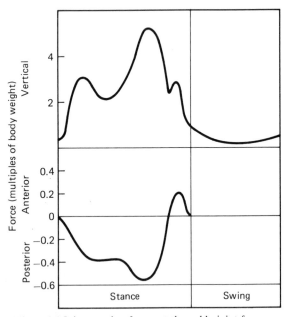

Figure 6.6 Joint reaction forces at the ankle joint for level walking in normal subjects

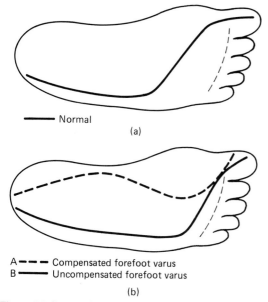

— Normal

(a)

A - - - Compensated forefoot varus
B —— Uncompensated forefoot varus

(b)

Figure 6.7 Centre of pressure pathways for an average foot (a) and two dysfunctions of the foot (b); compensated and uncompensated forefoot varus (see text for details)

pathway during its progression from heel to toe (Figure 6.7(a)). This may be displayed by a number of instruments the most commonly used being the dynamic pedobarograph and its derivatives (Betts *et al.*, 1980; Lord *et al.*, 1986). These devices have been used to demonstrate variations in this pathway and can be used to identify certain dysfunctions of the leg. For example, the usual pattern can be disrupted when the STJ pronates excessively to compensate for a forefoot varus (Figure 6.7(b), Trace A) or when the foot is uncompensated for a forefoot varus (Figure 6.7(b), Trace B). These results can be explained as follows.

In the first case (Figure 6.7(b), Trace A) the foot is pronated at heel-strike and remains so throughout stance when the foot is loaded. The second and third metatarsal heads are thus required to carry the forefoot loads and, because of the first ray position, at propulsion, the hallux cannot contribute as usual and so the forces move off to the medial side of the hallux.

In the second case (Figure 6.7(b), Trace B) the pattern of loading is normal initially but weight is concentrated on the lateral border of the foot during midstance due to a lack of medial forefoot contact. As the propulsion phase of gait is approached the foot abducts by

rotating on the fifth metatarsal head and then the force is transmitted through the medial border of the hallux as the tibia tilts to evert the foot.

Dynamically, the pressure distribution under specific areas of the foot whilst in the shoe can be a more clinically useful measurement (Soames et al., 1982; Barcroft, 1984; Cavanagh *et al.*, 1983). This approach has proved valuable in the assessment of diabetic and other neuropathic feet, with the successful resolution of their pressure-related problems (Boulton *et al.*, 1983) and for the assessment of foot orthoses (Hughes *et al.*, 1987).

The presence of shock loading during walking and running has been demonstrated by a number of workers (Light *et al.*, 1980; Lees and McCullagh, 1984). The foot is an important contributor to the overall shock attenuation in the lower limb (Salathe *et al.*, 1990). Shock due to the impact associated with walking and running is absorbed by the body by a number of mechanisms which can be termed either active or passive. Active mechanisms are related to joint motions. Upon ground contact, certain muscles undergo eccentric contractions, permitting controlled joint motions which can provide a delay in the load response of the limb (Collins and Whittle, 1989; Pratt, 1989) and can store energy for future needs (Bennett *et al.*, 1987). Particular active mechanisms are those of pronation at the STJ and controlled plantarflexion at the ankle joint at heel-strike. Passive mechanisms include the effect of the viscoelastic properties of the soft tissues in the foot and leg, particularly the calcaneal fat pad (Cavanagh *et al.*, 1984) and plantar fascia (Wright and Rennels, 1964).

6.4 Orthotic requirements for different pathologies

Three different types of foot pathology are amenable to orthotic management:

1. Foot instability or deformity due to muscle weakness or imbalance.
2. Foot instability or deformity due to structural malalignment.
3. Deformity arising from a loss of structural integrity within the foot.

In addition, the foot may function abnormally in order to compensate for proximal disorders.

These include genu valgum/varum, coxa valgum/varum or tibial and femoral torsions. Clearly the ideal way to manage such problems would be to correct the proximal malalignment as this would remove the need for specific foot orthotic management. However, such an approach is often impractical and the use of a foot orthosis can provide effective symptomatic relief. In assessing a patient presenting with a foot problem, it is thus important to examine the function of the whole limb.

Because it is usual for footwear to be used for everyday walking, the orthotic objectives, the biomechanical requirements and the description of the devices employed will be based upon the foot inside the shoe as a basic functional unit.

6.4.1 Foot instability or deformity due to muscle weakness or imbalance

Many different pathological conditions result in an upper motor neurone lesion which results in changes in muscle tone in the lower limb, resulting in rigid and difficult to correct deformities. As these deformities usually include the ankle, they are dealt with in the following chapter.

Simple muscle weakness may result from many pathological conditions, although pathologies specific to the foot alone are not as common as those affecting the lower limb generally. However, weakness within the intrinsic foot muscles does occur and leads to such problems as metatarsus adductus, hallux valgus (of which it may be one of many possible 'causes' (Miller, 1975)) and deformities of all the rays.

A foot which is unstable because of muscle weakness will not function as effectively as normal, as necessary and consequent compensatory motions will usually produce a less efficient, more energy consuming, and possibly painful, gait pattern. The general aim of orthotic intervention is to mitigate against the functional sequelae of the muscle weakness by attempting to replace the actions of the weak muscles or restricting but sometimes accommodating the out-of-balance deformities.

(a) Weak or absent supinators

A foot with weak or absent supinators will, upon weight bearing, adopt a pronated posi-

tion. This produces a pattern of deformity which is easily recognized, its most obvious feature being a calcaneovalgus deformity. This shifts the line of action of the tendo Achilles laterally, which reduces the supinating moment which can be produced by the triceps surae, further contributing to the imbalance. Similarly, the tendon of tibialis anterior is deflected laterally, reducing its supinatory ability particularly at the STJ, whilst stretching of the tendon of tibialis posterior impairs its function as a strong supinator at the STJ. The forefoot is unable to pronate because of the presence of the ground and thus is forced into a relatively supinated position and may also be slightly adducted.

The altered force distribution in both the rear- and the forefoot tends to produce secondary changes in the midfoot. The talonavicular joint is disturbed by the navicular being displaced medially and distally. In addition, the cuboid is displaced laterally and distally. The medial and intermediate cuneiforms are internally rotated and also displaced distally. In general there is a tendency for the bones on the medial side of the foot to be distracted while those on the lateral border are compressed.

The change in foot shape which results from this disruption causes the medial longitudinal arch to be depressed and the deltoid ligament to be stretched. Contractions occur in the ankle joint capsule and the calcaneocuboid ligament may also be similarly affected. The peroneal tendons, contracted as a result of the chronic malposition of the bones, tend to resist supination at the STJ. The short plantar muscles are stretched by the action of the depression of the arch and are thus less effective. Hence, once the deformity begins the tendency for depression of the arch and weakening of muscles leads to a reinforcement of the factors causing continued maintenance of the deformity. This is often erroneously referred to as a pes planus or flat foot (more properly called planovalgus).

Because of the strain that such a deformity can place upon the soft tissue structures of the foot, inflammatory reactions are not uncommon, leading to tonic spasms. However, these spasms can be relieved once the underlying condition is managed. Because of the interdependence of the various components of this deformity, it is possible to influence all of them by attempting to control one aspect. Since the principal problem in such a foot relates to STJ pronation, if this factor can be effectively dealt with, the other compensatory elements or sequelae of the excessive motion will be resolved. Pronation at the STJ has however been shown to be a normal and desirable part of the function of the foot and so total elimination of this motion is not indicated. Ideally an orthosis to correct this instability would need to hold the foot in STJ neutral and then allow it to move within predetermined limits in a controlled way, i.e. return function to the foot. Alternatively, the calcaneus could be encouraged to adopt a neutral position which would influence the STJ and MTJ, although this is less satisfactory as it does not address the main source of instability.

Because of the lack of supinator muscle activity, during swing phase the heel will adopt an abnormally valgus position. At heel-strike (Figure 6.8(a)), the line of action of the ground reaction force will be lateral to the line of the weight force, thus producing a valgus moment which forces the STJ further into pronation. This situation can be avoided by moving the point of initial foot contact medially so that the ground reaction force produces a correcting varus moment (Figure 6.8(b)) which swings the heel round into its correct alignment. In practice this is achieved by extending, or flaring, the heel of the shoe on the medial side.

The position of the foot can however only be effectively controlled by adapting footwear if the shoe is a close, intimate fit to the foot. To achieve this the shoe needs to:

1. Extend proximally on the foot to grip the hindfoot and hence control the subtalar joint.
2. Have some effective means of fastening with mechanical advantage (laces are preferable to elasticated supports).
3. Have a firm heel counter to control the position of the calcaneus.
4. Have a semirigid sole to help control the midfoot.
5. Have a broad heel for stability.

These factors in themselves will provide considerable stability to an unstable foot.

Correct shoe fitting involves more than matching the shoe to foot length and width and requires considerable practical experience since it is difficult to make a foot measuring device or instrument that will predetermine

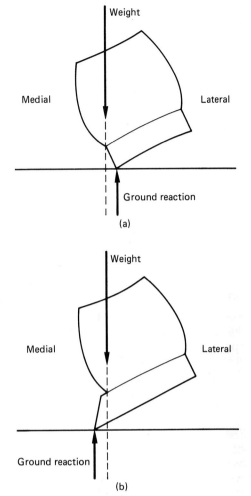

Figure 6.8 A foot which is pronated at heel-strike showing the deforming valgus moment generated with unadapted shoes (a) and the correcting varus moment produced when a flare is added to the medial side of the heel (b)

exact shoe size and fit (Rossi, 1983). Fitting checks should include depth at the level of the medial and lateral malleoli, depth at the toes, heel height, position of stitching relevant to the first MTPJ, heel width, absence of heel slip and a comfortable foot interface with the sole.

Court shoes which stay on the foot by wedging the forefoot into a triangular-shaped front and then compressing the foot longitudinally in order to achieve a snug fit, are not suitable for either shoe adaptions or orthoses. For a patient with foot pathology requiring a shoe adaption, starting from a correctly fitting, well-designed, comfortable shoe is essential.

Once an accurately fitting shoe has been provided, the corrective or stabilizing alterations may then be added. As already described, if the foot is pronated at heel strike, a medial flare will tend to cause the ground reaction force to turn the foot towards its correct functional position. The flare does not however have any effect on the final position of the foot relative to the ground. However, as the aim of biomechanical management of the foot is always to align the heel so that the STJ functions about its neutral position, it will often be necessary to wedge the calcaneus slightly to achieve this (Figure 6.9).

The simplest way to adjust the position of the calcaneus relative to the ground is to wedge the heel of the shoe (Figure 6.9(b)). However much more accurate control over the final heel position can be achieved if the wedging required is built into an in-shoe foot orthosis (Figure 6.9(c)). There are two reasons for this: first, the foot orthosis is manufactured to a cast of the foot from which the required angles can be obtained relatively accurately, and secondly, the presence of the orthosis, which is moulded to the plantar surface of the foot, adds significantly to the control of the foot within the shoe.

Wedging applied to a foot orthosis is referred to as posting. Posting can be either extrinsic or intrinsic. Extrinsic posting is that applied to the orthosis as a wedge of additional material after the main shell of the device has been formed. Intrinsic posting involves adding a wedge or making some similar alteration to the cast prior to moulding (Sanner, 1989), so that the required angulations are built into the orthosis when it is formed (Figure 6.10).

The orthosis will need to be rigid enough to support the foot as indicated but this requirement is contrary to the need for motion to take place within the foot during walking and running. As previously mentioned, an orthosis to correct a subtalar deformity would ideally need to hold the foot in STJ neutral and then allow it to move within predetermined limits in a controlled way. This controlled motion is sometimes called 'built-in' motion and can be achieved either by selecting materials for the rearfoot posting which have the required compressive properties or by removing sufficient material from a rigid rear post to allow for natural pronation. Both approaches have their

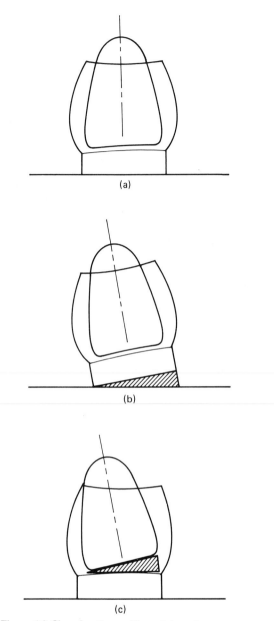

Figure 6.9 Changing the position of the calcaneus relative to the floor: (a) the uncorrected position; (b) corrected by wedging the heel of the shoe; (c) corrected by using a wedged orthosis

value and need to be matched to the individual requirements (Philps, 1990).

All of these orthoses are made from a cast taken of the foot in a reference position, (usually STJ neutral) and non-weight-bearing, which is then modified to take account of each individual's requirements (Burns, 1977). It is

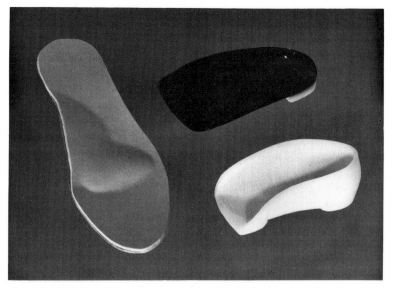

Figure 6.10 Three typical foot orthoses. From top right in a clockwise direction they are a functional foot orthosis with extrinsic rearfoot posting, a UCBL foot orthosis or heel cup with extrinsic rearfoot and forefoot posting and a flexible insole for accommodation or minor correction of the foot

well known that a normal foot changes shape during activity (Kapandji, 1970). It lengthens, the sustentaculum tali falls by about 4 mm and the forefoot spreads by up to 12.5 mm. Any orthosis which aims to correct a deformity and promote normal function must recognize these factors. This is particularly important when applying forces in the region of the medial longitudinal arch, otherwise the continuing natural motion could result in a problem at the patient–orthosis interface. Thus the orthosis needs to be rigid enough to provide control but must also be able to accommodate the natural change in foot shape during motion.

The positioning of the cast in neutral and the range and direction of the built-in motion is derived from a full biomechanical assessment of the foot (Root *et al.*, 1971a; Philps, 1990). The aim of such an assessment is to establish the relationship between the foot and the rest of the leg and between the forefoot and rearfoot. Two important angles are measured, the rearfoot angle (*r*) and forefoot angle (*f*), where *r* is the angle between a vertical to the ground and the calcaneal bisector when the leg is weight bearing in STJ neutral and *f* is the angle between the ground and a plane perpendicular to the calcaneal bisector. These angles are used to determine the values for the rearfoot and forefoot posting required to give a sound func-

tional foot orthosis (Root *et al.*, 1971a; Reigler, 1987; Philps, 1990).

Foot orthoses of this type have been the subject of some scientific assessment, particularly relating to material selection and posting guidelines (Weed *et al.*, 1978; Pratt and Rees, 1987; Tollafield and Pratt, 1990a,b). Tollafield and Pratt (1990b) used a Kistler force plate, pedobarograph and video analysis to compare the motion of the foot with different forefoot and rearfoot posting angles in selected subjects. The force plate demonstrated the illogicality of the often quoted rule that a 4° rearfoot post is appropriate for most foot pathologies because it is consistent with normal STJ motion (Weed, 1984). The results of the study did not confirm this and found that even greater angles of rearfoot posting, i.e. 8°, could still produce normal patterns of force in some cases.

The pedobarograph demonstrated that the use of a functional foot orthosis could result in a more normal forefoot loading pattern with the first metatarsal head retaining its functional loading even with an 8° post.

Ross and Gurnick (1982) considered the relevance of shoe heel height and the need to pitch a functional foot orthosis appropriately. This is because an orthosis pitched for, say, a 2-cm heel used in a shoe with a 3-cm heel will be less stable, as only the anterior part of the rear post will be in contact with the supporting shoe surface.

The restoration of normal forefoot function can be achieved by forefoot posting alone and can affect the foot/floor reaction forces much more significantly than a rearfoot post (Tollafield and Pratt, 1990b). It could be argued that a suitable forefoot post used simply to accommodate the forefoot position (which was a consequence of the pronated hindfoot) is sufficient to provide symptomatic relief. This is commonly practised but can adversely affect the overall function of the foot, whereas a rearfoot post will usually provide correction without such an effect. In addition, there is limited space in the front of a normal shoe for forefoot posting. Subjectively it has been found that a foot orthosis is also rendered more comfortable by including a stabilizing rearfoot post. A good description of posting can be found in Darrigan and Ganley (1985).

In-shoe orthoses are also useful for the treatment of feet with an abnormally high MTJ axis (Hice, 1984) and more complicated forms of posting are practised in some cases (Valmassy and Terrafranca, 1986; Lundeen, 1988). However, the alterations required to the cast for such complex systems need considerable skill. A biplanar posting technique, described by Dennis *et al.* (1985), achieves the application of the rearpost and the building in of motion in a single process.

The heel cup concept was first introduced by Helfet in 1956 and called the Helfet heel seat. Athough the earlier designs caused problems of skin rubbing particularly on the heels, modifications to these were proposed by Rose (1962) which eliminated this problem. Further changes have been made to this concept by Marvin and Brownrigg (1983) in what they term the negative anatomically modified foot orthosis or NAMFO.

In cases of more severe pronation, heel cups (UCBL, foot orthosis) can be used but have been accompanied by mixed success (Quigley, 1974) (Figure 6.10). These orthoses can provide more stabilization of the foot than purely plantar devices. With a foot orthosis the corrective moment is transmitted to the involved joint by means of a couple created between the shoe upper and the heel of the foot. With a UCBL orthosis, the greater intimacy of fit and its increased stiffness produce a more effective system to transmit corrective moments. Fore-

foot and rearfoot posting can be used with these in much the same way as for other functional devices. Increased stability can be achieved by filling in the medial arch with cork or foam. What is not acceptable functionally is a heel cup with a rounded plantar aspect as such an orthosis will be totally unstable within the shoe.

Foot orthoses function by changing the line of action of the ground reaction force so as to realign anatomical joints into their optimum functioning positions. Many practitioners claim that this realignment is achievable with great accuracy – to within 1° or 2° of the absolutely correct anatomical position. However, it is obvious to any bioengineer that to measure motions on a part of the human body using bisectors of segments drawn 'by eye' as the reference points and to claim the values to be within 1° of the actual motion is unrealistic. Nevertheless, all of the reported studies of the use of rigid functional foot orthoses illustrate their undeniable value in often returning the foot to an improved function.

(b) Weak or absent pronators

A foot with weak or absent pronators will, during swing phase and at foot contact, adopt a supinated position which may be maintained during stance. This is commonly observed secondary to paralysis of the peronei where the ankle dorsiflexes and the short flexors on the plantar surface of the foot contract. The talus is thus dorsiflexed and the plantar fascia tightens producing a high arched cavus foot. The angle of the MTJ is thus made more acute which leads to a tightness in the long extensors and this in turn causes the toes to become retracted and clawed, i.e. hyperextended, at the MTPJs and fixed at the IP joints (Boike *et al.*, 1990).

In the non-weight-bearing foot of this type, high longitudinal medial and lateral arches are evident together with an everted forefoot, plantarflexed first and sometimes fifth ray, tight plantar fascia and possibly metatarsus adductus. Upon weight bearing, the calcaneus adopts a varus posture, and the fifth ray is forcefully dorsiflexed and bears excessive weight. Because of the varus rearfoot, the triceps surae is able to more actively supinate the foot at the STJ. This effect is reinforced by the increase in the ability of the tibialis anterior to supinate the STJ and MTJ.

As with the pronated foot, malalignments of the bones lead to soft tissue inflammation and pain, resulting in protective tonic spasm. This may reinforce the supinatory tendency resulting in the development of a more rigid foot.

The area of the MTPJs is now overloaded by the hyperextension of these joints. The middle three metatarsals increase their angle of declination to the ground because of the raised arches together with retracted and sometimes subluxed MTPJs. The digital deformities all predispose to dorsal and apical corns which may be severe, as well as plantar callosities. In cases in which nutrition and sensation are deficient, skin metabolism is impaired and ulceration is prone to develop.

In the supinated foot, at heel-strike the calcaneal position gives rise to a destabilizing varus moment (Figure 6.11). To correct this a valgus moment is required and this can be produced by moving the point of initial calcaneus/ground contact, as previously described for pronation, but in this case, laterally.

By the use of wedging and flaring the heel of a shoe, a hindfoot corrective moment can be applied in a similar way to that already described for pronation (Figure 6.9). However, because of the direction of the axis of the STJ, the most effective point at which to apply a corrective ground reaching force to produce a supinatory moment is on the medial edge of the heel, whereas to create an effective pronatory moment the most effective point of application is along the entire lateral aspect of the foot, provided the shoe is suitably stiff. In practice however, as a supinated cavus foot is often rigid and uncorrectable (Lutter, 1981), orthopaedic surgical treatment is usually considered if the foot is symptomatic (Jahss, 1983).

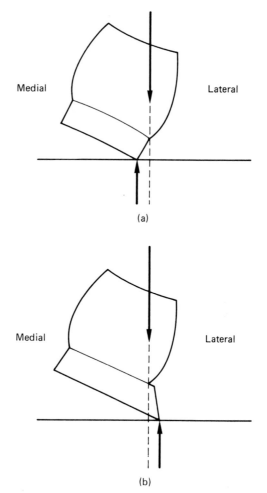

Figure 6.11 A foot which is supinated at heel-strike showing: (a) the deforming varus moment generated with unadapted shoes; (b) the correcting valgus moment produced when a flare is added to the lateral side of the heel

(c) Weak or absent toe extensors or flexors

Weakness of the toe extensors is usually associated with an inability to dorsiflex the foot at the ankle joint. Commonly, however, some digital deformities are also produced and the treatment of these is dealt with below.

Weakness of the toe flexor muscles, particularly those associated with the first ray and hallux, may cause significant foot pathology. Although this problem is often associated with an inability to plantarflex the foot at the ankle, the destabilization of the hallux during walking may lead to a number of sequelae.

Deformities of the MTPJs and the IP joints may result from the action of unopposed long toe flexors or extensors. Clawing of the toes may result from unopposed flexor activity, with subluxation of the MTPJs and an increase in pressure applied under the metatarsal heads. Associated dorsal lesions over the IP joints may also develop. This is more problematical when the hallux is involved because of the importance of the first ray for locomotion. Other deformities, such as hammer toes, which is a plantarflexion deformity of the proximal IP joint, or mallet toes (an abnormal

(a)

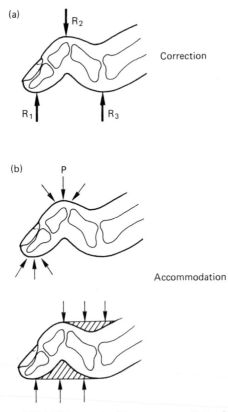

Correction

(b)

Accommodation

Figure 6.12 (a) Three-point force system applied to the distal IP joint to correct a flexion deformity. (b) The use of an interdigital orthosis to redistribute high pressure (P) on the apices of the flexed toes by spreading the loads over larger areas

urethane foams are the materials most frequently used to correct, or more usually accommodate, toe deformities.

Weakness in the flexors and extensors of the toes can lead to a malalignment of the metatarsal heads. This leads to the prominent heads being subjected to increased pressure and the creation of plantar callosities and discomfort. To relieve this pain, the prominent head may be re-aligned with the others by applying a corrective force under the shaft of the affected metatarsal using a metatarsal pad (Figure 6.13(a)). Secondary pronation may also occur to a limited extent and some medial arch support may also be required to alleviate the

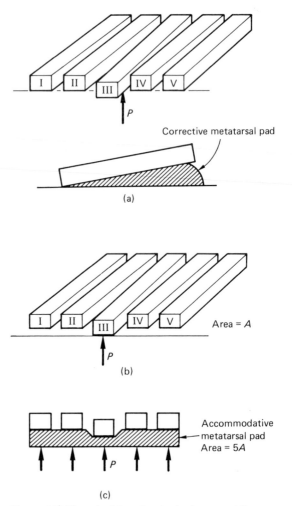

Corrective metatarsal pad

(a)

Area = A

(b)

Accommodative metatarsal pad
Area = 5A

(c)

Figure 6.13 The principles of orthotic plantar padding: (a) a corrective pad to realign a mobile metatarsal shaft; (b) an accommodative pad used to reduce plantar pressure under a fixed plantarflexed ray

plantarflexion of the distal phalanx only) can also be produced.

In all of the above cases it may be possible to correct the deformity by applying a three-point force system to the deformity as illustrated in Figure 6.12. In this case the forces are applied to correct a flexion deformity at the proximal IP joint of the hallux. Such an orthosis would need to be rigid enough to apply the corrective forces without being too thick to occupy the limited space inside the front of shoes. The point of application of the forces is often modified so the device can be fitted inside the shoe. Details of this group of digital orthoses can be found in Whitney and Whitney (1990a). The foundation for the use of digital orthoses was described in 1941 by Harry Budin in his book '*Principles and Practice of Orthodigita*'. His ideas have been brought up to date with better understanding of foot disorders and the introduction of new materials. Silicones and

effects of this. Figure 6.13a shows the usual method of correcting a plantarflexed metatarsal without causing a localized excessive pressure increase. To make such a correction tolerable however, the force needs to be applied using a semirigid material which is strong enough to give the correction but soft enough to allow some natural metatarsal motion. This result is usually achieved by trial and error. If the material is too soft there will be insufficient pain relief; if too hard it will be painful itself. A range of properties is required for the vast range of patient weights, deformity type and severity and tissue viability (Campbell *et al.*, 1984; Bradley and McDonald, 1987). No one material can satisfy all of these criteria in all cases.

If the deformity is only partially correctable or non-correctable then the area of increased pressure should be relieved (Figure 6.13(b)). In this case pressures are applied around the problem area so that the initially high pressure under, in this case, the third metatarsal head (P/A) is reduced (P/5A) and spread evenly under each head. This is too simplistic a picture, because there are often a number of problem sites and the tissue of the foot may be poor, preventing the application of pressure where it should ideally be placed.

At this point it is convenient to outline some limiting factors in the design of such insoles. With both of these types of foot orthosis the placement of the corrective/accommodative shapes requires care. Generally the use of stock orthoses for these conditions is only acceptable provided that they are adjusted appropriately before being used, as each individual is thought to need a slightly different shape or contour. It is convenient to consider the plantar surface of the foot divided into nine areas (Figure 6.14). For each of these regions there is a specific pad type that is appropriate (Whitney and Whitney, 1990b). With regard to placement, there are several rules that need to be observed, particularly in relation to the break line of the shoes and foot shape (Whitney, 1979).

Three factors govern the effectiveness of pads applied to the foot: material, foundation and design. The material is selected to perform a number of functions, the most important of which is pressure reduction and re-distribution. Soft foams can produce the same pressure as harder materials but require more bulk. Thus

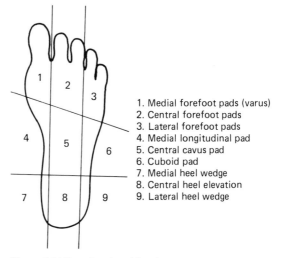

1. Medial forefoot pads (varus)
2. Central forefoot pads
3. Lateral forefoot pads
4. Medial longitudinal pad
5. Central cavus pad
6. Cuboid pad
7. Medial heel wedge
8. Central heel elevation
9. Lateral heel wedge

Figure 6.14 Functional padding is applied in one or more of nine areas of the foot. This kind of padding can be used to test the probable outcome of a more permanent orthosis and is quick and cheap to perform

within the confines of the shoe, firmer materials are generally preferred. The foundation relates to the support available in the shoe, which is often limited. The force which a pad can apply to the foot is limited by the rigidity of the surface with which it is in contact. Thus, in order for the orthosis to be effective the shoe into which it is fitted needs to be firm and supportive in the appropriate places.

The pad design is of importance in relation to its specific function. The need for space in the shoe must be appreciated and if necessary new shoes purchased. Each metatarsal pad will require to be contoured to the individual metatarsal length. The design of pads includes the use of cut-outs or apertures (Whitney and Whitney, 1990b) that permit a redistribution of forces over an area by suitable shaping.

6.4.2 Foot instability or deformity due to structural malalignment

Structural malalignments are often congenital and in general result in a foot in which the joints are mobile, but function about abnormal positions. Such a foot will be less capable of providing an energy-efficient gait pattern and the compensatory processes adopted by the body may result in long-term pain both in the foot and at sites remote from the foot itself. The aim of orthotic managment is to return more normal function to the foot and hence to reduce pain and the need for body compensation mechanisms. In children particularly, the foot can be readily realigned to function about a more normal neutral position. This approach would follow that already detailed in Section 6.4.1, and is well documented particularly in relation to pronated feet.

Powell (1983) has reported on the value of such devices in pes planovalgus in children and Mereday *et al.* (1972) studied ten children for 2 years using the UCBL design of orthosis. They found that these orthoses did relieve pain and improve gait although these changes were not maintained on removal of the device. Pennau *et al.* (1982) studied ten children and compared the UCBL orthosis with a Thomas heel and an over-the-counter device but found no radiographical difference between barefoot walking and any of the devices. Bleck and Berzins (1977) reported on a study of 71 childen comparing the UCBL device with a Helfet heel seat. They found a 1° improvement in pronation for every 2 months' use. Bordelon (1983) studied 50 children using UCBL devices with a Thomas heel and found about 5° of correction per year without loss of foot function.

If the deformity is not correctable then accommodatory orthoses are required. This, again, follows the methods already detailed in 6.3.1.

6.4.3 Foot deformity or instability due to a loss of structural integrity

The structural integrity of the foot is commonly compromised by an arthritic condition or by acute trauma, and may be associated with the chronic repetitive injury from high levels of sporting activity.

In rheumatoid arthritis the connective tissue is involved in the disease process with autodestruction: tendons become soft and therefore lose their mechanical stabilizing effect; cartilage becomes soft and eroded, and the joints start to dislocate, especially the MTPJs. Digital deformity leads to metatarsal overloading. The underlying skin becomes atrophic and susceptible to ulceration due to the occurrence of pressures of up to three times normal levels (Minns and Craxford, 1984).

The consequence of such instabilities is that the foot is painful even during normal activities. Orthotically the aim is to reduce the pain by controlling joint motion or by stress reduc-

tion and to compensate for either the reduced motion or other compensatory motions elsewhere within the foot.

(a) Pain resulting from joint instability or excess motion

The pain resulting from an unstable or excessively mobile joint is often such that the patient will try to eliminate the painful motion by changing their foot to ground orientation. This reorientation may produce secondary problems, such as excessive localized plantar pressure, and it is often for these secondary problems that the patient is initially referred.

Stabilizing the joints of the foot, which usually collapse into a pronated position, will make use of the principles already described for such a deformity. However, because extra stability is essential to limit the pain, the materials used for such an orthosis are usually stiffer. The final device would look very much like that shown in Figure 6.10, but extra stability may be achieved by having a wider than usual flare, medially or laterally as appropriate, incorporated into both the foot orthosis and the heel of the shoe. Additional support can be provided by the use of footwear which includes stiffeners around the rear counter and laced well proximally to maintain good contact between the foot and the orthosis.

(b) Pain on weight-bearing

If the joint surfaces are severely damaged or degenerate, then the only way in which pain relief may be obtained is to off load the joint either partially or totally and this will require the use of a lower limb orthosis as described in Chapter 7.

Pain on walking may however also be due to the transmission of shock to the affected joints. This problem may be related to a reduction in the amount of tissue, particularly under the calcaneus, or to the development of minor structural irregularities within the foot, or it may be idiopathic. Whatever the cause, the orthotic management is aimed at enhancing the natural shock attenuation mechanisms and thus reducing pain.

The selection of shock attenuating materials would seem to be simple. However, there are a number of factors which complicate the selection and use of such a material. Most important amongst these is the requirement for the material to absorb the shock sufficiently from one step to the next. It is not sufficient for the material to absorb the shock from the first step and then be unable to perform well subsequently. What needs to be optimized is the coefficient of restitution, a measure of the materials' ability to absorb shock at a certain frequency of impact. In the case of walking this is about 1 Hz. The material's abilities in this respect are related to its Young's Modulus or elastic modulus (E). The damping effect experienced by the body is inversely proportional to the modulus of the orthotic material, thus a high E is indicated. The material used needs to be placed under the area from which the excessive shock is generated, usually the heel. However, in running this may not be the appropriate area and the material selection may have to be altered (Oakley and Pratt, 1988).

Loss of structural integrity may also be responsible for painful conditions such as metatarsalgia and plantar fasciitis. This is a different problem from that of pain caused by a functional abnormality, such as pes cavus, for which treatment for the underlying pathology is required. Conditions producing this type of pain include arthritis, osteochondritis, digital neuritis and stress fractures, with the former being the most common. Frequently the cause is a loss of the normal adipose tissue under the metatarsal heads or the specialized tissue under the heel (Blechschmidt, 1933). Simply replacing the shock attenuation property lost as a result of this with a tissue equivalent material should be sufficient to relieve symptoms.

Overuse injuries are associated with the foot being repeatedly overloaded due to work or play and generally present as overpronation and pain. Pronation, a normal feature of shock attenuation at foot contact, may be abnormally prolonged in stance. The literature supports the view that excessive pronation causes a number of problems such as medial arch strain, plantar fasciitis, heel spurs, Achilles tendonitis, hallux abductovalgus and metatarsalgia (Smart and Edge, 1987). Excessive pronation may also affect the muscle balance in the leg causing shin splints, lateral knee pain and adductory twist, i.e. the heel adducts once

unloaded causing the forefoot to abduct (Subotnick, 1979).

The use of orthoses to control excessive shock at heel-strike has grown in popularity during the last few years. Although the tissue loading resulting from walking and running has been demonstrated by Light and colleagues (1980) and Lees and McCullagh (1984), the question as to whether such loading is injurious has only been satisfactorily answered in some specific instances (Simkin *et al.*, 1989). Radin *et al.* (1973) have suggested that it may be implicated in the development of idiopathic osteoarthritis resulting from microfractures of the trabeculae at the hip and knee, and Voloshin and Wosk (1982) have suggested an association with low back pain. Furthermore, it has been proposed by Light *et al.* (1980) that such loading may be associated with the loosening of orthopaedic implants – particularly hip replacements. This has resulted in an increase in interest in the problem and the development of polymeric materials which, it is claimed, can be used to reduce shock loading. Some benefit can also be obtained by gait training, which may augment orthotic intervention (Seliktar and Mizrahi, 1984).

The assessment of shock loading is usually carried out using an accelerometer. The study by Light *et al.* (1980) used an accelerometer attached to a pin inserted into the distal end of the tibia. They showed that the magnitude of the force transient was influenced both by the choice of footwear and the walking surface. Similar results were demonstrated by Voloshin and Wosk (1982) with transducers located at sites in the vertebral column. Further work by Johnson (1986) used a Fourier transform technique to measure the frequency pattern of acceleration at the ankle measured by an accelerometer attached to a specially designed splint around the malleoli. By defining shock acceleration as that lying in the spectrum above 50 Hz, it became possible to define a Shock Factor as the magnitude of the acceleration above 50 Hz expressed as a proportion of the total amplitude. Typical values for walking in normal footwear lie in the range 0.2–0.5. In order to remove the need for complex signal analysis a portable instrument was designed for this measurement. The repeatability of the system was found to be good and it was possible to discriminate a 10% change in Shock Factor (Johnson, 1990).

Table 6.3 Change in shock attenuating properties of some insoles with time

	Viscolas	PPT	Plastazote	Gait Aid
Days				
0	82.0 ± 2.2	83.5 ± 1.0	89.8 ± 3.6	97.7 ± 1.1
2	82.3 ± 2.6	85.9 ± 3.1	97.2 ± 2.5	98.0 ± 1.2
7	82.1 ± 2.1	85.7 ± 2.3	98.4 ± 1.3	97.6 ± 1.3
30	83.3 ± 2.5	86.6 ± 3.1	98.2 ± 1.2	98.3 ± 1.7
Months				
2	83.6 ± 2.9	85.9 ± 2.9	98.3 ± 1.3	97.9 ± 1.9
6	84.0 ± 2.2	86.2 ± 3.3	97.9 ± 1.9	98.1 ± 1.7
9	85.3 ± 3.3	90.1 ± 3.0	98.1 ± 1.1	98.3 ± 1.5
12	89.4 ± 3.1	93.5 ± 3.2	99.0 ± 1.0	98.5 ± 1.1

From Pratt (1990).

Using this technique Johnson (1988) evaluated the effectiveness of insoles during normal walking and found that polymeric insoles could decrease shock acceleration by up to 30%. Pratt (1990) has used the same technique to assess the long-term effectiveness of insoles over a 12-month period (Table 6.3).

(c) Rigid foot deformities

Rigidity in one or more joints of the foot can have a number of profound effects. There may be localized increases in pressures on the foot, both on the plantar and dorsal surfaces, or there may be gait alterations. The orthotic aim is not to correct the foot, as this is clearly impossible, but to alleviate the secondary effects. It may be useful to illustrate the general principles of this treatment by reference to some specific but frequently encountered problems.

With a rigid pronated or supinated foot the plantar surface is overloaded in specific areas. Here the aim is to reduce the plantar pressures using the techniques described earlier in this chapter. Sometimes however foot rigidity is associated with other factors which lead to an insensate or neuropathic foot. A common example of this is diabetes mellitus or, rarely in the UK, leprosy. In such feet the structure becomes somewhat immobile, generally with a reduction in muscular activity, and associated deformities develop in both the rearfoot and forefoot. Associated with such conditions are generally poor nutritional and metabolic states of the soft tissues which, together with the neuropathy, tend to lead to the development of ulcers which are commonly difficult to heal.

Orthotic management has two objectives in such individuals, assisting the healing of the ulcers and preventing their development in the future. In both cases the aim is to reduce pressure and shear stresses in the abnormally high loaded areas of the foot. These areas tend to be in the forefoot where peak loads are increased and have a tendency to move to the lateral side. In addition, because the heel tends to unload earlier during stance phase, the forefoot is loaded for longer, further exacerbating the problem. Load can be taken off the forefoot and transferred back to the heel and the midfoot structures using suitably shaped pads without treating excessive loading elsewhere because of the redistribution. The materials used should be soft enough to cushion the foot but firm enough to achieve the load redistribution. In relation to the shearing forces specifically, the material used should be capable of providing a reduction in shear stress at the foot–insole interface by shearing internally without rapidly degrading in service.

In addition, alterations can be carried out to footwear to reduce peak pressures on the susceptible metatarsal heads. A rocker sole slows down the forward progression of the centre of pressure of the ground reaction force, resulting in it 'hesitating' at the point of contact of the rocker with the ground (Figure 6.15). The rocker thereby reduces the moment about a stiff and painful MTPJ.

Studies of the peak pressures under diabetic or neurophatic feet confirm that these are up to

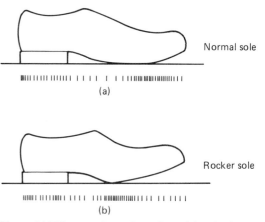

Figure 6.15 The use of a rocker sole to delay the forward progression of the foot/floor reaction force vector: (a) a normal progression; (b) that with a rocker sole. The tick marks indicate the point of progression of the force vector on the sole at equal time intervals

five times those found in the normal population (Baumann *et al.*, 1963; Ctercteko *et al.*, 1981; Cavanagh *et al.*, 1985). The value of footwear adaptions in managing this problem is well established (Tovey and Moss, 1987; Stess and Hetherington, 1990) and temporary shoes are often provided with insoles to 'off load' the ulcer prior to the provision of definitive, often custom-made shoes. These, together with the shoe adaptions described (Geary and Klenerman, 1987) and insoles (Block, 1981) are usually sufficient to prevent ulcer formation provided there is space for the foot which avoids excess dorsal pressure and provided that the insoles redistribute the pressures without creating an increase in pressure at another vulnerable site.

Hallux abductovalgus (HAV) is a common forefoot disorder often associated with arthritic conditions. Although included in this discussion of rigid deformities, some early HAV deformities can be partially or totally corrected. Usually orthotic management is not requested until this deformity has become well established. The biomechanical requirements for this situation include the relief of pressure between the foot and shoe and the prevention of overriding or underriding of the hallux on the second and third toes.

HAV has been thought to be due to a number of factors such as a pronation abnormality producing hypermobility of the first ray, metabolic disorders and congenital abnormalities. In addition, tight stockings or footwear have been cited as being responsible, although it is felt that these do not so much initiate the problem but exacerbate both its rate of development and severity (Noakes, 1981). Once fully developed, the first ray is adducted at its base, the hallux is abducted and impinges on or overrides the second toe and a medial bunion develops over the first MTPJ because of the shearing forces between the medial prominence of the metatarsal head and the overlying soft tissue.

This deformity leads to a displacement of the extensor and flexor tendons of the hallux which then tend to produce a further deforming adduction force in addition to their primary action. This 'bow stringing' of the tendons exacerbates the deformity as does the direction of the ground reaction vector applied during toe-off in gait. The normal function of the intrinsic muscles is disrupted with the control of the

transverse arch which later leads to metatarsalgia.

The orthotic management of this disorder encompasses a number of requirements. The hallux needs to be abducted and the first metatarsal shaft needs to be adducted. Abduction of the hallux at the first MTPJ can be produced by a three-point force system applied at the distal hallux (R1), the head of the fifth metatarsal (R2) and the medial border of the foot at a point more proximal than the head of the first metatarsal shaft (R3) (Figure 6.16(a)). The abduction of the first metatarsal shaft can be produced by employing forces R2 and R3 as part of a second three-point force system. The additional force needed (R4) would be applied

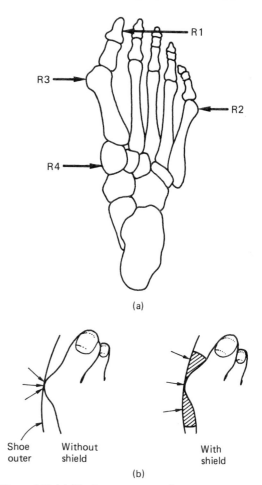

Figure 6.16 (a) The force system used to correct or maintain an HAV deformity using two three-point force systems (R1,R2 and R3) and R2,R3 and R4). (b) The use of a bunion shield to redistribute localized high pressures on a medial bunion related to an uncorrected HAV deformity

proximal to the base of the first metatarsal shaft (Figure 6.16(a)).

This approach would result in such a bulky device that it could not be fitted into normal footwear. The use of such devices however has been advocated for night use with some limited success, although the general opinion is that orthotic management of HAV has a poor record (Ross, 1986). There is a strong body of opinion that overpronation coupled with an unstable first MTPJ is the precursor to an HAV deformity (Root *et al.*, 1977), and thus by controlling pronation in the manner already described this deformity may be prevented or its progression prevented (Sperryn, 1983).

The most problematical aspect of HAV is the development of a medial bunion overlying the head of the first metatarsal. This, together with the increase in metatarsal width, leads to excessive pressure on the forefoot, pain, swelling and limitations in first MTPJ function. Many of these problems can be relieved by the provision of shoes with a wider metatarsal region than normal. In addition, padding around the medial bunion can be added to reduce the peak pressure and relieve pain (Figure 6.16(b)).

Where a prominent HAV exists leading to skin lesions a hole can be cut in the shoe upper and a soft matching leather stitched over the hole to provide extra room and relieve pressure. This adaption, known as a balloon patch, offers poor cosmesis even when carried out by a skilled craftsman and should only be used when no other option is available.

Another problem that causes significant gait abnormalities and discomfort is hallux rigidus or limitus. In this condition, usually associated with osteoarthritis, significant limitation in dorsiflexion of the hallux is termed limitus and total loss of dorsiflexion is termed rigidus. During the terminal stages of stance the hallux needs to dorsiflex up to 65–75°. If this is limited because of articular damage or by other factors, such as a congenitally plantarflexed first ray, pain and an apropulsive gait result. To compensate for the limitation of movement at the first MTPJ the distal phalanx may hyperextend which may lead to plantar callosities or damage to the hallux nail by repeated contact with the top of the shoe.

Orthotically the aim is to protect the painful joint and to compensate for the loss of toe extension. This is usually performed in mild

cases by simply stiffening the sole of the shoe a little and in moderate and severe cases by applying a rocker sole to the shoe as has been described for the management of diabetic foot (Figure 6.15). However, in this case the sole and shank of the shoe should be stiffened with a metal plate so that the MTPJs will not dorsiflex, because of the rigidity of the sole, but the foot will still provide a stable base for propulsion.

One condition not specific to the foot but which has a number of proximal effects, many of which can be serious, is that of a leg-length discrepancy. Leg-length discrepancy alters the natural symmetry of the body resulting in pelvic tilt which, if large enough, will produce an associated scoliosis and pain which may lead to early lumbar osteoarthritis (Figure 6.17). Raises used to correct the discrepancy should be lightweight and as cosmetically acceptable as possible. They should also allow the shoe to flex or they should incorporate a rocker sole. Care should be taken not to increase the height of a heel without also elevating the sole. As the heel height is increased the MTPJs are forced into dorsiflexion and the forefoot load increased. As heel height is increased from 25 mm to 100 mm the MTPJs require an additional 42° of dorsiflexion, i.e. 5° for each 9 mm of additional heel height (Sussman and D'Amico, 1984). This forced dorsiflexion may lead to pain if arthritis is already present.

Common practice suggests that up to 12 mm may be added to the heel before it is necessary to elevate the sole. Improved cosmesis may be

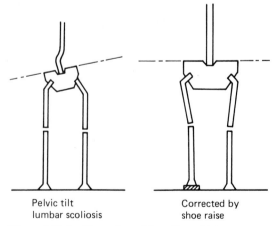

Pelvic tilt   Corrected by
lumbar scoliosis   shoe raise

Figure 6.17 An illustration of the effect of a leg-length discrepancy on pelvic tilt and lumbar scoliosis corrected by a suitable shoe raise

achieved by incorporating up to 6 mm inside the shoe and reducing the contralateral heel height by a similar amount. It is important to understand the importance of cosmesis to the user who can, in extreme cases, discard the raise because it is considered ugly.

In a study of athletes who had a leg discrepancy of less than 1.25 cm, Bandy and Sinning (1986) concluded that it was reasonable to employ a compensating raise on a trial basis to relieve symptoms but important to realize that all subjects do not respond in the same way, i.e. frequent monitoring is necessary.

6.5 Current and future developments

There is considerable interest in the use of foot orthoses which apply their corrective forces directly to the actual joints they aim to control. The main drawback of orthoses applying forces through the plantar surface of the foot is that they are applied some distance away from the joint. It is common knowledge that more effective control can always be provided by a total contact cast. In a study of this issue, the structure of a total contact cast was removed one piece at a time to establish at what point effective control was lost. The resulting shape is illustrated in Figure 6.18. Here the forces are applied via the dorsum of the foot and the plantar surface is left unsupported (Figure

6.19). This technique has also been reported as useful for ankle foot orthoses (AFO) (Brown *et al.*, 1987).

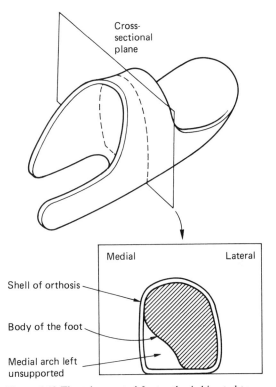

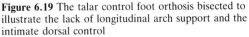

Figure 6.19 The talar control foot orthosis bisected to illustrate the lack of longitudinal arch support and the intimate dorsal control

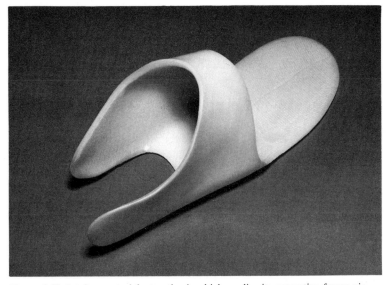

Figure 6.18 A talar control foot orthosis which applies its corrective forces via the dorsum of the foot

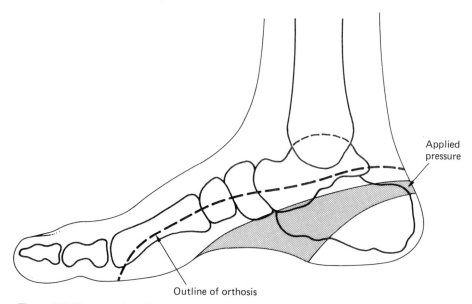

Figure 6.20 The area of applied pressure in a modified UCBL orthosis creating a supporting ledge under the sustentaculum tali

A more conventionally based technique finding favour more recently is the use of pressure applied under the sustentaculum tali to support the midfoot (Figure 6.20). This feature is introduced during casting and subsequently reinforced by modification of the positive cast and produces a ledge under the sustentaculum tali and a strong grip around the calcaneus. Sound support of pronation is achieved by this method without the pressure problems commonly experienced around the navicular using more conventional approaches. Once again, this design of orthosis may be used in an AFO with similar effects.

6.6 Alternative and complementary treatments

6.6.1 Operative solutions

As long as orthoses can provide the patient with a reduction of symptoms, offer greater mobility and confidence to the patient and improve foot stability, then surgery may not be necessary. So often the provision of orthoses is treated as entirely separate from surgical management because the surgical and orthotic team do not have an adequate liaison.

However, in a number of cases a combination of the two approaches may offer the best chance of a successful result.

Foot surgery involves either soft tissue or bone surgery, but more frequently a combination of both. Osteotomy, which is surgical division of bone, is used in a wide range of procedures; bone can be lengthened, shortened, rotated or the angle of deformity altered. Osteotomy is particularly applicable to the metatarsals, bones of the midfoot and the calcaneus.

Joint surgery ideally should reduce deformity and as a consequence the associated pain. Fixed deformities of joints will involve removal of cartilage and division of tight soft tissues which are hard to reduce by orthotic mechanics. The technique of choice varies between excisional arthroplasties (excision of joint) and joint arthrodesis (fixation of joint). Replacement arthroplasty involves the use of a synthetic implant and has been quite successful in selected patients with two stem implants at the first metatarsophalangeal joint, but Cracchiolo (1988) cites authors who have had disappointing results with prosthetic ankle implants.

STJ and ankle joint arthrodeses are practised as a last resort for pain at the ankle or where orthoses have failed to provide satisfactory pain relief. Often it is preferable to fuse only one joint in the hindfoot so that the remaining joint is capable of compensating for the subsequent loss of triplanar motion.

Ostectomy in the hindfoot and around the ankle is a less common procedure. Robbins (1976) describes excision of the navicular to reduce the effects of a vertical talus. Exostectomies can be performed for excrescences over the medial and dorsal first metatarsal, posterior heel (Haglund's deformity) and the dorsal first metatarsal-cuneiform. In each case the presence of an exostosis often makes shoe fitting with an orthosis difficult.

'-otomies' or surgical division can be applied to most tissues and include tenotomies, fasciotomies, capsulotomies and desmotomies (ligament). Tendons may be transferred from their sites of origin as a complete unit or division of the tendon may be used so that it still retains some of its original function. Transfers have been used largely where a correctable deformity due to muscle power being weaker of the one side needs stabilizing. Crawford-Adams (1986) has described the use of both tibialis anterior and tibialis posterior to reduce recurrence of deformity in congenital talipes equinovarus. Tendonplasty is valuable in providing additional length to a contracted tendon. The largest tendon in the foot, the achilles, may be associated with an equinus gait. A 'Z' shaped incision is a popular technique of lengthening. Overlengthening can however lead to weakness of the muscle. Long tendons can be shortened by plication or overlapping.

Deformities of the toes may be corrected by soft tissue surgery alone or combined with a bone procedure. Skin incisions should be carefully placed to avoid scar contractures. Lesions under the plantar surface may require bone excision or osteotomy. The excision of the hard keratinized mass produced by a callosity is generally unnecessary. If the high pressure pathology is removed then the callosity will disappear automatically. Wherever possible plantar surgery is avoided because of the risk of tender scarring.

Capsules of joints will become tight around any longstanding deformity. Incision will relieve tension, but frequently the desired joint position will be obtained only by bony realignment together with tendon and ligament division. The plantar fascia runs from the calcaneus to the digits and has a considerable effect upon the tightness across the arch. Various methods exist to divide the structure by transverse or longitudinal incision.

Skin lesions such as warty skin tags or fibroepitheliomata (fibrous outgrowths from the skin) can occur on the dorsum of the foot. While of little clinical importance, excision may be advisable to prevent irritation between the skin of the foot and the orthosis.

The most common nerve problem in the foot occurs between the third and fourth metatarsals. The intermetatarsal nerve is trapped by mechanical pressure and if this enlarges surgical excision remedies the pain in 95% of cases (Mann 1978). Tarsal tunnel syndrome, similar to carpel tunnel in hands, is the other neurological entrapment condition which may require surgical management.

6.6.2 Conservative solutions

With the current improved understanding of foot function and the relevance of the neutral joint position, orthotic management of the foot has advanced. However, in the past good results were obtained by the empirical application of tape. Whitney and Whitney (1990b) discuss this at length and continue to find it useful for rearfoot, STJ, MTJ and hallux problems but the disadvantage of this technique is the need to regularly re-apply the tape. Reports by Draper (1990) and by Rovert *et al.* (1988) found that such taping was less effective than moulded devices. The techniques of taping are specialized and should only be attempted by those who are aware both of the principles of application and the mechanics of the foot.

The management of foot ulcers in the early stages, prior to the provision of prescription footwear, has been successfully achieved by the use of total-contact plaster casts (Coleman *et al.*, 1984). This has the effect of redistributing forces over the widest possible area, thus relieving high pressure areas, and by holding the foot very still, excessive injurious shear forces are prevented. However caution and great care should be taken using this technique as amputation of the leg has resulted from poor supervision of patients treated by this method.

Bibliography

Frankel V.H. and Nordin M. (1980) *Basic Biomechanics of the Skeletal System.* Lea and Febiger, Philadelphia

Helal B. and Wilson D. (1988) *The Foot.* Churchill Livingstone, Edinburgh

Inman V.T. (1976) *Joints of the Ankle.* Williams and Wilkins, Baltimore

Tachdjian M.O. (1985) *The Child's Foot.* W.B. Saunders, Philadelphia

Yale I. (1980) *Pediatric Medicine,* 2nd edn. Williams and Wilkins, Baltimore

References

Bandy W. and Sinning W. (1986) Kinematic effects of heel lift use to correct lower limb length differences. *J. Orthopaed. Sports Phys. Med.* **7**, 173–179

Barcroft A.P. (1984) Gait analysis using a portable microprocessor based segmental foot force measuring system. *Br. J. Osteopathy* **16**, 20–23

Bates B.T., Osternig L.R., Mason B. *et al.* (1979) Foot orthotic devices to modify selected aspects of lower extremity mechanics. *Am. J. Sports Med.* **7**, 338–342

Baumann J.H., Girling J.P. and Brand P.W. (1963) Plantar pressures and trophic ulceration. *J. Bone Joint Surg.* **45B**, 652–673

Bennett M.B., Ker R.F., Bibby S.R. *et al.* (1987) Elastic properties of the human foot. In: Pratt D.J. and Johnson G.R. (eds), *Biomechanics and Orthotic Management of the Foot.* Derby: Orthotics and Disability Research Centre, Derby, pp. 69–78

Betts R.P., Austin I.G. Duckworth T. *et al.* (1980) Critical light reflection at a plastic/glass interface and its application to foot pressure measurement. *J. Med. Eng. Technol.* **4**, 136–142

Blake R.C. (1986) Inverted functional foot orthosis. *J. Am. Podiatr. Med. Assoc.* **76**, 275–276

Blechschmidt E. (1933) The structure of the calcaneal padding. *Foot Ankle* **2**, 260–283

Bleck E.E. and Berzins U.J. (1977) Conservative management of pes valgus with plantarflexed flexible talus. *Clin. Orthop.* **122**, 85–94

Block P. (1981) The diabetic foot ulcer: a complex problem with a simple treatment approach. *Milit. Med.* **146**, 644–649

Boike A.M., Johng B. and Hetherington V.J. (1990) Pes cavus. In: Levy L.A. and Hetherington V.J. (eds.) *Principles and Practice of Podiatric Medicine.* Churchill Livingstone, New York, pp. 931–952

Boulton J.M., Hardisty C.A., Betts R.P. *et al.* (1983) Dynamic foot pressure and other studies as diagnostic and management aids in diabetic neuropathy. *Diabetes Care* **6**, 26–33

Bordelon R.L. (1983) Hypermobile flatfoot in children. *Clin. Orthop.* **181**, 7–14

Bradley M.A. and McDonald W. (1987) The function and properties of metatarsal domes. In: Pratt D.J. and Johnson G.R. (eds) *Biomechanical and Orthotic Management of the Foot.* Orthotics and Disability Research Centre, Derby, pp. 69–78

Brown R.N., Byers-Hinkley K. and Logan L. (1987) The talus control ankle foot orthosis. *Orthot. Prosthet.* **41**, 22–31

Budin H.A. (1941) *Principles and Practice of Orthodigita.* Strathmore Press, New York

Burns M.J. (1977) Non-weight bearing cast impressions for the construction of orthotic devices. *J. Am. Podiatr. Assoc.* **67**, 790–795

Campbell G.J., McLure A. and Newell E.N. (1984) Compressive behaviour after simulated service conditions of some foamed materials intended as orthotic insoles. *J. Rehabil. Res. Devel.* **21** 57–65

Cavanagh P.R., Hennig E.M. and Bunch R.P. (1983) A new device for the measurement of pressure distribution inside the shoe. In: *Biomechanics VIIIB.* Human Kinetics, Illinois, pp. 1089–1096

Cavanagh P.R., Valiant G.A. and Miserich K.W. (1984) Biological aspects of modelling shoe/foot interactions during running. In *Sports Shoes and Playing Surfaces,* edited by E.C. Frederick, Human Kinetics, Illinois. pp. 24–46

Cavanagh P.R., Hennig E.M., Rodgers M.M. *et al.* (1985) The measurement of pressure distribution on the plantar surface of diabetic feet. In: Whittle M. and Harris D. (eds), *Biomechanical Measurement in Orthopaedic Practice.* Oxford University Press, Oxford, pp. 157–166

Close J.R. (1956) Some applications of the functional anatomy of the ankle joint. *J. Bone Joint Surg.* **38A**, 761–781

Coleman W.C., Brand P.W. and Birke J. (1984) The total contact cast. *J. Am. Podiatr. Assoc.* **74**, 548–551

Collins J.J. and Whittle M.W. (1989) Impulsive forces during walking and their clinical implications. *Clin. Biomech.* **4**, 179–188

Cracchiolo A. (1988) Operative technique of the ankle and hindfoot. In: Helal B. and Wilson D. (eds), *The Foot,* vol. 2. Churchill Livingstone, Edinburgh, pp. 1205–1244

Crawford-Adams J. (1986) *Outline of Orthopaedics,* 10th edn. Churchill Livingstone, Edinburgh, pp. 37–39

Ctercteko, G.C., Dhanendran M., Hutton W.C. and Le Quesne L.P. (1981) Vertical forces acting on the feet of diabetic patients with neuropathic ulceration. *Br. J. Surg.* **68**, 608–614

D'Amico B. (1986) The influence of foot orthoses on the quadriceps angle. *J. Am. Podiatr. Med. Assoc.* **76**, 337–340

Darrigan R.D. and Ganley J.V. (1985) Functional foot orthoses with intrinsic rearfoot post. *J. Am. Podiatr. Med. Assoc.* **75**, 619–624

Dennis K.J., Cooke R.A., Valmassy R.L. *et al.* (1985) Biplane posting elevator. *J. Am. Podiatr. Med. Assoc.* **75**, 272–274

Draper D.O. (1990) A comparison of shoe inserts to taping for painful arches. *J. Prosthet. Orthot.* **3**, 84–89

Ebisui J.M. (1968) The first ray axis and the first metatarsophalangeal joint. *J. Am. Podiatr. Assoc.* **58**, 160–168

Geary N.P.J. and Klenerman L. (1987) The rocker sole shoe: a method to reduce peak forefoot pressure in the management of the diabetic foot ulceration. In: Pratt D.J. and Johnson G.R. (eds), *Biomechanics and Orthotic Management of the Foot.* Orthotics and Disability Research Centre, Derby, pp. 161–173

Harris R.I. and Booth M.T. (1948) Hypermobile flatfoot with short tendo Achilles. *J. Bone Joint Surg.* **30A**, 116

Helfet A.J. (1956) A new way of treating flat feet in children. *Lancet* **i**, 262–264

Hice G.A. (1984) Orthotic treatment of feet having a high oblique midtarsal joint axis. *J. Am. Podiatr. Assoc.* **74**, 577–582

Hughes J., Klenerman L. and Foulston J. (1987) The use of a pedobarograph in the assessment of the effectiveness of foot orthoses. In: Pratt D.J. and Johnson G.R. (eds), *Biomechanics and Orthotic Management of the Foot*. Orthotics and Disability Research Centre, Derby, pp. 115–119

Inman V.T. (1969) The influence of the foot–ankle complex on the proximal skeletal structures. *Artif. Limbs* **13**, 59–65

Isman R.E. and Inman V.T. (1969) Anthropometric studies of the human foot and ankle. *Bull. Prosthet. Res.* Spring, 97–127

Jahss M.M. (1983) Evaluation of the cavus foot for orthopaedic treatment. *Clin. Orthop.* **181**, 52–63

Johnson G.R. (1986) The use of spectral analysis to assess the performance of shock absorbing footwear. *Eng. Med.* **15**, 117–122

Johnson G.R. (1988) The effectiveness of shock absorbing insoles during normal walking. *Prosthet. Orthot. Int.* **12**, 91–95

Johnson G.R. (1990) Measurement of shock acceleration during running and walking using the Shock Meter. *Clin. Biomech.* **5**, 47–50

Jones R.L. (1945) Functional significance of the declination of the axis of the subtalar joint. *Anat. Rec.* **93**, 151–159

Kapandji I.A. (1970) *The Physiology of the Joints*. Churchill Livingstone, Edinburgh.

Knittel G. and Stahili L. (1976) The effectiveness of shoe modifications for in-toeing. *Orthop. Clin. North Am.* **7**, 1019–1025

Lees A. and McCullagh P. (1984) A preliminary investigation into the shock absorbency of running shoes and shoe inserts. *J. Hum. Move. Studies* **10**, 95–106

Light L.H., McLellan G.E. and Klenerman L. (1980) Skeletal transients on heel strike in normal walking. *J. Biomech.* **13**, 477–480

Lord M., Reynolds D.P. and Hughes J.R. (1986) Foot pressure measurements: a review of clinical findings. *J. Biomed. Eng.* **8**, 282–294

Lundeen R.O. (1988) Polysectional triaxial posting: a new process for incorporating correction in foot orthoses. *J. Am. Podiatr. Med. Assoc.* **78**, 55–59

Lutter L.D. (1981) Cavus foot in runners. *Foot Ankle* **1**, 225–228

Mann R. (ed.) (1978) *Surgery of the Foot*, 4th edn. C.V. Mosby, St. Louis

Manter J.T. (1941) Movements of the subtalar and transverse tarsal joints. *Anat. Rec.* **80**, 397–409

Marvin R. and Brownrigg P. (1983) The negative anatomically modified foot orthosis (NAMFO). *Orthot. Prosthet.* **37**, 24–31

Mereday C., Dolan C.M. and Lusskin R. (1972) Evaluation of the University of California Biomechanics Laboratory shoe insert in 'flexible' pes planus. *Clin. Orthop.* **82**, 45–58

Miller J.W. (1975) Acquired hallux varus: a preventable and correctable disorder. *J. Bone Joint Surg.* **65A**, 923–931

Minns R.J. and Craxford A.D. (1984) Pressure under the foot in rheumatoid arthritis. A comparison of static and dynamic methods of assessment. *Clin. Orthop.* **187**, 235–242

Nicol A.C. and Paul J.P. (1988) Biomechanics. In Helal B. and Wilson D. (eds), *The Foot*. Churchill Livingstone, Edinburgh, pp. 75–86

Noakes T.D. (1981) The aetiology of hallux valgus. *S. Afr. Med. J.* **59**, 362

Oakley T. and Pratt D.J. (1988) Skeletal transients during heel and toe strike running and the effectiveness of some materials in their attenuation. *Clin. Biomech.* **3**, 159–165

Penneau K., Lutter L. and Winter R. (1982) Pes planus: radiographic changes with foot orthoses and shoes. *Foot Ankle* **2**, 299–303

Philps J.W. (1990) *The Functional Foot Orthosis*. Churchill Livingstone, London.

Powell H.D.W. (1983) Pes planovalgus in children. *Clin. Orthop.* **177**, 133–139

Pratt D.J. (1989) Mechanisms of shock attenuation via the lower extremity during running. *Clin. Biomech.* **4**, 51–57

Pratt D.J. (1990) Long term comparison of some shock attenuating insoles. *Prosthet. Orthot. Int.* **14**, 59–62

Pratt D.J. and Rees P.H. (1987) The use of second generation synthetic casting tape in the manufacture of functional foot orthoses. *Clin. Mater.* **2**, 207–212

Quigley M.J. (1974) The present use of the UCBL foot orthosis. *Orthot. Prosthet.* **28**, 59–63

Radin E.L., Parker H.G., Pugh J.W. *et al.* (1973) Response of joints to impact loading III: relationship between trabecular microfractures and cartilage degeneration. *J. Biomech.* **6**, 51–57

Riegler H.F. (1987) Orthotic devices for the foot. *Orthop. Rev.* **16**, 27–37

Robbins H. (1976) Naviculectomy for congenital vertical talus. *Bull. Hosp. Joint Dis.* **37**, 77–97

Root M.L., Weed J.H., Sgarlato T.E. *et al.* (1966) Axis of motion of the subtalar joint. *J. Am. Podiatr. Assoc.* **56**, 149–155

Root M.L., Orien W., Weed J.H. *et al.* (1971a) *Biomechanical Examination of the Foot*. Clinical Biomechanics Corp., Los Angeles

Root M.L., Weed J.H. and Orien W. (1971b) *Neutral Position Casting Techniques*. Clinical Biomechanics Corp., Los Angeles

Root M.L., Orien W. and Weed J.H. (1977) *Normal and Abnormal Function of the Foot*. Clinical Biomechanics Corp., Los Angeles

Rose G.K. (1962) Correction of the pronated foot. *J. Bone Joint Surg.* **44B**, 642–647

Ross F.D. (1986) The relationship of abnormal foot pronation to hallux abductovalgus: a pilot study. *Prosthet. Orthot. Int.* **10**, 72–78

Ross A.S. and Gurnick K.L. (1982) Elevator selection in rearfoot posted orthoses. *J. Am. Podiatr. Med. Assoc.* **72**, 621–624

Rossi W.A. (1983) The enigma of shoe sizes. *J. Am. Podiatr. Assoc.* **73**, 272–274

Rovert G.D., Clarke T.J., Yates S.C. *et al.* (1988) Retrospective comparison of taping and ankle stabilizers in preventing ankle injuries. *Am. J. Sports Med.* **16**, 228–232

Salathe E.P., Arangio G.A. and Salathe E.P. (1990) The foot as a shock absorber. *J. Biomech.* **23**, 655–659

Sanner W.H. (1987) Midtarsal joint contribution to transverse plane leg rotation. In: Pratt D.J. and Johnson G.R. (eds), *Biomechanics and Orthotic Management of the Foot*. Orthotics and Disability Research Centre, Derby, pp. 141–149

Sanner W.H. (1989) The functional foot orthosis prescription. In: Jay R. (ed.), *Mechanical Therapy in Podiatric Surgery*. Decker, Philadelphia, pp. 302–307

Seliktar R. and Mizrahi J. (1984) Partial immobilization of the ankle of talar joints complex and its effects on the ground-foot force characteristics. *Eng. Med.* **13**, 5–10

Shereff M.J., Bejjani F.J. and Kummer F.J. (1986) Kinematics of the first metatarsophalangeal joint. *J. Bone Joint Surg.* **68A**, 392–398

Simkin A., Leichter I., Giladi M. *et al.* (1989) Combined effect of foot arch structure and an orthotic device on stress fractures. *Foot Ankle* **10**, 25–29

Smart J.H. and Edge L.H. (1987) Control of pronation with prefabricated inserts. In: Pratt D.J. and Johnson G.R. (eds), *Biomechanics and Orthotic Management of the Foot*. Orthotics and Disability Research Centre, Derby, pp. 128–140

Soames R.W., Stott J.R.R., Goodbody A. *et al.* (1982) Measurement of pressure under the foot during function. *Med. Biol. Eng. Comput.* **20**, 489–495

Sperryn P.N. (1983) *Sport and Medicine*. Butterworths, London

Stauffer R.N., Chao E.Y.S. and Brewster R.C. (1977) Force and motion analysis of the normal, diseased and prosthetic ankle joint. *Clin. Orthop. Rel. Res.* **127**, 189–196

Stess R.M. and Hetherington V.J. (1990) The diabetic and insensitive foot. In: Levy L.A. and Hetherington V.J. (eds), *Principles and Practice of Podiatric Medicine*.

Churchill Livingstone, Edinburgh, pp. 523–548

Subotnick S.I. (1979) *Cures for Common Running Disorders*. Anderson World Inc., Mountain View, California.

Sussman R.E. and D'Amico J.C. (1984) The influence of the height of the heel on the first metatarsophalangeal joint. *J. Am. Podiatr. Med. Assoc.* **74**, 504–508

Tollafield D.R. and Pratt, D.J. (1990a) The control of known triplanar forces on the foot by forefoot orthotic posting. *Br. J. Podiatr. Med. Surg.* **2**, 3–5

Tollafield D.R. and Pratt D.J. (1990b) The effects of variable rearposting of orthoses on a normal foot. *Chiropodist* **8**, 154–160

Tovey F.I. and Moss M.J. (1987) Specialist shoes for the diabetic foot. In: Connor, H., Boulton A.J.M. and Ward J.D. (eds), *The Foot in Diabetes*. Wiley, Chichester, pp. 97–107

Valmassy R.L. and Terrafranca N. (1986) The triplane wedge: an adjunctive treatment modality in pediatric biomechanics. *J. Am. Podiatr. Med. Assoc.* **76**, 672–675

Voloshin A. and Wosk J. (1982) An *in-vivo* study of low back pain and shock absorption in the human locomotor system. *J. Biomech.* **15**, 21–27

Weed J.H. (1984) *Lecture Notes*. College of Podiatric Medicine, California

Weed J.H., Ratliff F.D. and Ross B.A. (1978) A biplanar grind for rearposts on functional foot orthoses. *J. Am. Podiatr. Med. Assoc.* **68**, 35–39

Whitney A.K. (1979) *Biomechanical Footwear Balancing*. Pennsylvania College of Podiatric Medicine, Philadelphia

Whitney K.A. and Whitney A.K. (1990a) Orthodigita techniques. In: Levy L.A. and Hetherington V.J. (eds), *Principles and Practice of Podiatric Medicine*. Churchill Livingstone, Edinburgh, pp. 697–708

Whitney A.K. and Whitney K.A. (1990b) Padding and taping therapy. In: Levy L.A. and Hetherington V.J. (eds), *Principles and Practice of Podiatric Medicine*. Churchill Livingstone, Edinburgh, pp. 709–746.

Wright D.G. and Rennels D.C. (1964) A study of the elastic properties of plantar fascia. *J. Bone Joint Surg.* **46A**, 482–492

Wright D.G., Desai S.M. and Henderson W.H. (1964) Action of the subtalar and ankle joint complex during the stance phase of walking. *J. Bone Joint Surg.* **46A**, 361–382

7

Ankle–foot orthoses

David N. Condie and C. Barry Meadows

7.1 Introduction

Ankle–foot orthoses (AFOs) are amongst the most commonly prescribed categories of lower limb orthoses and, despite their small size and apparent simplicity, have proved disproportionately effective in enhancing the function of a wide range of patient groups of all ages. This functional influence may extend beyond the joints of the ankle and foot customarily encompassed by an AFO to include other more proximal joints. Indeed, in some situations it is this 'indirect' effect upon these joints which is the most important and may even be the principal reason for prescribing the AFO. Thus AFOs may be prescribed not only to compensate for problems encountered during the swing phase of gait, e.g. 'drop foot', but also to influence the characteristics of the stance phase of gait.

The design and construction of AFOs has undergone significant changes in recent years due to the impact of modern materials and technology. The use of thermoplastic materials has resulted in the production of lighter and more cosmetically acceptable devices offering, most significantly, improved function (Yates, 1968). These devices are relatively cheap to produce, can be manufactured quickly and require less maintenance than orthoses constructed using conventional materials.

One of the incidental disadvantages of thermoplastic devices relates to the fact that their function and hence their effectiveness is critically dependent on the correctness of both construction and fit. Thus the adverse consequences of poor manufacturing and fitting are more severe than with conventionally constructed orthoses. This consideration should however be regarded as an incentive to achieve the highest possible quality of orthotic practice.

Thermoplastic AFOs are also apparently less readily adjustable to accommodate for growth or other anthropometric changes. This limitation however may be substantially reduced by the skilled practitioner using simple techniques during the cast rectification and subsequent fabrication process, thereby extending the life of the orthosis.

The footwear which is worn with an AFO is an essential and integral part of the orthotic fitting. For example, the upper of the footwear provides the counter pressure on the dorsum of the foot which is an essential component of the three-point force system required to resist inappropriate ankle plantarflexion. Similarly, during the stance phase of gait, the characteristics of the shoe, e.g. the heel height and sole profile, will significantly influence the pattern of motion of the shank of the limb and the relationship of the ground–foot reaction force to the foot. This in turn will influence the nature of the external moments being generated at all joints of the lower limb and hence the demand placed upon the neuromuscular system.

Footwear design therefore plays a crucial role in overall function and must be considered fully at the time of prescription and monitored

fully at the time of prescription and monitored along with all other aspects of the orthosis at the fitting stage.

As with all orthoses it is desirable that the biomechanical function of the AFO should match exactly the required need of the patient. Unfortunately this is rarely possible. For instance, an AFO designed to prevent inappropriate plantarflexion may also inadvertently restrict dorsiflexion. Recent advances in the design and choice of materials used in AFO construction have addressed this problem with some success, although it must be remembered that any increase in the complexity of an orthosis will have implications both for the training of staff and the cost of the device and its speed of supply.

7.2 Relevant anatomy

The ankle and foot anatomy relevant to the understanding of this chapter have been described in Chapter 6.

7.3 Pathology

AFOs are potentially applicable to virtually every pathological condition which results in a locomotor disorder. For the purposes of this chapter, the description of the objectives of orthotic management, the biomechanical requirements and the specification and description of the appropriate orthosis will be divided into three sections based on the nature of the principal impairment which is being addressed. These are:

1. Conditions which result in weakness of the muscles which control the ankle–foot complex (and in selected cases the knee).
2. Upper motor neurone lesions which result in hypertonicity or spasticity of the muscles.
3. Conditions which result in pain or instability due to a loss of integrity of the structure of the lower leg and ankle–foot complex.

7.3.1 Muscle weakness

Simple muscle weakness may result from a number of pathological conditions including injury to a nerve or tendon, a prolapsed intravertebral disc or a lower motor neurone condi-

tion such as poliomyelitis. Muscle weakness resulting from a spinal lesion such as occurs in spina bifida may be complicated by impaired or absent sensation.

Muscle weakness affecting the foot and ankle alone will seldom immobilize a patient totally, however the resultant loss of joint control and the consequent compensatory manoeuvres will usually result in a hazardous, less efficient and more energy-consuming gait pattern. In general the objective of the orthotic management of this group of patients will be to attempt to replace the functions of the weakened or absent musculature and thereby mitigate the functional consequences.

The specific treatment objectives, the biomechanical requirements and the appropriate orthotic designs will be described for each of the commonly encountered forms of muscle weakness.

(a) Weak or absent dorsiflexors

When a limitation or absence of the power to dorsiflex the ankle occurs in isolation, the commonly encountered functional problems are easily recognized. Mild weakness may result in a foot slap following heel contact due to inadequate control of initial ankle plantarflexion. Total absence of dorsiflexor power will result in a foot drop which will imperil foot clearance during swing and will require compensatory increases in hip and knee flexion. Initial foot contact will occur with the forefoot.

The orthosis–body force system necessary to control these gait abnormalities may be determined by the application of the biomechanical principles described in Chapter 2. Considering, first, the normal leg during midswing, the principal external force present is that from the weight of the lower leg and foot (W) (Figure 7.1(a)). Equilibrium requirements dictate that the effects of this force at the level of the knee joint are resisted by axial and normal components of force at the joint and a flexion moment resulting from activity of the knee flexor muscles.

If the foot is now separated from the leg to create two separate free body diagrams it is possible to deduce the internal forces and moments occurring at the ankle joint (Figure 7.1(b)). Thus considering first the foot it may be seen that the effect of the weight of the foot alone (WF) requires axial and normal

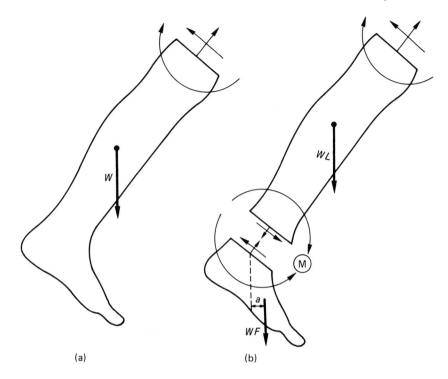

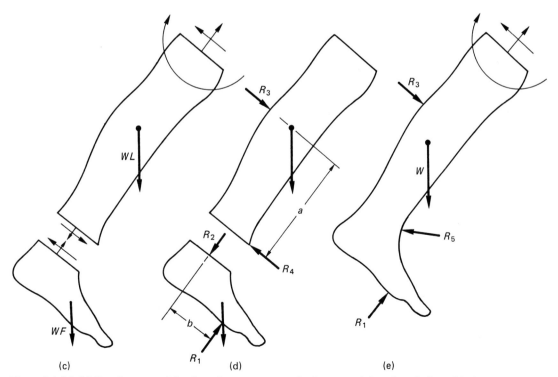

Figure 7.1 (a)–(e) Development of the three-force system required to control drop foot during midswing

components of force at the joint and in addition a dorsiflexion moment (M), where $M = (WF \times a)$. The internal forces and moment acting on the leg alone may also be deduced by a similar process. It should be noted that this internal force/moment system will be in every aspect equal but opposite in direction to the internal foot force/moment system and that the internal force/moment system at the knee remains unchanged.

Considering now the pathological situation where the dorsiflexor muscles are paralysed, it will be apparent that the external plantarflexion moment resulting from the weight of the foot is unopposed (Figure 7.1(c)). As a result and assuming unlimited ankle mobility the foot will drop until the line of action of the foot weight force passes through the ankle joint axis of motion thus eliminating its moment effect.

It is now possible to propose additional external forces, which might be provided orthotically, which would replace the action of the dorsiflexors (Figure 7.1(d)). Considering first the foot, a pair of forces (or couple) of equal magnitude but opposite direction (R_1 and R_2) positioned as shown such that $R_1 \times b = M$ will satisfy equilibrium requirements for this segment alone. Similarly considering the leg, a second couple (R_3 and R_4) positioned as shown such that $R_3 \times c = -M$ will satisfy equilibrium requirements for this segment.

If finally the force body diagram for the foot and leg together is considered it can be seen that the complete additional external force system will comprise R_1 and R_3 plus R_5, which is the vector sum of R_2 and R_4 positioned as shown on the anterior aspect of the ankle such that its line of action passes through the ankle joint axis of motion (Figure 7.1(e)). This 'three force system' identified as being appropriate to the control of drop foot during swing, will also satisfy the requirement for preventing foot slap at heel contact.

Obviously this 'static' analysis does not take into account the inertia forces which occur during walking. However it can be demonstrated that the addition of these forces does not change the configuration of the basic force system required to restore ankle joint equilibrium.

In order to complete the biomechanical specification of the appropriate orthotic solution for the case of weak or absent dorsiflexors,

it is necessary to consider the inclusion of an orthotic 'ankle' joint which will resist abnormal plantarflexion and ideally assist normal dorsiflexion during the appropriate phases of the walking cycle.

Conventionally constructed orthoses for this purpose seek to achieve these requirements by virtue of the forces generated on the calf band of the orthosis and the upper and sole of the attached shoe. The structure of these orthoses will include a mechanical ankle joint preferably located at the level of the anatomical ankle joint, but in many instances created by 'tubing' the heel of the patient's shoe. Joint control is achieved by incorporating a spring mechanism acting about the joint which will permit resisted plantarflexion when subjected to an external plantarflexion moment and which will return the joint to its neutral position when this moment is removed (Figure 7.2).

Alternative contemporary moulded plastic designs of orthoses, such as the Ortholen Posterior Leafspring Orthosis, rely for their

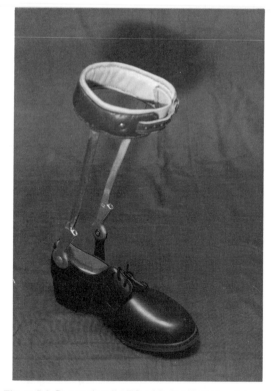

Figure 7.2 Conventional AFO with dorsiflexion assist mechanism

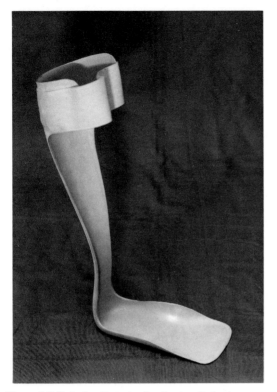

Figure 7.3 Ortholen Posterior Leafspring Orthosis

function on the manner in which they are formed and trimmed and the mechanical properties of the resulting structure (Figure 7.3). Thus the three forces required are achieved through the contact of the calf section and the footpiece of the orthosis acting in concert with the shoe upper. These devices achieve ankle joint control by virtue of the flexibility/stiffness of the posterior strut of the orthosis which is specifically designed to bend and hence permit resisted plantarflexion, but then to return to its neutral attitude when this loading is relieved.

The only published scientific study which has investigated this form of orthotic treatment (Lehmann *et al.*, 1980) concluded that an appropriately designed orthosis can susbstitute for the weakened musculature with the only serious residual gait abnormality being a 'shortened, modified push-off phase'. Clearly the moulded plastic designs are more cosmetically acceptable, lighter and, since they do not require a formal shoe attachment, they permit shoe interchangeability.

Neither design is capable of providing active dorsiflexion beyond the plantigrade position,

indeed the moulded design will actually resist this motion although only to a minor degree.

(b) Weakness or absent plantarflexors

The functional consequence of weakness of the ankle plantarflexors is most apparent during the second half of the stance phase of walking and will present as excessive dorsiflexion prior to heel-off (resulting in so-called 'drop-off' in the gait pattern) accompanied by a total absence of push-off. The patient will simply lift his entire foot off the ground in one instant rather than pressing downwards with his forefoot as is normal. This gait pattern will result in a significantly reduced walking speed.

Using the same biomechanical approach as employed in the previous section, it may be deduced that the orthotic management of this problem requires the application of a three-force system as illustrated in Figure 7.4. Control of joint motion will additionally require the use of an orthotic 'ankle' joint which will resist

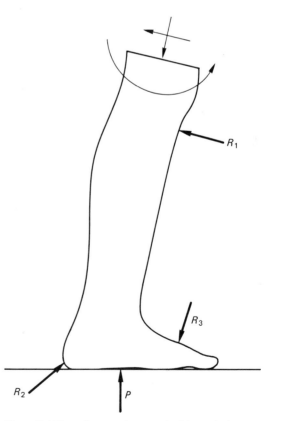

Figure 7.4 Three-force system required to control excessive dorsiflexion during midstance

excessive dorsiflexion and ideally assist active plantarflexion during the appropriate periods of the stance phase.

Conventionally constructed orthoses seek to achieve these requirements through the contact between the calf band and the shoe upper on the leg and foot and by the inclusion of a mechanical orthotic ankle joint of an appropriate design. In this instance the most common practice is to employ a joint whose freedom of motion is limited to plantarflexion.

Contemporary moulded plastic designs such as the Floor Reaction Ankle–Foot Orthosis (Glancy and Lindseth, 1972) achieve their desired function once again by virtue of the forces generated between the moulded structure of the device and the shoe and the enclosed limb segments (Figure 7.5).

A report of a biomechanical study conducted by the developers of this orthosis has confirmed the importance of preventing any ankle dorsiflexion if the required function of assisted plantarflexion is to be achieved (Lindseth and Glancy, 1974). This study also emphasized the critical nature of the alignment of the orthosis,

i.e. the angle of the leg section relative to the foot section. This finding was supported by a detailed study of its use with a series of normal subjects whose plantarflexors were paralysed using a tibial nerve block, which concluded that the best gait pattern was achieved when the ankle was held in 5° of dorsiflexion (Lehmann *et al.*, 1985).

Restricting ankle dorsiflexion in this manner will, however, have the inevitable consequence of inducing premature loss of heel contact causing a sudden forward progression of the centre of pressure of the ground–foot reaction force and an associated marked increase in the external knee extension moment. This undesirable effect may be addressed by the addition of a 'rocker' sole adaptation of the patient's shoe which will have the effect of smoothing the rate with which the ground–foot reaction force moves forward. The influence of the shape and position of such adaptations has been investigated by Hullin and Robb (1991) in a study of normal subjects wearing rigid below knee casts.

The Floor Reaction Ankle–Foot Orthosis has a further feature which is a disadvantage in that its rigid construction totally prevents plantarflexion. One recent manufacturing innovation which has attempted to address this problem entails creating an articulation in the AFO which, while still limiting dorsiflexion, does allow free plantarflexion as is the case in the conventionally constructed designs (Figure 7.6). The functional advantages of this feature are as yet scientifically unproven.

It is perhaps worthwhile noting at this juncture that in both this and the preceding category of ankle muscle weakness the orthotic solutions proposed inadvertently to a greater or lesser extent also restrict the normal functioning of the subtalar joint. The functional consequences of these restrictions will be examined in the following discussion of the treatment of general ankle-subtalar weakness.

(c) General ankle weakness with subtalar instability

The final form of ankle–foot weakness which will be discussed in this section relates to those conditions in which the gait problems arising from weakness or absence of the power to dorsiflex or plantarflex the ankle are compounded by weakness or absence of the

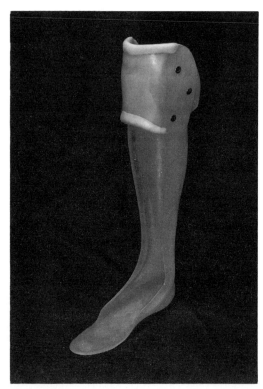

Figure 7.5 Floor reaction AFO

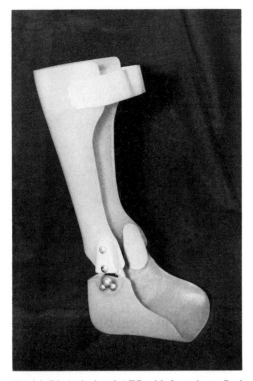

Figure 7.6 (a),(b) Articulated AFO with free plantarflexion

muscles which control the supination and pronation movements of the subtalar joint, as is commonly the case in a variety of neurological disorders.

Such patients may present with the gait problems already described for weakness of the dorsiflexors or plantarflexors. However, additional weakness of the pronators will result in a varus position of the foot during swing with the associated danger of ligamentous injury following foot contact. Alternatively, weakness of the supinators will result in a valgus position of the foot during weight bearing, creating an abnormally high and potentially damaging stress in the structures of the medial longitudinal arch of the foot.

The biomechanical requirements for the treatment of this group of disorders will include both those features necessary to compensate for the ankle muscle weakness and additional features appropriate to the type and degree of subtalar muscle weakness. Thus the force systems necessary to control weakness of the pronators or supinators comprise three forces positioned as illustrated in Figure 7.7.

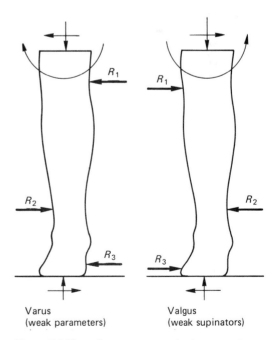

Varus
(weak parameters)

Valgus
(weak supinators)

Figure 7.7 Three-force system required to control varus/valgus

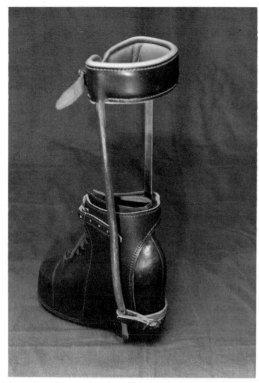

Figure 7.8 Conventional AFO with T-strap

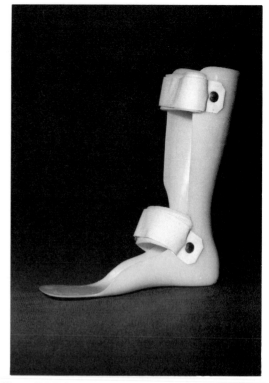

Figure 7.9 Polypropylene AFO

Conventionally constructed orthoses seek to achieve this requirement by virtue of the contact between the calf band and the shoe upper with the addition of a third central force generated by contact with the so-called T-strap which is positioned over the appropriate malleolus and fastened around the contralateral iron (Figure 7.8). Ideally such a system should incorporate an orthotic joint which provides only the appropriate degree of subtalar joint control. In practice no such system is commercially available with the result that this design of orthosis totally eliminates normal subtalar motion.

The contemporary moulded plastic design of orthosis normally used for this situation is the simple Polypropylene Ankle–Foot Orthosis (Figure 7.9). The controlling force system is easily obtained by contact between the moulded structure and the enclosed segments. Care must be taken to ensure that the central force is directed onto the shaft of the tibia or fibula rather than directly upon the prominent surfaces of the malleoli. The relatively rigid nature of the structure which results from the trim lines which are necessary to provide ef-

fective subtalar control means that this device also eliminates virtually all subtalar motion, normal or otherwise. However, subtalar motion forms an essential part of the lower limb mechanism necessary for the absorption of the longitudinal rotations which occur during walking, and the restriction of these movements by an orthosis will necessitate adjustments in the pattern of movement of more proximal joints, notably the hip joint.

One contemporary plastic design of orthosis which was designed specifically with this type of functional requirement in mind is the Spiral Ankle–Foot Orthosis (Lehneis *et al.*, 1972) (Figure 7.10). Manufactured from Plexidur, a nylon-acrylic 'alloy', and comprising, as the title suggests, an integral spiral leg and footpiece section attached to a moulded calf band, this design permits controlled motion about both ankle and subtalar joints in both directions. The force system responsible for controlling ankle motion consists of two force couples (R_1 and R_2 and R_3 and R_4) generated between the calf band and the leg and the footpiece–shoe combination and the foot (Figure 7.11).

The derivation of these force systems is

exactly the same as explained in detail for the case of weak or absent dorsiflexors with the exception that R_2 and R_4 have not been combined to produce a single equivalent force. Thus the requisite force system comprises *four* forces and not *three*. Similarly, the force system responsible for controlling subtalar motion consists of two force couples (R_5 and R_6, and R_7 and R_8) located as illustrated in Figure 7.11.

Unfortunately this design of orthosis has proved time consuming and difficult to fit successfully and extremely prone to breakage, with the result that it quickly fell from favour. More recently a report on the use of this design for children using a Plexidur/Polypropylene hybrid material for its construction describes much improved durability (Hodgins, 1985).

(d) Weak knee extensors

Patients with unilateral weakness of the knee extensors will commonly be successful in overcoming this problem by adopting an anteriorly flexed posture of their trunk to bring the line of action of the ground–foot reaction force in front of their knee, thus creating a stabilizing knee moment. The success of this manoeuvre requires sufficient plantarflexor

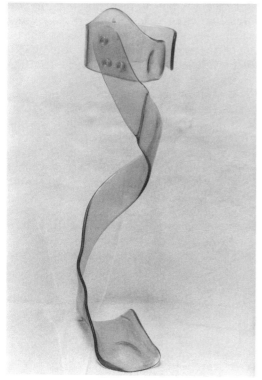

Figure 7.10 Spiral AFO

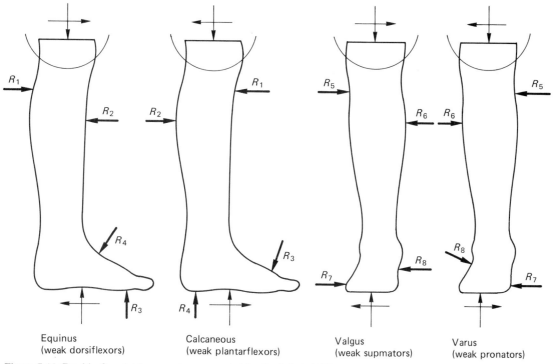

Equinus (weak dorsiflexors) — Calcaneous (weak plantarflexors) — Valgus (weak supmators) — Varus (weak pronators)

Figure 7.11 'Double Couple' force system generated by the Spiral AFO

power to prevent the ankle dorsiflexing as the patient leans forward. Where this is not the case it may be necessary to employ a knee-ankle-foot orthosis as will be described in the following Chapter. However in some few cases of moderate weakness where the patient is of light stature, an AFO may be sufficient to provide the necessary resistance to dorsiflexion.

Spina bifida children with sacral lesions typically present with a combination of knee extensor and plantarflexor weakness resulting in a flexed or 'crouched' standing posture and gait pattern.

The AFO provided for this group of patients is the same as that offered for isolated plantarflexor weakness, i.e. the Floor Reaction Ankle–Foot Orthosis. However, in this application the function of the orthosis results from the combination of the direct action of the orthosis upon the ankle joint and its indirect action upon the knee joint.

As previously described, following foot-flat as the leg attempts to pivot anteriorly over the supporting foot, the rigidity of an orthosis which prevents dorsiflexion will cause the centre of pressure of the ground–foot reaction force to move quickly forward such that its line of action passes in front of the knee joint resulting in a stabilizing knee extension moment. The time of the onset of this effect is determined by the position in which the ankle joint is held by the orthosis. This may be demonstrated by considering the external knee moment which will arise with the same hip and knee attitudes when the AFO is constructed first to hold the ankle in a plantigrade position and secondly to hold the ankle in a few degrees of plantarflexion (Figure 7.12). Clearly in the latter case, the knee stabilizing effect will occur earlier in the gait cycle than in the former situation.

However, as previously mentioned in the section on the treatment of isolated plantarflexor weakness, a disadvantage of this design

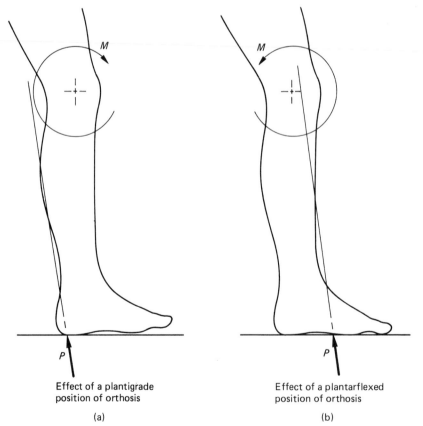

Effect of a plantigrade position of orthosis

(a)

Effect of a plantarflexed position of orthosis

(b)

Figure 7.12 Knee stabilizing effect of the Floor Reaction AFO: (a) with the ankle plantagrade; (b) with the ankle plantarflexed

of orthosis is the rapid forward progression of the centre of pressure of the ground–foot reaction force after heel-off which results in a sudden increase in the knee extension moment. With this group of patients this effect may result in overstabilization of the knee causing hyperextension sometimes accompanied by pain and difficulty in initiating knee flexion in preparation for the swing phase of the gait cycle. Hullin *et al.* (1991) have demonstrated, through a biomechanical study of this form of treatment, how a rocker sole adaptation may be utilized to control the rate of forward progression of the ground–foot reaction force, thereby optimizing the knee stabilizing effect of the orthosis throughout the latter stages of the stance phase.

It is also important to note that it has been experimentally demonstrated that the restriction of plantarflexion also inadvertently imposed by this extremely rigid design of AFO will actually prejudice knee stability at heel contact and during early stance (Finley *et al.*, 1966; Lehmann *et al.*, 1970; Lee and Johnson, 1974; Lehmann 1979). This effect is due to the prolonged period of weight bearing on the heel which results in an external knee flexion moment. Techniques proposed to address this problem include the use of heel cushioning (Wiest *et al.*, 1979) and a novel hydraulic ankle system (Finley *et al.*, 1966). As previously mentioned, an alternative approach which has been clinically practised but not yet scientifically evaluated is the use of an articulated plastic AFO which allows free plantarflexion but resists dorsiflexion.

(e) *Alternative and complementary forms of treatment*

The only alternative or complementary form of treatment for muscle weakness affecting the ankle–foot complex is surgery. This may take two forms: *arthrodesis* and *tendon transfer*. The primary objective in both cases is to achieve a stable plantigrade position of the foot.

The term *arthrodesis* means the surgical fixation of a joint by fusion of the joint surfaces. *Ankle arthrodesis* may be performed in cases of weakness of the ankle musculature, although it has been observed that this procedure is not appropriate if the subtalar joint is also unstable. *Triple arthrodesis* which entails the fusion of

both the subtalar and midtarsal joints is performed when there is instability on pronation/supination movements of the subtalar joint in adults. Finally in those cases where both ankle and subtalar midtarsal stability is impaired a *pantalar* arthrodesis may be performed involving the fusion of the ankle, subtalar and midtarsal joints.

The disadvantage of all these procedures is that they result in total joint immobilization. They should therefore be reserved for situations when there is no alternative means available of stabilizing the ankle–foot complex.

A more attractive surgical alternative is to transfer tendons of normally acting muscles. Procedures have been described to deal with weakness or paralysis of the dorsiflexors, plantarflexors, supinators and pronators and various combinations of these impairments. For example, significant weakness of the tibialis anterior resulting in an equinovalgus form of instability may be treated by transposing the peroneus longus tendon to the dorsum of the foot. A posterior transfer of both the tibialis anterior and the peroneus tertius has been proposed for the management of weakened plantarflexors in the presence of normal dorsiflexors. The loss of the pronating power of the peroneal muscles may be treated by transposing either part or the whole of the tendon of the tibialis anterior laterally.

When considering a tendon transfer, the importance of a detailed and accurate assessment of the patient and the remaining muscle function must be stressed. Factors which require to be considered include:

1. The pathology and natural history of the disease.
2. The presence of bony deformities and soft tissue contractures.
3. The effect of growth in children.
4. The effect of the loss of the normal action of the muscle transferred.
5. The likelihood of some loss of power in the transferred muscle.

In contrast to an arthrodesis, muscle transfers may actually restore a degree of joint function. However, at worst they should restore the balance of the musculature about the joint, thereby avoiding the likelihood of deformities developing due to unopposed muscle activity.

The obvious advantage of surgery in the

management of muscle weakness is the avoidance of the weight incumbrance, and inconvenience of doffing and donning associated with the use of an orthosis.

7.3.2 Upper motor neurone lesions

Many different pathological conditions will result in an upper motor neurone lesion. These include cerebral palsy, head injury, multiple sclerosis and cerebrovascular accidents. This type of neurological lesion will result in abnormal muscle tone. In some cases the tone may fluctuate with periods of markedly increased tone, resulting in the typical spasticity, and periods of reduced tone. This may occur instantaneously due to mechanical influences such as the patient being moved or orientated differently in space or other influences such as anxiety or stress. Alternatively, tone may gradually increase over a period of weeks or months following the initial trauma, or as the disease progresses.

The uses of AFOs described in the previous sections of this chapter relate to the control of abnormal or undesirable joint movements resulting from the inability of muscles to resist the external moments generated by the ground–foot reaction force. This situation will also exist in patients with upper motor neurone lesions. In these cases, however, because of the potential for high muscle tone to occur, abnormal internal moments caused by muscle action may also be generated, resulting in abnormal patterns of motion of the joints.

AFOs used in the management of these patients will therefore also be required to resist these internal moments, in order to obtain the required functional objectives. This will be further complicated by the possible fluctuation of the abnormal muscle tone significantly altering the demand placed on the AFO.

AFOs can, in some instances, reduce excessive tone in the ankle musculature by maintaining the ankle in an appropriate position. This local tone reduction may also induce a reduction of tone generally, throughout the body. A badly fitting, uncomfortable AFO on the other hand, may stimulate reflex activity with high tone being generated throughout the body. It is important that the clinic team managing patients with neurological lesions are fully aware of the complex nature of the factors influencing muscle tone, including the effect of applying an orthosis. (Meadows *et al.*, 1980).

During locomotion, AFOs and the associated footwear will influence the nature of the ground–foot reaction force being generated, altering the centre of pressure, its line of action and its magnitude. Obviously the external moment generated at the ankle will be influenced by this, however it is important to recognize that the external moments at the hip and the knee will also be affected. The demand on the hip and knee muscles will thus be influenced and, depending on the patient's neuromuscular capacity, this may or may not be beneficial. This factor will be considered further in the following discussion on the orthotic management of patients whose problems are due predominantly to hypertonicity of the plantarflexors causing equinus.

The biomechanical function of the AFOs used for this category of patient, and hence their design and construction, are similar to those described in the previous section for muscle weakness. The force systems applied by the AFO are also similar, although varying possibly in magnitude and timing either throughout the gait cycle or over longer periods. The reason for the prescription of the AFO will however differ, e.g. to resist overactive plantarflexors as opposed to assisting weak or absent dorsiflexors.

For convenience, the three most commonly encountered problems with upper motor neurone disorders will be described separately, namely those which result in equinus, equinovarus and valgus positions of the ankle–foot complex. It must be remembered, however, that these problems will not necessarily exist in isolation.

(a) Equinus

Increased tone in the plantarflexor muscles, if unresisted, will result in an equinus position of the foot. Depending on the severity of the condition, this will create a range of problems. In mild cases initial foot contact with the ground may occur through the forefoot, followed by foot-flat contact as the external moment dorsiflexes the ankle to a neutral position. High tone may prevent the further dorsiflexion required later in the stance phase resulting in either the heel lifting off the ground early or secondary hyperextension of the knee as the femur continues forwards over the stationary tibia or a combination of the two. If the muscle tone is very high, a plantarflexed attitude may persist, with no heel contact, preventing an adequate gait pattern from being achieved or even independent standing balance being attained.

The orthotic device to solve this problem must be designed to resist plantarflexion and hence maintain the ankle in a functional position which may be plantigrade, or perhaps slightly dorsiflexed. The force system required is the same as that described for weak dorsiflexors (Figure 7.1); however the magnitudes of the forces generated will be higher and accordingly a stiffer design of AFO will be required.

Conventional orthoses or calipers, comprising a calf band, double side steels and an appropriate mechanical joint, if correctly fitted, may achieve adequate control of the ankle joint. An alternative and preferable prescription is the simple Polypropylene Ankle–Foot Orthosis with a design and construction similar to that described earlier in this chapter.

It should be remembered that with upper motor neurone lesions the interface forces generated will be influenced by the ankle angle at which the AFO is set. Clinical experience suggests that the plantarflexor tone may be reduced if a position of 10–20° of ankle dorsiflexion is adopted. This effect is possibly due to the elongation imposed on the plantarflexor muscles, although this theory has not yet been proven scientifically. Setting the AFO in this 'quiet zone' should make controlling the ankle–foot complex easier due to the resultant relaxation of muscle tone.

It is important in this situation, even when optimal positioning is still associated with high tone, that good control of the position of the ankle is maintained. To achieve this it is considered more appropriate to use an ankle strap attached to the front of the AFO rather than to rely on the vamp of the footwear. The analysis of the force system described earlier (Figure 7.1) indicates that this strap must be aligned at approximately 45° rather than being horizontal, if it is to function optimally. This ankle strap also facilitates donning footwear by maintaining control of the ankle during this operation, which can often stimulate high tone.

In some patients the toes may tend to flex either because of high tone in the toe flexors or

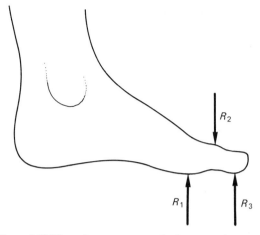

Figure 7.13 Three-force system required to control toe flexion

because of stimulation of the plantar grasp reflex, particularly if the trimline of the AFO is behind the metatarsal heads. In these cases the footpiece of the AFO should be extended beyond the toes, thus avoiding this stimulation and permitting control of the toes even if flexion persists.

Reducing toe flexion orthotically will require the application of a three-force system (Figure 7.13) with one force located under the metatarsal heads and a second located distally under the distal phalanges of the toes; both generated by the AFO footpiece. The third force must be distributed over the dorsal aspects of the toes and is usually generated by the shoe upper, however in severe cases and with 'night' AFOs an additional toe strap might be necessary.

Polypropylene AFOs may be designed to be sufficiently rigid to resist the undesirable plantarflexion moment which occurs during use but also, by buckling outwards around the ankle, they will permit limited dorsiflexion with little resistance.

This characteristic can be useful for those patients whose neurological condition is such that whereas high tone exists at initial foot contact, the tone is sufficiently low in late stance that passive dorsiflexion can occur usefully. Other functions such as squatting may also be facilitated.

An alternative approach to this situation is to utilize an articulated AFO which will allow passive dorsiflexion while resisting plantarflexion (Figure 7.14). Some of these designs feature a screw adjustment to alter the maximum

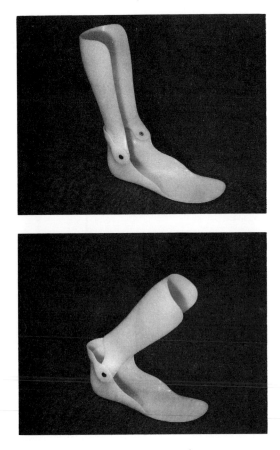

Figure 7.14 (a),(b) Articulated AFO with free dorsiflexion

permissible plantarflexion angle. While these designs offer the potential of improved function, their use may also result in increased problems with service provision due to the additional complexity of the entailed fabrication and fitting procedures.

Middleton *et al.* (1988) have described a case study of a patient with cerebral palsy fitted with a pair of rigid polypropylene AFOs and a pair of articulated polypropylene AFOs. They concluded that the articulated AFOs provided more natural ankle motion during stance, greater symmetry of segmental lower extremity motion and decreased knee moments during stance compared with the rigid AFOs.

One of the potential dangers of using an articulated AFO is the production of the 'rocker bottom foot', often seen in cerebral palsied children, where excessive forefoot loading results in deformation of the midfoot. (This is described in the section on valgus, later

in this chapter.) If the child has a limitation of passive ankle dorsiflexion, due for example to muscle contracture, the dorsiflexion of the AFO itself may result in dorsiflexion motion taking place at the midfoot instead. Weber (1991) stated that articulated AFOs may be prescribed in cases where the midfoot is either stable or unstable but correctable. In cases where the midfoot is unstable and contractions are present, producing a non-correctable deformity, articulated AFOs are contraindicated.

As mentioned earlier, the use of AFOs with appropriate footwear will influence the external moments generated at the more proximal joints of the legs. Research has shown that these influences may be very significant (Meadows, 1984, 1986). Persistent uncontrolled plantarflexor activity will restrict passive dorsiflexion of the ankle during midstance and will result in forward progression of the centre of pressure of the ground–foot reaction force onto the forefoot. As a consequence an external extension moment will be generated at the knee resulting in the knee being forced into full extension (Figure 7.15(a)). This in turn will prevent smooth forward progression of the lower leg and will thus disrupt the gait cycle. Knee hyperextension deformities are a possible longer-term consequence.

An appropriately designed AFO set possibly in slight dorsiflexion, with, if necessary, footwear incorporating heel wedges and/or rocker soles, may be used to achieve a reduction in the knee extension moment, or even to create a flexion moment if considered desirable (Figure 7.15(b)). It is important that the two mechanisms whereby this effect is achieved should be understood fully to enable problems with individual patients to be solved. First, the dorsiflexed setting of the AFO or the use of a heel wedge pushes the knee forwards. Secondly, this measure, assisted if necessary by the use of a rocker sole, ensures that the centre of pressure of the ground–foot reaction force is prevented from moving anteriorly and that as a result the line of action of the force is no longer far in front of the knee and may even be kept behind the knee if desired.

Studies of the gait of cerebral palsied children, typically those who demonstrate an equinus problem, has shown that some seem to be unable to sustain their body weight in late stance and hence tend to collapse (Meadows,

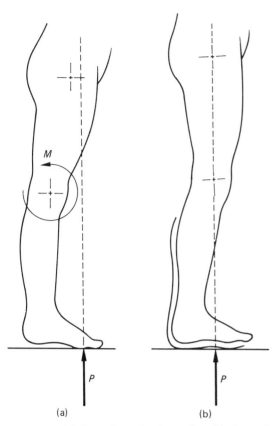

Figure 7.15 (a) Ground reaction force aligned in front of the knee resulting in an external knee extension moment forcing the knee into full extension. (b) AFO–footwear combination alters the alignment of the ground reaction force thus reducing the external knee extension moment

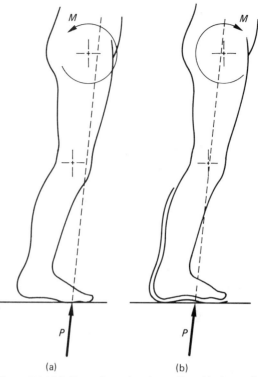

Figure 7.16 (a) Ground reaction force aligned in front of the hip resulting in an external hip flexion moment resisting hip extension. (b) AFO–footwear combination alters the alignment of the ground reaction force sometimes resulting in an external hip extension moment thus assisting hip extension

1984). This appears to be due largely to weakness of their hip extensors, exacerbated by the external hip flexion moment which results from the anterior position of the ground–foot reaction force which occurs as a consequence of excessive forefoot loading (Figure 7.16(a)). An appropriately designed AFO–footwear combination, by aligning the limb segments and controlling the forward progression of the centre of pressure of the ground–foot reaction force will reduce the external flexion moment at the hip (Figure 7.16(b)). The orthotic effect may even generate a hip extension moment which will therefore assist the weakened extensor muscles.

Thus the child is then able to support his body weight and also to generate adequate push-off forces. Now that the impending disaster of collapse has been averted he will be able to slow down his walking cycle and to

learn to walk in a more controlled and less energy consuming fashion. The AFO–footwear combination may thus be regarded as a powerful and relatively easily adjustable tool for influencing knee and hip kinetics.

Mossberg *et al.* (1990) described the effect of AFOs on the energy expenditure of gait in spastic diplegic children using calculated physiological cost indexes (PCI) as described by MacGregor (1981). They indicated that the PCI calculated for their patient sample of 18 was three to four times greater than normal values reported by others. Of the 18 children studied, 13 had reduced PCIs when using AFOs, four had reduced PCIs when not wearing AFOs and in one case there was no change. They concluded that their study supports the use of AFOs for reducing the energy demands of gait in spastic diplegic children. However, they mentioned that the large variability within the sample studied emphasized the need for individual assessment.

It should be borne in mind that if the AFO–footwear combination chosen is not bio-mechanically optimal for a given child it is likely that the energy expenditure will be higher than if a biomechanically optimal prescription is achieved. It may even be the case that an inappropriate AFO–footwear combination may result in more energy consumption than a barefooted gait to which the child is accustomed, however bad the appearance of the gait might appear to the observer!

There is significant interest, particularly amongst physiotherapists, in the use of tone-inhibiting or tone-reducing casts. These are below-knee applications using plaster or other synthetic materials such as Baycast or Scotch-cast. As the name suggests these casts are intended to inhibit unwanted muscle tone and hence improve function. They may also be used to reduce contractures of the plantarflex-ors in order to permit improved walking after their removal, or as a precursor to the supply of AFOs. Many claims are made regarding their efficacy, however, there is little scientific evidence available to support this practice at the present time.

Cusick and Sussman (1982) described their extensive experience with the use of short-leg casts in the management of cerebral palsy. They indicated that below-knee casts could function as an 'extra pair of hands' for the therapist who, during therapy sessions, re-quired more normal alignment of the foot, toes and ankle, particularly in the standing position, while inhibiting toe grasp which may occur as a compensatory stabilizing reflex. They saw the casts as an adjunct to therapy rather than a substitute for it, but with the additional advant-age of maintaining the positioning of the foot, ankle and toes between therapy sessions. They indicated that by setting the ankle angle of the cast in slight dorsiflexion or by using heel wedging they could address the problems of genu recurvatum secondary to equinus. Simi-larly, choosing a slightly plantarflexed attitude could be useful in managing mild crouch gait. The use of the casts as a night splint to prevent contracture of the heel cord, the tibialis poste-rior, the peroneals and the toe flexors was also considered to be appropriate.

It should be appreciated, however, that these various devices are themselves a form of AFO. The preceding discussions relating to the design and use of AFOs are therefore equally valid and should not be ignored.

(b) Equinovarus

Neuromuscular disorders rarely result in prob-lems which are restricted to one joint and hence one type of motion. More commonly there will be multiple joint involvement and the orthotic management will need to address a number of problems simultaneously.

Cerebrovascular accidents (CVAs) may cause an increase in tone in a number of the muscles of the lower limb resulting in an equi-novarus position of the foot (Figure 7.17). When managing the equinus component of this problem, the solutions described in the pre-vious discussion of isolated equinus are equally relevant. Management of the varus component is similar to the management of subtalar insta-bility discussed earlier in this chapter. A three-point force system therefore needs to be applied by the orthosis about the subtalar joint (Figure 7.7). Due to the hypertonicity of the

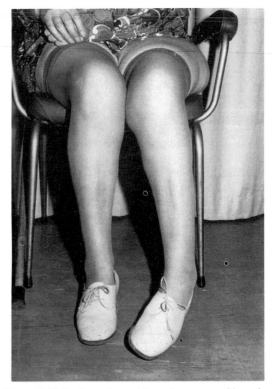

Figure 7.17 Stroke patient with equinovarus position of the foot

muscles involved, however, the magnitude of the forces generated will usually be higher than those required to control subtalar instability due to pronator weakness. The design of the AFO will consequently need to reflect this.

A conventionally constructed AFO, as described earlier, will incorporate a T-strap located over the lateral malleolus. This design has the advantages of the compliance of the leather against the leg which should ensure comfort and the potential for adjusting the amount of correction imposed upon the joint. Thermoplastic AFOs in general do not have these advantages, however, because of the intimacy of their fit, if correctly shaped, they will in most circumstances provide superior joint control.

Several types of plastic AFOs exist designed specifically to control equinovarus. The so-called Three-Point-Pressure Polypropylene AFO is a variation of the simple Polypropylene AFO used to control general ankle and sub-talar weakness, with additional specific rectification of the cast to achieve particular load application and load relief in the desired areas of the leg and foot (Figure 7.18) (Condie and Meadows, 1977). The Hemispiral Ankle–Foot Orthosis, produced from Plexidur, is designed to control varus while allowing some resisted plantarflexion and dorsiflexion (Lehneis, 1974). It incorporates an upright section located laterally on the lower leg to distribute the central of the three necessary forces. This orthosis can result in good function particularly for more active patients, however the problems of fabrication, breakages and donning common to the Spiral AFO remain and clinical experience suggests that the modified polypropylene AFO is more appropriate, particularly for elderly hemiplegic patients.

A large number of investigators have reported on the benefits of this type of orthotic treatment (Smith *et al*, 1982; Hale and Wall, 1987; Lehmann *et al*., 1987; Burdett *et al*., 1988). There appears to be general agreement that the principal advantage is the improved patient security deriving from assured foot clearance during swing and subtalar stability during stance. Indeed it has been demonstrated (Lehmann *et al*., 1983) that if a more flexible design of AFO is used with these patients, problems of toe dragging are likely to occur. Reductions in the energy cost of walking

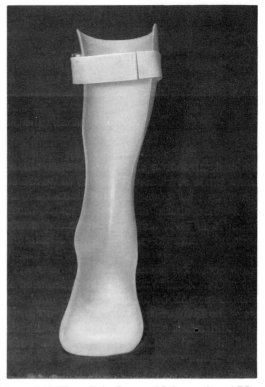

Figure 7.18 'Three-Point-Pressure' Polypropylene AFO

and an increase in the comfortable walking speed have also been reported (Dasco *et al*., 1963; Corcoran *et al*., 1970) and a reduction in body sway (Mojica *et al*., 1988) has also been demonstrated.

The AFOs described above are designed on biomechanical principles to control the position of the joints of the ankle–foot complex. They may of course have effects at the more proximal joints of the leg due to alterations in the ground reaction force. By reducing or altering the biomechanical demand on the neuromuscular system they may have a direct influence on muscle tone. More direct influence on muscle tone may be obtained by paying attention to the trimline of the footpiece, for example, to avoid stimulation of the plantar grasp reflex.

Recently some interest has been shown in the design of AFOs incorporating neurological as well as biomechanical features. Ford *et al*. (1986) described the design and production of a polypropylene 'Neurophysiological' AFO intended to use both biomechanical principles to limit calcaneal varus and neurophysiological principles (of facilitation and inhibition) to obtain dynamic ankle dorsiflexion and plantarflexion. They argued that as more patients have increased lifespan following a CVA, treatments and orthotic care which assure prolonged quality of life become increasingly important.

Neurophysiological treatment attempts to do this through an emphasis on normal movement patterns and integration of the affected and unaffected sides. To date none of these designs, with rectifications and trimlines designed to impose or reduce forces to facilitate or inhibit muscle tone, have been objectively evaluated. They are certainly very interesting and may prove to be very significant clinically, however improvements in performance may need to offset the inherent increase in complexity of fabrication and associated costs.

(c) Valgus

Hypertonicity of the evertor muscles, particularly the peroneal muscles, may result in a valgus position of the foot (Figure 7.19). This problem, which may be accompanied by a calcaneus deformity of the ankle, is less common than either equinus or equinovarus, but when it does occur it can cause significant problems.

Children with cerebral palsy may present with increased tone in their peronei. The pronated position of their feet which results means that load bearing on the foot is painful and may cause pressure on the medial aspect including, in extreme cases, the medial malleolus. Walking ability may also be seriously restricted. Load bearing will exacerbate this problem and in the long term severe deformities may result.

Any orthosis used to treat this problem needs to impose a three-force system as described in the previous discussion of subtalar instability (Figure 7.7). The central force will in this case be located on the medial aspect of the leg. Once again, thermoplastic AFOs are likely to be more efficacious than conventionally constructed devices for similar reasons to those described in the discussion of varus control.

Clinical experience has shown that stretching the peroneal muscles sufficiently (perhaps by imposing a slight varus attitude) may reduce tone and therefore the magnitudes of the forces required to maintain a corrected position. This aspect should be investigated fully with each patient since this may have an influence on the degree of function which is achievable and the degree of acceptance by the patient due to the greater comfort thus attained. The neurological mechanism underlying this phenomenon has not been investigated but it may be similar to the 'quiet zone' described previously for hypertonic plantarflexors.

The valgus problem described above should not be confused with the 'rocker-bottom foot' seen in some children with cerebral palsy (Figure 7.20). This is a secondary deformity, comprising laxity and deformation of the midfoot accompanied by excessive pronation of the

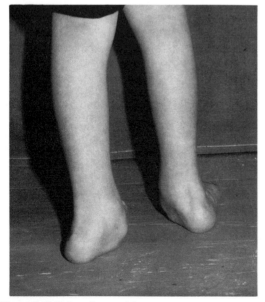

Figure 7.19 Valgus foot position

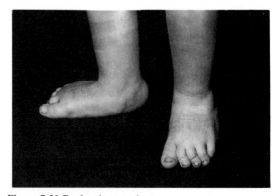

Figure 7.20 Rocker-bottom foot

forefoot (sometimes called an 'escape valgus') produced as a result of a persistent equinus position of the ankle and excessive forefoot loading. In this case, treatment (and hopefully prevention) is best achieved by controlling the initial ankle equinus as discussed earlier.

(d) Alternative and complementary forms of treatment

In addition to the use of orthoses, the other treatment methods employed in the management of the physical problems of patients with upper motor neurone lesions include physiotherapy, chemotherapy, functional electrical stimulation, orthopaedic surgery and neurosurgery. As described earlier in this chapter the management of these patients is complex and the outcome of many of these methods of treatment is uncertain. Good objective methods of patient assessment have not yet been devised and hence the problem of the evaluation of the various forms of treatment still remains.

Many different approaches to the physiotherapy management of patients with upper motor neurone lesions have been proposed over the past few decades. They include, for example, Bobath, Vojta, Temple Fay, Doman Delacato and Peto. These differ significantly in the details of the types and intensity of the therapy methods involved. There are differences too in the perceived effects of treatment on the patient and the neurological reasons for these. Many of these approaches, however, are aimed at the reduction of abnormally high muscle tone and the development of controlled voluntary movement. Over the years the attitudes of physiotherapists to the use of AFOs have varied. These range from the view that AFOs may be of considerable assistance either as an 'extra pair of hands' during therapy sessions, or as a means of maintaining the ankle in an acceptable position between therapy sessions, to the view that AFOs are totally contraindicated for patients with upper motor neurone lesions.

Drugs such as diazepam (Valium) and more recently baclofen (Lioresal) have been used in attempts to overcome some of the physical problems resulting from increased muscle tone. The effects of these drugs are unpredictable and vary from patient to patient. While some benefits may be obtained, the results can often be disappointing. Sometimes the drug has little effect on muscle hypertonicity even with relatively high doses, and in some cases undesirable side-effects may be experienced. Smaller doses however may usefully lower muscle tone sufficiently to facilitate the wearing of AFOs.

Functional electrical stimulation (FES) has been in use clinically for many years. The most extensively used system is the Functional Electronic Peroneal Brace (FEPB) designed to control equinovarus problems in adult hemiplegia (Vodovnik, 1971). With this system electrodes are applied over the peroneal nerve close to the head of the fibula. A stimulator is worn on a waist belt and operated by a heel switch in the shoe on the affected side. Stimulation of the peroneal nerve is triggered appropriately to provide dorsiflexion and eversion of the foot during the swing phase of gait. A number of centres worldwide have acquired significant experience with the FEPB (Gracinin, 1972; Murdoch *et al.*, 1978) and found it useful, however, despite this it has yet to be adopted generally as a routine method of patient management.

Orthopaedic procedures which have been developed to address the physical problems of patients with upper motor neurone lesions include both soft tissue procedures and bony surgery. Soft tissue procedures employed include *tendon lengthening* (and similar procedures applied to the muscle itself) to compensate for the shortening secondary to high muscle tone, *tenotomy* to remove the unwanted effects of selected muscles whether simply overactive or contracted, and of course *tendon transfers* with the objective of redistributing the muscle power around a joint to achieve a more balanced function. Bony procedures employed include *arthrodesis* to fix a joint in an acceptable position of function and *osteotomy* which may be performed to realign the leg bones often with additional surgery to the muscles and tendon.

During the 1980s interest in the surgical treatment of cerebral palsy was stimulated by the research and surgery carried out by Dr Jim Gage then working in Newington, Connecticut who has carried out 'one stage' surgery to correct multiple deformities and improve function in children with cerebral palsy.

There remains considerable controversy within the orthopaedic profession as to both the relative merits of different procedures and their timing in relation to the age of a child or the time since the onset of the neurological problem in an adult. This is due largely to the fundamental complexity of upper motor neurone disorders, the variability of outcome of the same surgical procedures applied to apparently similar patients, and the difficulty of objective evaluation previously referred to.

Surgical procedures may be used either as a means of overcoming a physical problem directly or as a precursor to other forms of treatment. For example, lengthening of the Achilles tendon may enable a patient to obtain heel contact with the ground during standing or walking, or may simply facilitate the fitting and use of an AFO to achieve the same goal.

Neurosurgical techniques employed in the past in the management of patients with upper motor neurone disorders include *nerve blocks*, using for example alcohol or phenol, and *neurotomies* (surgical division of nerves) intended to partially or completely denervate muscles whose activity may be precluding or hindering the rehabilitation process.

More recently, selective *dorsal rhizotomy* has been performed to reduce spasticity in children with cerebral palsy. This procedure was designed to reduce spasticity by cutting selectively posterior-nerve rootlets on the basis of intraoperative stimulation and electromyographic recordings (Gros, 1979). Instrumented gait analysis has been conducted by Cahan *et al.* (1990), who concluded that while in some instances this procedure may improve walking performance by reducing spasticity and improving gait dynamics, the patterns of muscle activation during walking are not changed.

It should be borne in mind, when discussing the different methods of treatment of patients with upper motor neurone lesions, that the underlying biomechanical principles remain the same irrespective of which treatment method is chosen. For instance, the reduction of excessive ankle plantarflexion to achieve heel contact will have the same biomechanical effects at knees and hips (as described earlier in this chapter) whether obtained by AFOs, physiotherapy, drugs or surgery. There will however be physiological differences between the different treatment methods. Thus there may be significant similarities between the outcomes of different treatment methods and hence a potential

potential for mutual compatibility. For certain patients therefore the optimum management programme may be developed, and the biomechanical objectives achieved, by combining aspects of several treatment methods.

7.3.3 Impaired structural integrity

The structural integrity of the ankle joint may be impaired following trauma or more commonly as a result of an arthritic condition. This may take the form of damage to either the ligamentous structure of the joint and/or the joint surfaces themselves resulting in joint stiffness, instability and ultimately deformity. The principal functional consequence of such a situation is pain resulting from normal ranges of movement and loading levels. The general objectives of orthotic treatment will therefore be to provide relief from the pain-inducing mechanisms and to compensate for the resulting limitations of the normal joint functions. The specific objectives, the biomechanical requirements and the orthotic designs appropriate to this situation may be described for two variants of this group of patients.

(a) Pain resulting from joint motion or instability

When pain is experienced as a result of a particular form of joint motion normal or otherwise, the patient will naturally attempt to minimize or eliminate this motion. This will in turn require compensatory adjustments in the overall pattern of limb motion which may reduce the efficiency of walking.

The biomechanical requirements for an orthosis to treat this situation will depend on the severity of the situation and the precise nature of the movements which give rise to pain. In general however it will entail applying the appropriate three-force system(s) in conjunction with an orthotic joint system which limits the painful motion.

Conventional orthoses constructed for this purpose will therefore need to incorporate joints which restrict these motions in conjunction with perhaps a T-strap, most commonly on the medial side, if movement in the coronal plane is a source of pain. The contemporary moulded plastic AFO which is customarily employed for this situation is the Solid Ankle–Foot Orthosis, (sometimes referred to as an ankle blocking AFO). This device is essentially a simple Polypropylene AFO formed from a thicker than normal sheet of polypropylene and trimmed such that the resulting structure is capable of resisting motion in either the sagittal or coronal planes depending on the pathology. When, as a result of deformity, it is impossible to achieve a neutral position of either the ankle or subtalar joints it will be necessary to employ compensatory wedges either on the sole of the AFO or on the sole and heel of the footwear to accommodate these limitations and thus ensure an acceptable weight-bearing pattern.

The most obvious disadvantage of these designs of orthoses is the restriction of normal joint movement implicit in their designated function. Footwear adaptations commonly practised to address this problem include cushioning of the heel of the patient's shoe to compensate for the loss of shock-absorbing plantarflexion following initial heel contact and the addition of a rocker bar to the sole of the shoe to compensate for the loss of dorsiflexion from midstance, hence permitting a more natural rollover prior to toe-off. It is however worthwhile reporting that some orthotists (Schuh, 1988) report no need for these adaptations if a shoe with a soft sole and heel construction is used with the orthosis.

An AFO designed to overcome this problem with one specific patient category is the Cherwell splint (Abery and Harris, 1983). This moulded plastic design is intended for use by patients with rheumatoid arthritis who require valgus control only and incorporates an articulation to permit some free ankle motion.

The developers of this orthosis are one of the few groups to present information on the pressure levels encountered at the orthosis–body interface when wearing an AFO (Gant *et al.*, 1984) (Figure 7.21). Whilst the relative magnitude of the pressures recorded at the calf, ankle and foot regions are perhaps predictable from a theoretical consideration of the clinical and biomechanical function of the orthosis, the absolute values may come as a surprise to many clinicians and serve to reinforce the importance of accurate fitting when using plastic moulded designs.

(b) Pain on weight-bearing

In some instances where the joint damage or degeneration is more severe simple immobili-

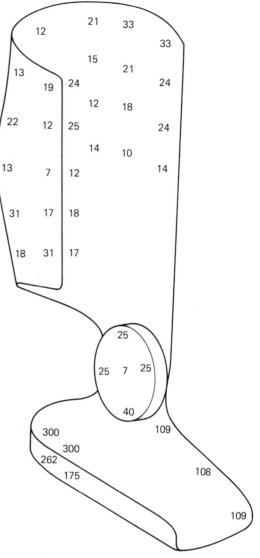

Figure 7.21 Orthosis–body pressure distribution (mmHg) recorded with arthritic patient requiring valgus control wearing a Cherwell splint

zation is insufficient to provide relief of pain and it may be appropriate to consider totally relieving the joint of the weight-bearing forces.

The biomechanical requirements for this situation entail the identification of an alternative area of the skeleton proximal to the ankle joint onto which these forces may be transferred. In order to complete the system it will be necessary to link this support area rigidly to the patient's shoe. The conventional orthotic design employed for this situation is the traditional Thomas splint with its ischial bearing

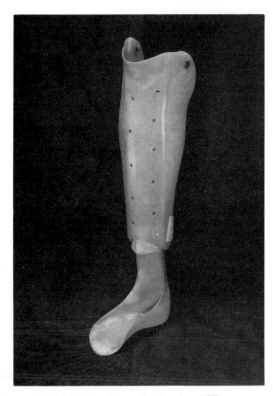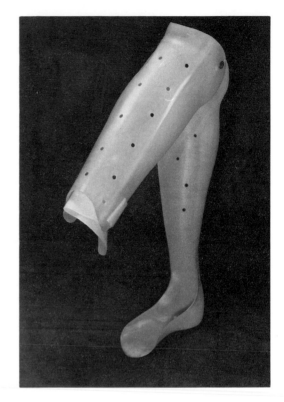

Figure 7.22 (a),(b) Patellar-tendon-bearing AFO

ring located under the pelvis connected by unjointed metal uprights attached to the toe.

An alternative preferable solution which allows uninhibited knee motion is the Patellar Tendon Bearing Ankle–Foot Orthosis (Figure 7.22). (McIlmurray and Greenbaum, 1958). This moulded plastic design consists of a rigid posterior ankle–foot shell extending proximally to the level of the knee crease with a hinged anterior tibial shell extending from mid patella to the ankle joint. The proximal support area is achieved by moulding the proximal regions of the two sections of the orthosis intimately anteriorly over the flares of the tibial condyles and into the patellar tendon and posteriorly onto the popliteal region. The effective transfer of the weight-bearing forces is achieved by virtue of the rigidity of the posterior section created during the moulding and trimming process.

It is important to stress that no design of AFO, or indeed KAFO, is capable of totally relieving the external loading on the leg. Experimental studies (Lehmann *et al.*, 1971; (Lehmann and Warren, 1973) have demon-strated that 50% relief of axial loading is the maximum attainable. This result was achieved by holding the ankle in a position of 5° dorsi-flexion and compensating for the resulting restriction of ankle motion by using cushion heel and rocker sole adaptations.

(c) Alternative and complementary forms of treatment

The only realistic alternative or complementary form of treatment for impairments to the structural integrity of the ankle and foot joints is surgical *arthrodesis*. *Ankle*, *triple* and *panta-lar arthrodesis* are all employed to provide relief of pain resulting from severely damaged and stiff joints. Many of these cases will already exhibit deformities and the success of the arthrodesis is critically dependent on the realignment of the bony segments being fused. All of these procedures therefore entail the removal of 'wedges' of bone designed to restore normal joint alignment.

In general, orthotic treatment is regarded as the first and preferable form of treatment for these patients, with surgery only being considered for those whose symptoms cannot be relieved by orthotic treatment or who reject orthoses. Surgery is less desirable for those patients with multiple joint involvement, such as may occur with rheumatoid arthritis where fusion of a distal joint may place additional stress on the more proximal joints.

Finally the outcome of arthrodesis is somewhat unpredictable. Indeed in some instances an apparently successful procedure may still require continuing use of an orthosis to achieve an acceptable degree of pain relief.

7.4 Current and future developments

The single most significant development in the evolution of designs for AFOs has been the application of thermoplastic materials in their construction. More recently the functional limitations imposed by this method of construction have been recognized by the emergence of a range of articulated AFOs with simple joint control features. Developments will continue both in the refinement of the properties of the plastic interface elements and the design of joint components resulting in more sophisticated orthotic designs with enhanced benefits for the users.

Investigations of the use of AFOs with cerebral palsied children (Meadows, 1984) have revealed the significant influence that these apparently simple devices can have on the entire locomotor process, and thereby have focused attention on the importance of 'tuning' the orthosis to achieve optimal function.

Further investigations are continuing in this area, some of which entail the use of readily adjustable 'assessment' AFOs which may be used in conjunction with gait measurement systems to allow the prescriber to refine the prescription before embarking on the fabrication of a definitive orthosis (Awais, 1987). This work has also reawakened interest in the concept of modular orthoses whereby a very specific individual prescription may be achieved by assembling appropriate components selected from a 'kit' of standard components. Attractive though this proposition may be from a supply viewpoint, it must be stressed that its success will depend on the ability of the modular orthoses to emulate the close, accurate fit, attainable with bespoke orthoses, which is essential for their effective function.

Considerable interest is being expressed in current designs of AFO which incorporate 'neurological' features. It is hoped that clinical experience and appropriate research will indicate whether these designs are really beneficial, and guide their further development in the future. Despite the additional complexity of their production, AFOs which incorporate both optimum 'neurological' and biomechanical features are an attractive proposition.

Reference has already been made to the use of functional electrical stimulation in the design of the Functional Electronic Peroneal Brace. A further extension of this concept has led to the development of a number of so-called 'hybrid' orthotic systems which combine electrical stimulation with a mechanical orthotic system. One of these based on the Floor Reaction AFO (Andrews *et al.*, 1988) has been used experimentally to provide knee stability for carefully selected paraplegic patients. The principal obstacles to the future development and application of these systems relate to the unreliability and limitations imposed by the use of surface electrodes and the lack of sensitivity of the present stimulation control systems. Extensive research and development work is proceeding in both these areas and it seems likely that further improved substitutes for the existing range of 'mechanical' AFOs will inevitably emerge from these activities.

References

Abery J.M. and Harris J.D. (1983) The Cherwell splint: an ankle and foot orthosis for rheumatoid arthritis. *Br. J. Rheumatol.* **22**, 183–186

Andrews B.A., Baxendale R.H., Barnett R. *et al.* (1988) Hybrid FES orthosis incorporating closed loop control and sensory feedback. *J. Biomed. Eng.* **10**, 189–195

Awais S.M. (1987) Development of Modular Ankle Foot Orthosis in the Management of Cerebral Palsied Children. MSc Thesis, School of Biomedical Engineering, University of Dundee

Burdett R.G., Borello-France D., Blatchly C. *et al.* (1988) Gait comparison with subjects with hemiplegia walking unbraced, with ankle–foot orthosis, and with air-stirrup brace. *Phys. Ther.* **68**, 1197–1203

Cahan L.D., Adams J.M., Perry J. *et al.* (1990) Instrumented gait analysis after selective dorsal rhizotomy. *Dev. Med. Child Neurol.* **32**, 1037–1043

Condie D.N. and Meadows C.B. (1977) Some biomechanical considerations in the design of ankle–foot orthoses. *Orthot. Prosthet.* **31**, (3), 45–52

Corcoran P.J. *et al.* (1970) Effects of plastic and metal leg braces on speed and energy cost of hemiparetic ambulation. *Arch. Phys. Med.* **51**, 69–77

Cusick B. and Sussman M.D. (1982) Short leg casts: their role in the management of cerebral palsy. *Phys. Occup. Ther. Pediatr.* **2**, 93 –110

Dasco M.M. *et al.* (1963) Bracing and rehabilitation training effect on energy expenditure of the elderly hemiplegic. *Postgrad. Med.* **34**, 42–47

Finley F.R., Appoldt N.V. and Fishman S. (1966) *The Effect of Posterior Ankle Stops on Knee Stability During Early Stance.* New York University, School of Engineering and Science, New York

Ford C., Grotz, R.C. and Shamp J.K. (1986) The neurophysiological ankle–foot orthosis. *Clin. Prosthet. Orthot.* **10**, 15–23

Gant C., Chase A. and Harris D. (1984) *The Cherwell Ankle–Foot Orthosis,* vol. 11. Annual Report, Oxford Orthopaedic Engineering Centre, University of Oxford, pp. 82–83

Glancy J. and Lindseth R.E. (1972) The polypropylene solid-ankle orthosis. *Orthot. Prosthet.* **26**, 14–26

Gracinin F. (1972) *Use of Functional Electrical Stimulation in Rehabilitation of Hemiplegic Patients.* Final Report. The Institute of SR Slovenia for Rehabilitation of the Disabled, Ljubliana

Gros C. (1979) Spasticity – clinical classification and surgical treatment. *Adv. Tech. Stand. Neurosurg.* **6**, 55–97

Hale S. and Wall J.C. (1987) The effects of different ankle–foot orthoses on the kinematics of the hemiplegic gait. *Orthot. Prosthet.* **41**, (3), 40–49

Hodgins J. (1985) Hybrid spiral ankle–foot orthosis. *J. Assoc. Child. Prosthet. Orthot. Clin.* **20**, 47 (abstract)

Hullin M.G. and Robb J.E. (1991) Biomechanical effects of rockers on walking in a plaster cast. *J. Bone Joint Surg.* **73B**, 92–95

Hullin M.G., Robb J.E. and Loudon I.R. (1992) Ankle--foot orthosis function in low level myeolomeningocele. *J. Paediatr. Orthop.* **12**, 518–521

Lee K.H. and Johnson R. (1974) Effect of below-knee bracing on knee movement: biomechanical anlaysis. *Arch. Phys. Med. Rehabil.* **55**, 179–182

Lehmann J.F. (1979) Biomechanics of ankle–foot orthoses: prescription and design. *Arch. Phys. Med. Rehabil.* **60**, 200–207

Lehmann J.F. and Warren C.G. (1973) Ischial and patellar-tendon weight-bearing braces: function, design, adjustment and training. *Bull. Prosthet. Res.* **10**, (19), 6–19

Lehmann J.F., Warren C.G. and Delateur B.J. (1970) A biomechanical evaluation of knee stability in below knee braces. *Arch. Phys. Med. Rehabil.* **51**, 688–695

Lehmann J.F., Warren C.G., Pemberton D.R. *et al.* (1971) Load bearing functions of patellar tendon bearing braces of various designs. *Arch. Phys. Med. Rehabil.* **52**, 366–370

Lehmann J.F., Ko M.J. and Delateur B.J. (1980) Double stopped ankle–foot orthosis in flaccid peroneal and fibral paralysis: evaluation of function. *Arch. Phys.*

Lehmann J.F., Esslemann P.C., Ko M.J. *et al.* (1983) Plastic ankle–foot orthosis: evaluation of function. *Arch. Phys. Med. Rehabil.* **64**, 402–407

Lehmann J.F. *et al.* (1985) Ankle–foot orthoses: effect on gait abnormalities in tibial nerve paralysis. *Arch. Phys. Med. Rehabil.* **66**, 212–218

Lehmann J.F., Condon S.M., and Price R. *et al.* (1987) Gait abnormalities in hemiplegia: their correction by ankle–foot orthoses. *Arch. Phys. Med. Rehabil.* **68**, 763–771

Lehneis H.R. (1974) Plastic spiral foot–ankle orthoses. *Orthot. Prosthet.* **28**, 3–13

Lehneis H.R., Frisina W. and Marx H.W. (1972) *Plastic Spiral Below-knee Orthosis.* New York University Medical Center, Institute of Rehabilitation Medicine, New York

Lindseth R.E. and Glancy J. (1974) Polypropylene lower extremity braces for the paraplegic due to myelomeningocela. *J. Bone Joint Surg.* **56A**, 556–563

MacGregor J. (1981) The evaluation of patient performance using long-term ambulatory monitoring technique in the domiciliary environment. *Physiotherapy* **67**, 30–33

McIllmurray W.J. and Greenbaum W. (1958) A below-knee weight-bearing brace. *Orthot. Prosthet. J.* **12**, 81–82

Meadows C.B. (1984) The influence of Polypropylene Ankle–Foot Orthoses on the gait of CP children. PhD Thesis, University of Strathclyde

Meadows C.B. (1986) *An Investigation into the Mobility of the Cerebral Palsied Child.* Final Report to the Committee for Research on Equipment for the Disabled, Scottish Home and Health Department Project Ref. R/LIM/14/75

Meadows C.B., Anderson D.M., Duncan L.M. *et al.* (1980) *The Use of Polypropylene Ankle–Foot Orthoses in the Management of the Cerebral Palsied Child.* A Guide Based on Clinical Experience in Dundee, Tayside Rehabilitation Engineering Services

Middleton E.A., Hurley G.R.B. and McIlwain J.S. (1988) The role of rigid and hinged polypropylene ankle–foot orthoses in the management of cerebral palsy: a case study. *Prosthet. Orthot. Int.* **12**, 129–135

Mojica J.A.P., Nakamura R., Kobayashi T. *et al.* (1988) Effect of ankle–foot orthosis (AFO) on body sway and walking capacity of hemiparetic stroke patients. *Tohoku J. Exp. Med.* **156**, 395–401

Mossberg K.A., Linton K.A. and Friske K. (1990) Ankle–foot orthoses: effect on energy expenditure of gait in spastic diplegic children. *Arch. Phys. Med. Rehabil.* **71**, 470–494

Murdoch G., Condie D.N. and Van Griethuysen C. (1978) *A Clinical Evaluation of the Ljubliana Functional Electronic Peroneal Brace.* Final Report to the Chief Scientist office, Scottish Home and Health Department.

Schuh C.M. (1988) Orthotic management of the arthritic foot. *Clin. Prosthet. Orthot.* **12**, 51–60

Smith A.E., Quigley M. and Waters R. (1982) Kinematic comparison of Bicaal orthosis and the rigid polypropylene orthosis in stroke patients. *Orthot. Prosthet.* **36**, (2), 49–55

Vodovnik L. (1971) *Development of Orthotic Systems using Functional Electrical Stimulation and Myoelectric Control.* Final Report, University of Ljubliana, Faculty for Electrical Engineering

Weber D. (1991) Use of a hinged AFO for children with spastic cerebral palsy and midfoot instability. *J. Assoc. Child. Prosthet. Orthot. Clin.* **4**, 61–65

Wiest D.R., Waters R.L., Bontrager E.L. *et al.* (1979) The influence of heel design on a rigid ankle–foot orthosis. *Orthot. Prosthet.* **33**, (4), 3–10

Yates G. (1968) A method for the provision of lightweight aesthetic orthopaedic appliances. *Orthopaedics* **1**, 153–162

8

Knee orthoses

Peter Bowker and David Pratt

8.1 Introduction

The knee is the largest and most complex synovial joint in the human body. Because of the incongruence of the surfaces of articulation, its principal motion, flexion-extension, occurs about a continually changing joint centre and consists of a combination of rolling and sliding – the precise motion pattern being controlled by the interactive effects of bony and soft tissue joint structures. However, if one considers the bone geometry alone, relative motion between the femur and tibia is also potentially possible in the other 5 degrees of freedom. These additional, unrequired motions are normally prevented by the fibrous structures surrounding the joint, principally the joint capsule and ligaments. Consequently, derangement of one or more of these structures gives rise to a looser, less stable joint which, in severe cases, leads to severe functional impairment. Management of the joint with a knee orthosis aims to restore its stability by eliminating unrequired motions.

The essential anatomy and biomechanics of the joint are summarized below. For more detailed treatments the reader is directed to Kapandji (1970), Muller (1983), Maquet (1984), Palastanga *et al.* (1989), Segal and Jacob (1989) and Cox (1990).

8.2 Knee joint anatomy

The knee joint (Figure 8.1) is formed in the first instance by the articulation of two in-congruent surfaces: the femoral condyles and the tibial plateau. In addition, a plane joint exists between the patella and the femur. The articulating surfaces are covered with a thin layer of hyaline cartilage which is bathed in a lubricating synovial fluid contained in the surrounding fibrous articular capsule. This capsule, which forms a cuff around the joint and contributes to its mechanical stability, usually shows a number of localized thickenings, termed ligaments, which are named according to their position or attachment. In addition, the knee joint possesses numerous accessory ligaments which are thick fibrous bands of tissue standing clear of the fibrous capsule, either within or outside it. Of these, four are key joint stabilizers: the medial and lateral collateral ligaments and the anterior and posterior cruciate ligaments.

8.2.1 The tibiofemoral joint

The tibiofemoral joint is the articulation between the two disparately sized convex condyles of the femur and the two slightly concave condyles of the tibial plateau. It acts as a 'modified hinge', the principal motion of which is flexion-extension, but also allows some adduction/abduction and internal and external rotation, the extent of this motion depending upon the degree of flexion of the joint (Table 8.1). Additionally, the axis of rotation moves posteriorly in flexion due to the variable radius arcs of the femoral condyles. Two menisci (lateral and medial), which are essentially semilunate in plan and triangular in

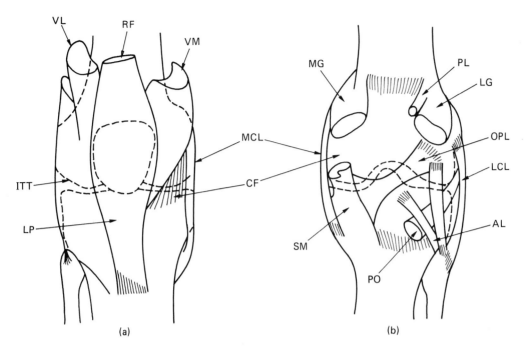

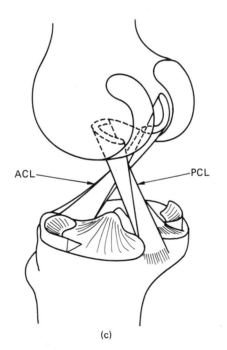

Figure 8.1 Anatomy of the knee joint showing: (a) the anterior aspect of the capsule; (b) the posterior aspect of the capsule; (c) a perspective view of cruciate ligaments and menisci showing their triangular cross-section. VL = vastus lateralis, VM = vastus medialis, RF = tendon of rectus femoris, ITT = iliotibial tract, LP = ligamentum patellae, MCL = medial collateral ligament, CF = capsular fibres, MG = medial head of gastrocnemius, LG = lateral head of gastrocnemius, PL = plantaris, SM = semimembranosus, OPL = ob' popliteal ligament, LCL = lateral collateral ligament, Po = popliteus, AL = arctuate ligament, ACL = anterior cruciate ligament, PCL = posterior cruciate ligament

Table 8.1. Full ranges of motion of tibiofemoral joint and ranges used during various activities

	Degrees
Total available range of motion	
Flexion	0–140
At full extension	
Internal rotation	0
External rotation	0
At 90° of flexion	
Internal rotation	0–30
External rotation	0–45
At full extension	
Abduction	0
Adduction	0
At 30° of flexion	
Abduction	Few degrees
Adduction	Few degrees
Range of flexion required in common activities	
Walking	0–67
Climbing stairs	0–83
Descending stairs	0–90
Sitting down	0–93
Tying a shoelace	0–106
Lifting an object	0–117

Data from Frankel and Nordin, 1980.

cross-section, are interposed between the femoral and tibial surfaces.

8.2.2 The patellofemoral joint

The patellofemoral joint is the articulation between the posterior surface of the patella and the anterior aspect of the femoral condyles. The patella, the largest of the body's sesamoid bones, is a flattened, triangular bone situated in front of the knee joint in the tendon of the quadriceps femoris muscle. The patella has, on its posterior aspect, an oval articular surface with a ridge running vertically on its midline. Either side of this ridge are concave facets which articulate with the convex condyles of the femur, the ridge itself fitting into the groove between the two femoral condyles. Flexion-extension of the knee leads to relative sliding between the femur and the patella, the pathway of motion being guided by the tracking of the patella ridge in the femoral intercondylar notch.

8.2.3 Joint musculature

Knee extension is mainly provided by the four muscles which form the quadriceps group –

rectus femoris, vastus lateralis, vastus medialis and vastus intermedius. These four muscles all overlie the femur anteriorly and their four distal tendons unite just proximal to the patella to form the quadriceps tendon. This tendon then continues from the distal apex of the patella as the flat, tapering patellar tendon, and attaches to the upper end of the tibia. Because of the axial deviation of the quadriceps tendon in its course across the patella (known as the Q angle) and the angled pulls of rectus femoris and vastus intermedius, extension of the knee tends to be accompanied by a secondary internal rotation of the tibia.

Knee flexion is controlled by a number of muscles, some also cause internal rotation of the joint, and others give rise to an associated external rotation. In the former group are gastrocnemius, which consists of medial and lateral heads and spans both knee and ankle joints (the latter via the tendo Achilles), and a group of four muscles which span both hip and knee, semimembranosus, semitendinosus, sartorius and gracilis. In the latter group are two muscles, fascia lata and biceps femoris, which also both span hip and knee. Of these seven muscles, the most powerful flexors are the three which form the posterior femoral muscle group, or hamstrings – the biceps femoris, semimembranosus and semitendinosus. These three muscles all arise principally from the pelvis and have distal tendons which insert posteriorly at the upper ends of the tibia or fibula.

8.2.4 Joint stabilizers

Although cradled on the menisci, the femoral condyles essentially simply rest on the almost flat tibial condyles. As a result the knee has little inherent bony stability and relies on fibrous structures within and around the joint to maintain its alignment. Whilst some of this stability is provided by the menisci and by the synovial capsule and its integral ligaments, it is principally the two collateral ligaments and two cruciate ligaments which stabilize the joint.

The collateral ligaments reinforce the articular capsule and are principally responsible for the stability of the knee in the coronal plane. The medial collateral ligament, which resists excessive abduction, runs from the medial aspect of the femoral condyle to the upper end of the tibia, whilst the lateral collateral ligament, which prevents adduction, spans the joint from the lateral femoral condyle to the fibular head. These ligaments are generally in tension during extension and are slack during flexion, as a result of the combined rotation and translation of the knee joint during these motions.

Anteroposterior stability of the knee, although contributed to by the collateral and posterior capsular ligaments, is principally attained through the action of two ligaments lying in the centre of the joint, the anterior and posterior cruciate ligaments. The anterior cruciate ligament, which resists excessive anterior motion of the tibia relative to the femur, runs obliquely, superiorly and laterally from the anterior horn of the medial meniscus to the internal aspect of the lateral femoral condyle. The posterior cruciate ligament, which prevents excessive posterior tibial motion, runs obliquely, medially and anteriorly from the posterior aspect of the tibial intercondylar fossa to the femoral intercondylar notch. These two ligaments touch each other where they cross in the centre of the joint, with the anterior cruciate ligament running laterally to the posterior cruciate ligament. The cruciate ligaments also act to limit extension and thereby prevent hyperextension and, if forced into the latter, the weaker anterior cruciate ligament often suffers damage.

In addition to these passive structures, there are also a number of dynamic stabilizers of the knee. The iliotibial band or tract originates in the ilium and passes down the lateral surface of the thigh, inserting into Gerdy's tubercule on the anterolateral aspect of the tibia. At its distal end it acts as an accessory collateral ligament of the knee providing extra adduction stabilization. Both fascia lata and gluteus maximus are external rotators of the knee via this band. Additionally, this dynamic stabilizer acts as an extensor beyond about 30° extension and as a flexor beyond about 30° flexion. Finally, a number of dynamic ligaments, such as pes anserinus, contribute to the stability of the joint. These are fibrous structures protected from overstretching by attachment to a muscle either directly or indirectly via fascia (Muller, 1983).

8.3 Knee joint biomechanics

8.3.1 Kinematics

For walking, the knee needs about 70° flexion, which is usually considerably less than the full range of motion, and to extend to full extension or often into slight hyperextension just before heel-strike. Some internal/external rotation and adduction/abduction also takes place during gait (Table 8.1). The centre of rotation of the knee in the sagittal plane does not lie at a single point, but on a curve, the pathway of which can be reproduced by using a crossed four-bar mechanism which emulates the cruciate ligaments in producing the combined rolling and sliding of the knee (Goodfellow and O'Connor, 1978). From full extension the femoral condyle begins to roll without sliding but as flexion continues, the anterior cruciate ligament, in effect, prevents the femur from rolling off the back of the tibia by pulling it anteriorly (Figure 8.2). Thus motion between the articulating surfaces becomes a mixture of rolling and sliding. Because of the geometry of the femoral condyles and positioning of the anterior cruciate ligament, sliding becomes increasingly more predominant as flexion proceeds and ultimately tibiofemoral motion consists of pure sliding. The action of the posterior cruciate ligament produces the reverse sequence of motion on re-extension of the joint.

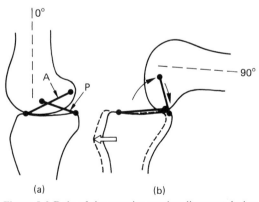

Figure 8.2 Role of the anterior cruciate ligament during knee flexion. (a) With a straight knee both cruciate ligaments (A = anterior, P = posterior) are in tension and lie approximately horizontally. (b) At 90° of flexion the anterior cruciate is horizontal and the posterior cruciate is nearly vertical. Note that if the anterior cruciate is ruptured the tibia can be displaced anteriorly for all positions of the joint

In addition, flexion-extension of the knee is accompanied by transverse plane axial rotations of the tibia or femur, the most important aspect of which is the 'screw home' mechanism which occurs during the last few degrees of extension. For a non-weight-bearing limb, this involves a relatively large external rotation of the tibia relative to the femur, or, for a weight-bearing limb, an internal rotation of the femur relative to the tibia. This rotational motion again arises as a result of the restraint of the cruciate ligaments which actually lie at about 15° to the sagittal plane, and has the effect of 'locking' the knee to provide a joint which is stable in weight bearing with little or no muscular activity.

8.3.2 Kinetics

The force passing through the tibiofemoral joint during walking reaches a maximum of around seven times body weight (Figure 8.3), with principally the hamstrings, quadriceps femoris and gastrocnemius muscles providing the control. In the stance phase, when the peak forces occur, the majority of the load is carried by the medial plateau, whilst during swing, the lateral plateau takes most of the (reduced) load.

In a normal knee the joint reaction force is shared between the articular cartilage and the

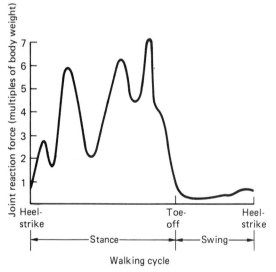

Figure 8.3 Resultant knee joint reaction force, in multiples of body weight. (Adapted from Seireg and Arvikar, 1975)

menisci. Seedholm *et al.* (1974) found from cadaveric studies that in menisci-deficient knees, the stresses in the tibiofemoral joint during weight bearing were up to three times higher. This is because without the cushioning menisci present, the contact area of the joint is reduced to a small area in the centre of the plateau.

The patellofemoral contact force is dependent upon quadriceps force but is independent of flexion angle (Hehne, 1990). The action of the joint has been likened by many to a simple pulley (Morrison, 1969; Perry *et al.*, 1975), but this view is now felt to be too simplistic as it has been found that the quadriceps (F_q) and patellar tendon (F_p) forces are not equal, as they would be in a simple frictionless pulley, but have relative values which are a function of the angle of knee flexion (Bishop and Denham, 1977). Cox (1990) has shown that the ratio F_p/F_q in fact decreases from unity at full extension to 0.5 at 80–90° flexion and then increases again at higher flexion angles due to changes in force directions and modifications to the effective lever arm as knee motion takes place.

The patella itself, as well as distributing the force exerted by the tensioned quadriceps tendon on the femur, also has the important biomechanical function of lengthening the lever arm of the quadriceps muscle. This effect varies with knee angle, increasing from a minimum of about 10% at full extension (when the patella is in the intercondylar groove) to a maximum of 30% at about 45°, further flexion then causing it to fall slightly (Nordin and Frankel, 1980).

Estimations of muscle and ligament forces in the knee have been made by a number of workers, most techniques being based on those of Morrison (1967). As with all biomechanical studies certain approximations had to be made to produce equilibrium equations which were statically determinate. These typically involved grouping together muscles having similar action into a single unit and making simplifying assumptions regarding lines of action of muscles, phasic or antagonistic muscle activity, and the location of joint centres. Nissan (1980) reviewed some of the common assumptions and, whilst he found that most were acceptable, concluded that more consideration needs to be given to agonistic/antagonistic muscle activity and the definition of the knee joint centre, especially in the anteroposterior direction.

8.4 Orthotic requirements for different biomechanical deficits

Knee orthoses are prescribed for four types of biomechanical deficit. Three of these are associated with a loss of structural integrity in the joint: (i) a tendency to collapse into valgus or varus on weight bearing, as commonly occurs in rheumatoid and other types of arthritis; (ii) excessive anteroposterior translation of the tibia typically arising from joint trauma; (iii) significant hyperextension of the joint. The fourth biomechanical deficit is a loss of muscular control which places the knee at risk of collapsing in flexion on weight bearing.

Knee orthoses are additionally used prophylactically to prevent knee injuries during sporting activities. This practice is widespread in the USA amongst baseball players and is increasingly being adopted by rugby and soccer players in the UK. The value of knee orthoses in this application is however doubtful, with several studies concluding that such usage is either of unproven benefit (Garrick and Requa, 1987) or even dangerous (Tietz *et al.*, 1987), with France *et al.* (1987) concluding that ' . . . the majority of prophylactic knee braces available appear biomechanically inadequate'.

8.4.1 Abduction/adduction instability (valgus/varus collapse)

Abduction instability, or valgus collapse, of a knee is most commonly seen in rheumatoid arthritis in which there is a generalized destruction of joint structures including erosion of the articulating bone ends. This leads to a progressive collapse of the joint with an associated loosening of the supporting structures. Significant instability results with the joint normally deforming into valgus on weight-bearing. Thus, for the patient with arthritis, the aims of orthotic management are likely to be the control of pain and the improvement of function through the correction of the varus or valgus angulation of the knee. This correction will have the effect of realigning the limb close to the line of action of the body's weight force, reducing the coronal plane bending moment at the joint to its normal value and reducing the

abnormally high load within the medial or lateral compartment of the joint, i.e. re-equilibrating the medial and lateral contact loads. Realignment of the limb will also have the effect of restoring its correct functional length and hence reducing the high energy costs of walking with a limb-length discrepancy. If the valgus or varus angulation is fixed, some benefit may accrue from an accommodative knee orthosis which will relieve some of the load on the more highly stressed knee structures – in valgus, the medial collateral ligament and the lateral joint bearing surfaces – and thus may be effective in reducing pain. However, as the knee joint deviates from its normal alignment in the frontal plane by an increasing angle, the forces required to support the joint rise rapidly and soon become very large. In these cases, in which frontal plane angulation at the knee exceeds around 20°, the required orthosis/skin loadings may be unacceptable and the possibility of pain relief through off-loading weight from the limb using a knee-ankle-foot orthosis (KAFO) may present a more practicable approach. Alternatively, surgical realignment of the limb using a femoral wedge osteotomy, followed by bracing if valgus/varus instability remains may, in some cases, be the preferred solution.

Biomechanical requirements and orthosis design

Figure 8.4(a) shows a lower limb with coronal plane rotatory instability at the knee, tending to collapse into valgus on weight-bearing. The free body diagrams of the shank and thigh (Figure 8.4(b)) confirm the tendency of the segments to rotate on weight-bearing such as to increase the angulation at the knee. Figure 8.4(c) then shows the limb with the three-point fixation system required to prevent the unwanted rotation at the knee.

The simplest design of brace which would apply the required force system to the limb is shown in Figure 8.5. Three pads mounted on a rigid framework, which encircles the limb, contact it laterally over the joint centre and medially proximal and distal to the joint. It has been seen that biomechanical advantage is gained by making the brace as long as possible, but clearly this has implications for both the weight and bulk of the orthosis and

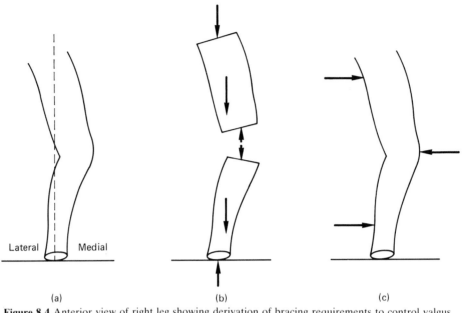

Figure 8.4 Anterior view of right leg showing derivation of bracing requirements to control valgus angulation of the knee: (a) lower limb collapsing into valgus on weight bearing; (b) free body diagram of thigh and shank; (c) required orthotic forces

compromises have to be sought. Careful design is also required to prevent the orthosis impinging on the contralateral limb during gait. Finally, knee joint flexion must be facilitated by incorporating pivots and, because of the involvement of more than one joint in many rheumatoid patients, often including the upper limb joints, and particularly the hands, the need for an orthosis which is easy to don and doff is paramount.

The foregoing discussion has related to a knee which is collapsing in valgus; a similar analysis reveals that a brace which is a mirror image of that in Figure 8.5 would be indicated for a knee which collapses in varus.

8.4.2 Anterior/posterior instability of the knee

Joint instability can appear as the principal sequela of trauma in many circumstances, but is most commonly seen in young, active men and women who have damaged their knees playing football or undertaking other sporting activities. However, within this group, both the nature and magnitude of the injury, and hence of the resulting instability, are highly variable. In the most severe cases, a number of the ligaments and other soft tissue structures surrounding the joint may be ruptured or contused leading to a significant, often complex

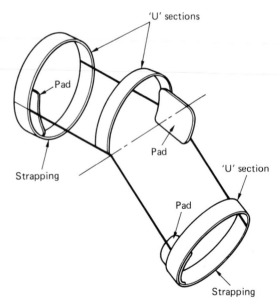

Figure 8.5 Theoretical three-point fixation brace required to control valgus angulation of the knee

instability pattern; this is discussed in the next section. In less severe cases, however, damage will apparently be restricted to a single ligamentous structure and a single clearly defined mode of instability will result. In many subjects this will lead to minor functional impairment with the joint performing satisfactorily most of the time but giving way unpredictably, often when turning or negotiating stairs. Clinically, the most commonly observed type of injury is rupture of the anterior cruciate ligament leading to excessive anterior translation and internal rotation of the tibia with respect to the femur (Marquette, 1988; Maltry *et al.*, 1989). Ruptures of the posterior cruciate ligaments, which lead to excessive posterior draw and external rotation of the tibia, are very much less common.

Thus, in this case the aim of orthotic management is to improve function by preventing excessive anterior or posterior motion of the tibia relative to the femur during walking and other weight-bearing activities. The orthotic requirements for prevention of anterior motion of the tibia relative to the femur are dealt with below: the case of posterior motion is examined similarly and yields a mirror-image solution.

Figure 8.6(a) shows the free body diagrams of the shank and thigh of a normal weight-bearing lower limb at the instant at which its long axis is vertical. The limb is subjected to a ground reaction force with vertical and posteroanterior components and is free to rotate on the ground in the sagittal plane. The hip and knee are maintained in extension by fixing moments generated by muscular forces and passive restraints. The shear forces F at the knee required to maintain the limb in equilibrium are provided by the anterior cruciate ligament.

Figure 8.6(b) presents the free bodies of the shank and thigh under the same conditions but for a limb without a functioning anterior cruciate ligament. It can be seen that the segments are now not in equilibrium but tend to translate, the shank anteriorly and the thigh posteriorly. Figure 8.6(c) then shows the four-point fixation system required to prevent this translation. Thus, an orthosis which is effective in controlling the unwanted motion in an anterior cruciate ligament deficient knee will consist of a rigid framework incorporating pads or straps which apply the four controlling forces R_1–R_4 to the limb.

However, to allow knee flexion to occur, this rigid brace must be hinged at the joint centre.

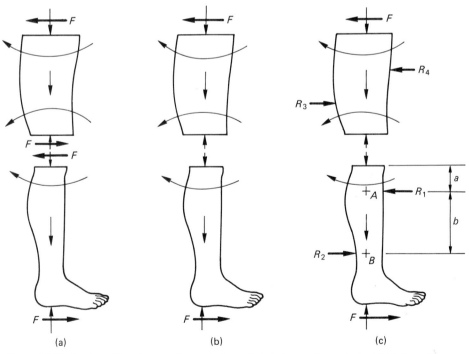

Figure 8.6 Derivation of bracing requirements for restraint of excessive anterior tibial draw. The figure shows the mechanics of a weight-bearing lower limb with knee extended for: (a) normal knee joint; (b) anterior cruciate ligament deficient knee; (c) orthotically stabilized knee

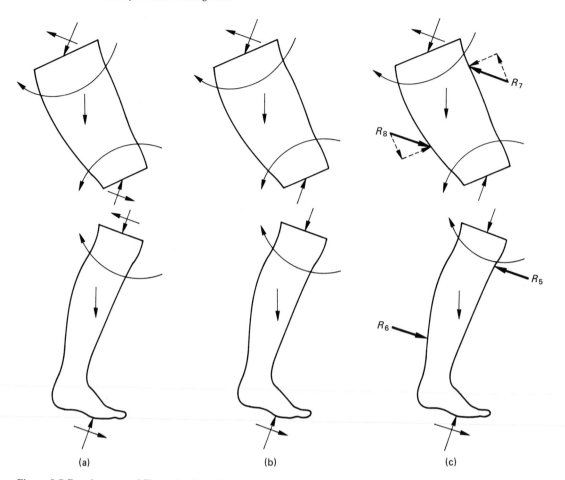

Figure 8.7 Development of Figure 8.6 for a flexed knee: (a) normal knee joint; (b) anterior cruciate ligament deficient knee; (c) orthotically stabilized knee

Looking first at the mechanics of the normal lower limb with the knee partially flexed leads to the free body diagrams in Figure 8.7(a), in which the reactions at floor, knee and hip are represented as components parallel and perpendicular to the longitudinal axis of the tibia. Figure 8.7(b) shows the corresponding diagrams for a limb with a ruptured anterior cruciate ligament which has resulted in there being no restraint at the knee to motion of the calf anteriorly perpendicular to its long axis. The analysis is then similar to that for the straight leg and leads to the four-point fixation system shown in Figure 8.7(c). It should be noted however that in this case, the two controlling forces on the thigh have both normal and tangential components. As knee flexion increases, their tangential components progressively increase until at 90° of flexion, anterior draw of the calf is prevented entirely by

shear forces at the orthosis–thigh interface. As these shear forces are generated through friction between the brace and the thigh, a good grip between the orthotic pads or straps and the skin surface is required if the brace is to be maximally effective for all angles of knee flexion.

The resulting brace required to deal with excessive anterior motion of the tibia, is thus illustrated in Figure 8.8. The corresponding orthosis required when there is excessive posterior tibial motion would have each of the four pads transposed through 180°.

8.4.3 Rotatory instability

Whereas injury to a single ligamentous structure will tend to cause a single clearly defined mode of instability (as in a ruptured anterior cruciate ligament giving rise to excessive ante-

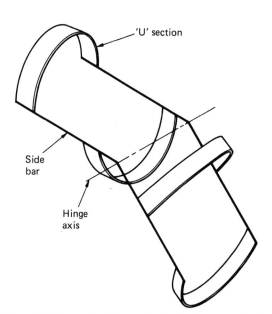

Figure 8.8 Theoretical four-point fixation brace required to restrict anterior draw

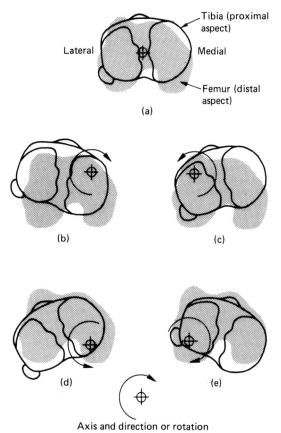

Figure 8.9 Patterns of rotatory instability: (a) normal position of left knee, no rotation; (b) anterolateral instability; (c) anteromedial instability; (d) posterolateral instability; (e) posteromedial instability. (Adapted from Nicholas, 1973.)

rior translation of the tibia), after more severe trauma, in which multiple ligamentous injuries have occurred, more complex patterns of instability result. These are generally known as rotatory instabilities and permit rotation of the tibia in a transverse plane relative to the femur about a centre which shifts from the region of the tibial spine in the geometric centre of the knee, the so-called pivot shift (Figure 8.9). The pattern of rotatory instability observed in a joint depends upon the combination of ligaments which have been torn. The most severely injured knees may exhibit more than one form of rotatory instability (Nicholas, 1973; Kennedy, 1979).

In this case the aim of the orthotic management is to control rotation of the tibia about its longitudinal axis. This is perhaps the most difficult aim to achieve as far as orthotic control of the knee is concerned, both because of the problems of interfacing an orthosis to the limb in such a way that it is effective in preventing this form of motion, and also because even very small rotations may be painful and extremely disabling.

Figure 8.10(a) shows the free body diagrams of the shank and thigh of a normal limb with a straight knee subjected to a pure transverse plane moment applied distally. Weight forces and their reactions have been omitted for clarity. Figure 8.10(b) presents the free bodies of the shank and thigh under the same conditions but now with a knee which is unable to resist rotation. In this case application of the moment tends to cause rotation of the shank about its longitudinal axis relative to the thigh. In order to control this abnormal rotation, an orthosis must restore the reaction moment at the knee, that is return the limb to the normal conditions of Figure 8.10(a). In practice this may be achieved by using a brace of high torsional stiffness which interfaces to the shank via a snug-fitting cuff and is similarly secured to the thigh. Note that this brace depends entirely on tangential, i.e. shear, forces, at the orthosis–skin interface for its effectiveness. Again, however, in order to allow knee flexion to occur, this rigid brace must be hinged at the joint centre. In the flexed position, the longitudinal axis of the thigh is no longer coincident

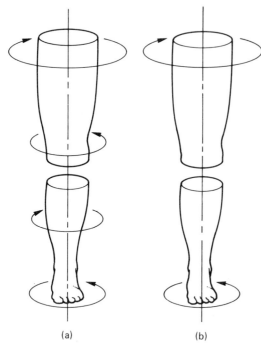

Figure 8.10 Derivation of bracing requirements to control internal rotation of right leg: (a) the normal limb; (b) a limb with ligamentous injury unable to resist rotation at the knee

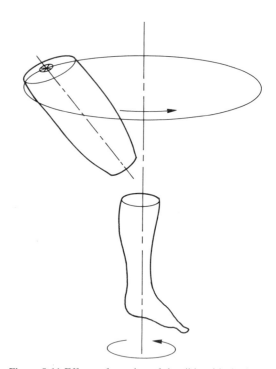

Figure 8.11 Effects of rotation of the tibia with the knee flexed

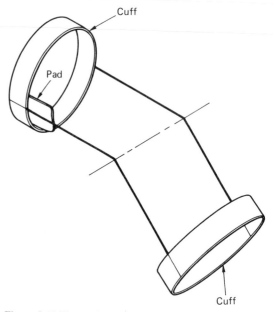

Figure 8.12 Theoretical brace design for control of internal tibial rotation in right leg

with that of the shank but is inclined to it at the angle through which the joint has been flexed. A pure moment applied to the shank will therefore be transmitted to the thigh as a moment plus a force: the hip will in fact tend to travel around the circular path as shown in Figure 8.11. In this case, the fixation to the thigh will be easier to achieve as the cuff is resisting both rotation and translation, and thus it achieves its effectiveness through the action of both tangential and normal force at the orthosis–skin interface. It may however be helpful to include an appropriately positioned pad, as in Figure 8.12, in order to reduce the normal contact force between the soft tissues of the thigh and the cuff.

The basic design of brace shown in Figure 8.12 would be appropriate for controlling internal tibial rotation in the right leg. To control external tibial rotation in the same leg or internal rotation of the other (left) leg, the pad would be placed medially rather than laterally. Effective rotational fixation of the brace to the limb is in practice difficult. A high friction inner surface to the cuffs is helpful but in itself does nothing to fix the skin surface relative to

the underlying bone. Using rigid cuffs shaped to lock against the femoral condyles and around the tibial spine would further contribute to the effectiveness of the orthosis.

8.4.4 Hyperextension of the knee

An orthosis may also be used to prevent or limit abnormal hyperextension of the knee in order to improve function or to reduce its destructive effects on the structures of the joint.

Hyperextension, although not normally considered to be an instability type, is often experienced clinically, frequently in combination with generalized knee looseness. In controlling hyperextension orthotically, the first requirement is to mechanically block the hinges of any brace so that it cannot itself hyperextend. The problem is then again identical to that of controlling abduction or adduction but with the angulation occurring in the sagittal plane. In this case, the analysis indicates the ideal brace to contact the limb posterior to the knee joint centre and anteriorly as distal and as proximal to the joint as is practicable.

8.4.5 Weakness of the muscles controlling knee flexion

Orthotic management of the knee may also be of value for patients who have paralysis of the muscles controlling the joint – and particularly of the quadriceps group. In walking, paralysis of these muscles will have its greatest effect just after heel-strike. During this period the effect of gravity and the forward momentum of the body will cause the knee to bend. In the absence of the quadriceps, the knee would collapse unless stability was maintained through compensation (e.g. use of hip extensors or forward bending of the trunk in early stance), or through the use of an orthosis. Hamstring paralysis, whilst also requiring gait compensations (such as hip hiking or increased hip flexion) to obtain clearance of the swinging foot, is not amenable to orthotic intervention.

For quadriceps weakness the aim of the orthosis will be to hold the knee in full extension during dynamic weight bearing. The biomechanical analysis of this requirement is again identical to that of the brace to prevent abduction or adduction of the joint but with the angulation occurring in the sagittal rather than the coronal plane. In this case the ideal brace will contact the limb anterior to the knee joint centre and posteriorly as distal and as proximal to the joint as is practicable. It will not, of course, include knee hinges.

8.4.6 Patellar instability

Malalignment within the lower limb can lead to patellar instability usually resulting in recurrent patellar subluxation or dislocation. There is associated pain at variable times but often occurring when subluxation or dislocation takes place. The causes of malalignment fall into two distinct groups, although features of both can be found in the same patient (Insall, 1984).

Rotational malalignment is characterized by excessive femoral anteversion with internal rotation of the femur and compensatory external rotation of the tibia (Figure 8.13). This results in an internally rotated knee relative to both hip and ankle and the typical patella 'squint'. This produces an increase in the Q angle and a consequent rise in the lateral force on the patella.

In patella alta (high-riding patella), the fact that the patella is not correctly positioned within the femoral sulcus results in an inability to resist lateral force and subsequent patellar

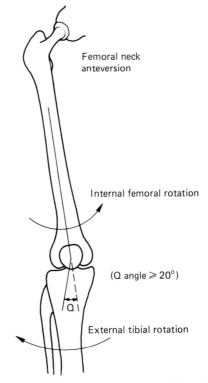

Femoral neck anteversion

Internal femoral rotation

(Q angle ⩾ 20°)

Q

External tibial rotation

Figure 8.13 Malalignment in the lower limb including femoral neck anteversion, internal rotation of the distal femur and external rotation of the tibia leading to an increase in the Q angle

instability. This can be seen as a lateral patellar deviation when the knee is actively extended (Insall *et al.*, 1972). The lack of congruence has been confirmed by radiographic measurements from over 250 knees (Aglietti *et al.*, 1983).

The aim of orthotic management is to return stability to the patella and to aid pain-free and less damaging tracking. This is difficult to achieve because of the problems at the orthosis–skin interface and those associated with soft tissue interposition which have been highlighted earlier in this chapter. However, some control may be sufficient to reduce the pain as the correction required is quite small.

Figure 8.14(a) shows the free body diagram for the patella of a normal knee with the forces in the quadriceps (F_Q), the patellar tendon (F_P) and that resulting from contact with the lateral border of the femoral sulcus (R). Other patellofemoral forces have been omitted for clarity. Figure 8.14(b) shows the same free body but with the forces positioned corresponding to the unstable situation illustrated in Figure 8.13. In Figure 8.14(a), assuming the normal Q angle to be 15°, the only force producing the lateral reaction is $F_Q \sin 15°$, which gives $R = 0.26F_Q$. In the unstable situation of Figure 8.14(b), the rotational malalignments have resulted in an increase in Q angle and an angular deviation of R. This time $R = F_Q \sin 20° = 0.34F_Q$, a significant increase of 31% which is such that the restraining mechanisms, principally bony, cannot reliably contain the patella in its correct position at all knee flexion angles.

During knee motion the patella moves both in translation and rotation in a pathway which

a rigid orthosis would not be able easily to follow and provide the necessary corrective medial force. Thus an elastic device would be indicated which would be capable of snug attachment to the limb both above and below the knee. This orthosis would rely upon shear forces to transmit the medial force to the patella. By being elastic, padded or reinforced areas strategically placed around the patella would be able to exert some force on the patella and move with it during motion. However, the inherent elasticity will restrict the absolute force that can be applied as will the tightness with which the orthosis can be attached to the limb.

The basic design of the orthosis would be able to provide, via a padded or stiffer area, a medially directed force to the patella in an elastic sleeve. A high friction inner layer would aid the transmission of forces at the orthosis–skin interface and some form of adjustment to the tightness of the leg, via straps, would facilitate the optimization of the fit.

8.5 Detail design considerations

Having established the outline designs for each of the four types of knee orthoses, the other requirements which must be taken into account in compiling the detail designs must be considered. The most significant of these are the problems of attaching the orthosis securely to the leg. As the lower limb essentially tapers from hip to ankle, knee orthoses have a tendency to slip distally under the action of gravity and the inertial forces generated at heel-strike. This will lead to misalignment of knee joint hinges with a subsequent reduction in knee flexion and sometimes also significant discomfort. A compromise therefore needs to be sought between attaching the orthosis too lightly to the limb and hence risking slippage of the device, and strapping the orthosis so firmly that it is uncomfortable. It has been in an attempt to circumvent such difficulties that techniques such as suspension from a hip or waistband, or the attachment of the orthosis to below-knee elements anchored in the shoe have been tried.

However, even if secure fixation of the orthosis on the limb can be satisfactorily

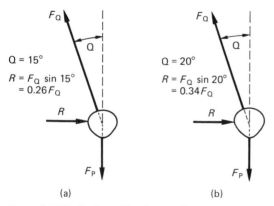

Figure 8.14 Derivation of bracing requirements to control patellar instability for: (a) the normal limb; (b) the malaligned limb

achieved, there will always be a layer of soft tissue interposed between the orthosis and the underlying bone which it is attempting to control. This will inevitably reduce the effectiveness of the brace. In some of the designs described, the pads which interface with the limb can be placed so as to lie directly over bony prominences. If this can be done, soft tissue movements will be minimized. In addition, it will sometimes be possible to 'lock' the orthotic pad onto the limb by shaping the pad so that it forms a snug fit over the bony prominence. This strategy will also help to reduce contact pressures and improve comfort.

In some instances, however, it will not be possible to position orthotic pads over bony prominences, an example being the anterior thigh pad of the hyperextension brace. In these cases, pads should be as large as practicable to facilitate tight strapping without causing excessively high contact pressures and should be contoured to the limb profile to assist fixation. Soft lining on orthotic pads to improve comfort will of course reduce fixation rigidity, although this may be small compared with soft tissue effects.

Turning to the structural members of knee orthoses, these clearly require to be sufficiently stiff to carry the loads imposed upon them without significant deformation whilst keeping weight and bulk to an absolute minimum. The hinges in the side bars should ideally be polycentric to allow the normal pattern of joint motion to occur during flexion and extension, although there is no evidence of either discomfort or long-term damage resulting from the use of uniaxial hinges. It is also important that, as far as possible, the required support is provided without impeding normal and desirable joint motions. Thus, a brace to provide adduction/abduction stability or to prevent anterior/posterior translation should allow knee joint flexion/extension and the transverse plane internal/external rotations required for normal knee function and especially for the locking of the joint in extension.

Finally, there are two further requirements not previously referred to. These are that the orthosis should be easy to don and doff, and of reasonable appearance. Whilst aesthetics will often not be of prime importance, as the orthosis will be hidden under clothing, this factor acquires greater significance if it is to be used for sporting activities.

8.6 Description of current orthoses

Although there are very many different knee orthoses currently available, there are really only three different basic types of construction: knee sleeves, stabilized knee sleeves, and frame braces.

The knee sleeve is the simplest type of device, consisting of a tube of stretch cotton or neoprene which is pulled lightly over the joint (Figure 8.15(a)). A hoop stress is developed in the sleeve which then exerts a radial pressure on the limb. With the orthosis in place, the joint can flex and extend, although flexion may be partially restricted by bunching of the material behind the knee and resistance to stretching over the patellar region. Some designs therefore have cut-outs at the front and/or rear to avoid these problems (Figure 8.15(b)). Transverse motions in the joint are restrained through the longitudinal fibres of the brace resisting elongation, as are internal/external rotations. However, as the sleeves allow flexion of the joint, they must also allow adduction and abduction.

The simple sleeve is usually the basis for the orthosis chosen to control patella tracking. Here a cut-out around the patella is formed and a reinforced padded edge is located in a horseshoe shape, usually around the lateral border and the upper part of the patella, (Figure 8.16(a)). This relies upon the elastic properties of the sleeve to provide the stabilizing force. Alternatively, air cells have been used to provide stability and an added dynamic 'milking' which is claimed to help relieve pain and resist swelling (Figure 8.16(b)). Straps

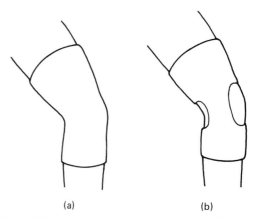

(a)   (b)

Figure 8.15 (a) A simple knee sleeve orthosis. (b) A similar device with front and rear cut-outs

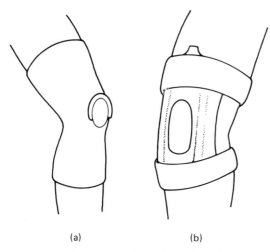

Figure 8.16 Knee orthoses to control patellar instability:
(a) with padded horseshoe borders; (b) pneumatic cells

have also been added such that, when they are tightened they move the cells so that the patella is further encouraged to move medially.

Stabilized knee sleeves consist of simple neoprene sleeves incorporating hinged bars or closely coiled helical springs on their medial and lateral aspects (Figure 8.17). The sleeve may be either a continuous tube of material or in the form of a sheet which is wrapped around the limb and closed with laces or some other fastening device. The stabilizing members are normally located in pockets sewn longitudinally onto the neoprene sleeve, as shown. Hinges may be uniaxial or multiaxial and may incorporate a hyperextension stop. These are supplied flat and will normally be bent to the contours of the limb by the fitting orthotist.

The orthosis may also incorporate straps which pass around the limb with the intention of increasing its fixation around the joint.

The addition of the hinged bars or springs to the simple sleeve provides, in effect, very stiff longitudinal fibres which bestow additional stability against transverse joint motions and internal/external rotations. Hinges will also help to restrict adduction and abduction since they rotate only in the sagittal plane, although this will not be the case for orthoses stabilized with springs which will flex in adduction/abduction as in flexion-extension.

The third group of knee stabilization orthoses, the frame braces, are by far the most supportive. These devices, rather than using stabilizing elements to strengthen a knee sleeve, consist of rigid hinged frameworks which carry strapping by means of which the orthosis is secured to the limb (Figure 8.18). Some frame braces are manufactured in a range of standard sizes for supply 'off the shelf', whilst others are custom made to a cast of the patient's knee. The frames may be fabricated from a polymer, aluminium alloy or carbon fibre. Braces of this type, having a rigid framework to which pads can be attached as required, are usually constructed specifically for a particular instability type, or alternatively are available in several variants to suit a number of different instability patterns. It is therefore possible to prescribe a frame brace which has been specifically designed to control a particular type of instability.

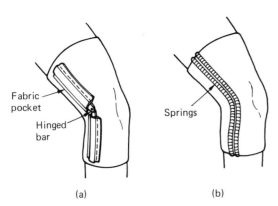

Figure 8.17 Knee sleeves stabilized with hinged bars (a) and helical springs (b)

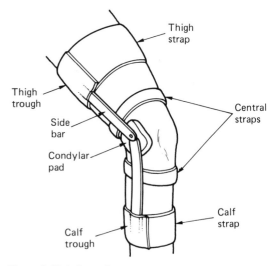

Figure 8.18 A frame brace

8.6.1 Static evaluation

In the most extensive series of static tests reported (Liggins, 1989; Liggins and Bowker, 1991), 24 orthoses (Table 8.2) were compared in a specially designed jig. This consisted of an instrumented limb substitute with a completely free knee to which the orthoses could be attached and the resulting load/displacement characteristics of the joint determined in anterior/posterior draw or in adduction/abduction or internal/external rotation. The results of the tests are summarized in Figure 8.19 for anterior/posterior draw and in Figure 8.20 for adduction/abduction rotation: in each case steeper lines indicate less stiff orthoses.

The wide range of results obtained from different braces has also been reported by Wojtys *et al.* (1990), although the latter authors made no attempt to relate performance to design.

The data indicated three factors which contribute to the effectiveness of an orthosis in controlling hypermobility of the knee. Firstly, the mechanical characteristics of the individual components of the orthosis, which in turn depended on both the material and cross-sections used, were of major importance; perhaps the most striking finding here was the significant superiority of neoprene rubber over woven materials. Secondly, the structural integrity of the orthosis design was an important

Table 8.2. Braces included in study and brief details of their construction: the symbols ((o) = open and (c) = closed) indicate whether the sleeve-based braces had an opening over the patella

Knee sleeves	
Tubigrip	Elasticated fabric, tubular (c)
Promedics Knee Sleeve	Neoprene, tubular (o)
Sprung sleeves	
Juzo J1222	
Juzo J3222	Elasticated fabric, tubular (c)
Juzo J1002 (tubular)	
Camp 8656 Spirex	Elasticated fabric, tubular (o)
Juzo J1002 (wrap)	Elasticated fabric, wrap-round (o)
Promedics Stabilised Knee Sleeve	Neoprene, tubular (o)
Hinged sleeves	
Juzo 1402 (tubular)	Elasticated fabric, tubular (c)
Camp Cinch	Elasticated fabric, wrap-round (c)
Juzo 1402 (wrap)	
Camp K-Line	Elasticated fabric, wrap-round (o)
Camp Fastwrap	Fabric covered foam, wrap-round (o)
Zimmer Ultraglide	
Paraprene NP 110	Neoprene, tubular (o)
Promedics Hinged Knee Sleeve	
Promedics SK	
Promedics VK	Neoprene, wrap-round (o)
Zimmer Flex 10	
In-Care	Long hinged arms with plastic wings strapped over foam wraps (o)
Adjustabrace	
Frame braces	
Lenox Hill Derotation	Customized, aluminium frame
Remploy Remmedi De-Rotation	Customized rigid thermoplastic
Donjoy ACL	Ready-made, aluminium frame
Lerman Multi-Ligamentous	Ready-made, steel and thermoplastic frame

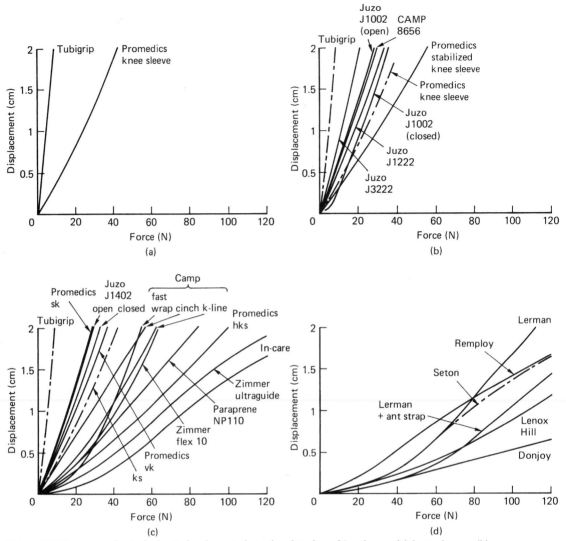

Figure 8.19 Summary of anterior/posterior draw static testing data from 24 orthoses: (a) knee sleeves; (b) sprung sleeves; (c) hinged sleeves; (d) frame braces. (Reproduced with permission from Liggins and Bowker, 1991)

contributor to its performance; discontinuities and holes in sleeves, looseness between components or in fasteners all reduced stiffness. Thirdly, the interaction between the orthosis and the limb was critically important; this factor included both the magnitudes and the points of application of the controlling forces applied to the limb by the orthosis, and the effectiveness of the design in preventing relative motion between the two. Thus in anterior draw (Figure 8.19) the Donjoy brace, which has a frame specifically designed to produce the required four-point fixation system, was superior to all the others tested, with the

Lenox Hill brace, which achieves effective four-point fixation via its system of patella and cross straps, rated as second, these results being in general agreement with those of Beck *et al.* (1986). The adduction/abduction data, (Figure 8.20), confirmed that brace effectiveness increased as the length of the orthosis was increased, as previously demonstrated by Carlson and French (1989). Thus, the long arm In Care orthosis gave a good performance which, even amongst the frame braces, only the customized Lenox Hill could equal. Finally, in internal/external rotation, the results confirmed that effectiveness was improved by

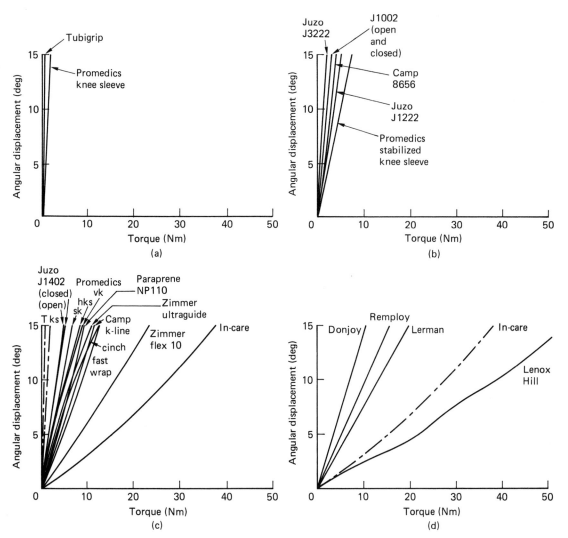

Figure 8.20 Summary of valgus/varus rotation static testing data from 24 orthoses: (a) knee sleeves; (b) sprung sleeves; (c) hinged sleeves; (d) frame braces. (Redrawn with permission from Liggins, 1989)

maximizing brace stiffness and by customizing its manufacture to the limb.

8.6.2 Dynamic evaluation

Dynamic comparisons of knee orthoses have been carried out by Knutzen *et al.* (1983), Pratt (1990) and Liggins (1989). In the first two of these, in which only rotational knee motions were recorded, the performances of two and six orthoses using the CARS-UBC and TRIAX electrogoniometers respectively were examined. The two studies differed in that the former investigated running whereas the latter examined walking. The orthoses studied were:

Knutzen *et al.* (1983)	Lenox Hill derotation brace, a 'support' brace	
Pratt (1990)	Zimmer Drop-Lok	Group 1
	Zimmer Flex 10	Group 2
	Camp Fastwrap	Group 1
	Camp Cinch	Group 1
	Lerman Multi-Ligamentous	Group 2
	Donjoy 4 Point	Group 2

The study by Pratt (1990) showed that the performance of the two groups of orthoses tested was very different. The action of Group 1 orthoses was particularly variable, leading to unwanted restriction of knee flexion and no significant control of abduction/adduction or internal/external rotation. In fact, for all the group 1 orthoses there was an apparent increase in abduction and for Drop-lok and Cinch an increase in internal rotation, Fastwrap having no measurable effect. The group 2 orthoses were generally better, giving less restriction in knee flexion and useful control of abduction and rotation, with the Donjoy and Flex 10 performing well overall.

Liggins (1989), who used a custom-built six degree of freedom transducer to measure the effects of four orthoses on healthy knees, found that the orthoses were better able to control translational displacements than rotational, perhaps because they were unable to control soft tissue movements between the orthosis and the leg. He also found that despite a wide variation in the constructions of the orthoses (and their stiffnesses) there was no apparent relationship between mechanical stiffness and dynamic action of the orthosis. It would appear that the soft tissue of the leg reduces the stabilization that the orthosis provides to about the same level for each orthosis. This finding is in agreement with that of Knutzen *et al.* (1984) who compared the ability of two orthoses to control tibial rotation and found that despite different constructions, the results were similar for both orthoses. Cook *et al.* (1989) have cautioned prescribers that the C.Ti brace, although aiding function, does not prevent abnormal anterior translations within the knee and that the long-term effects of orthosis use are unknown. As patients do nevertheless derive real benefits from these devices, and it is known that the anterior cruciate ligament contains a sophisticated network of mechanoreceptors (Schutte *et al.*, 1987), and that its rupture leads to a significant proprioceptive loss (Barrock *et al.*, 1989), orthoses may be effective through the provision of an alternative proprioceptive pathway rather than through restoring the original mechanical characteristics of the joint. Some recent EMG work by Branch *et al.* (1989) does not however support this hypothesis.

Insall (1984) finds that patellar instability due to malalignment syndromes in the lower limb responds well to elastic patellar braces with horseshoe padding. They seem to provide added stability and significantly reduce discomfort. He also finds that these orthoses do not benefit people suffering from disorders not associated with malalignment except for occasional value in patellofemoral osteoarthritis.

Ultimately however, the most meaningful assessment of orthoses must be that made by the users. Fisher and McLellan (1989) surveyed a group of patients who had been supplied with five different sorts of orthosis (sleeve type, T.V.S., Lenox Hill, Swedish knee cage and bespoke). They found that 42% of users were dissatisfied, the most common criticisms of the orthoses being: heavy, cumbersome and cosmetically unacceptable, tends to slip, chafes opposite leg, and difficulty in applying device (especially in the presence of upper limb problems such as arthritis). It should be stressed however that this dissatisfaction could largely arise from poorly fitted orthoses rather than poorly designed ones.

8.7 Current developments

The results quoted above clearly indicate that there is a great deal of scope for the development of knee orthoses. Whilst it is essential to develop research on the dynamic action of braces to confirm their mode of operation, perhaps the most urgent requirements revolve around improving the design of braces through more sophisticated engineering and the use of modern materials to make them lighter and less cumbersome – and hence of improved cosmesis, with better fixation mechanisms and improved ease of donning and doffing. If these qualities can be combined with designs which are biomechanically sound, orthotic management of the disordered knee will become very much more attractive and effective than it has hitherto been.

8.8 Alternative and complementary treatments

For many of the patients with the knee joint pathologies described in this chapter, surgery will offer an alternative, and sometimes more attractive, approach to conservative management using an orthosis.

For the patient with rheumatoid or other forms of arthritis, the surgical possibilities include total joint replacement, joint arthrodesis or some form of osteotomy. The decisions as to whether or not to proceed with such surgery are dependent upon a number of factors, including age, and the extent of joint involvement and deformity (Waugh, 1984). In cases of mild arthritis an osteotomy or unilateral replacement would often be carried out. Only in the case of post-traumatic arthritis in the young patient, or other severe conditions (such as a failed joint replacement), would an arthrodesis be considered. However, the outcome of many such procedures is unpredictable as a technically successful procedure does not necessarily lead to a rehabilitated patient, often for psychological reasons. Surgical approaches do not therefore provide guaranteed success and some patients, despite very poor knees, do not want an operation.

For soft tissue injuries to the knee, i.e. ligamentous injuries, many surgical techniques are available. Ligamentous reconstructions have been carried out for many years using both intra- and extra-articular procedures (Zarins and Rowe, 1986; Clancy *et al.*, 1982; Lam, 1968). More recently a number of techniques have been developed which enable a damaged ligament to be replaced by a prosthetic device or augmented by the use of a Ligament Augmentation Device (LAD) (Dahlstedt *et al.*, 1990; Aragona *et al.*, 1981; Jenkins, 1980). However, apart from the usual operative risks there is the risk of a reaction to the implant and effusions plus a long rehabilitation period (Indelicato *et al.*, 1989). There is also the problem of the stiffness of the prosthetic ligament, a matter examined by Amis (1989). He found that small changes to the tightness of an implant caused significant differences in both stability and range of motion but that stiff implants did not cause abnormal behaviour (the benefits of particular elasticities remaining unproven). He also found that the use of tensiometers was not helpful in determining the effectiveness of the implant. It was found that the positioning of prosthetic ligaments is critical and could have profound consequences upon knee motion and the life of the implant. This could account for the observations that whilst the short-term results of surgical replacement of the ruptured ligament are generally good, longer-term outcomes are questionable (Noyes *et al.*, 1983; Odensten *et al.*, 1985; Clancy *et al.*, 1988).

Recurrent patellar subluxation or dislocation can be treated surgically by what is termed a proximal realignment. This is a major procedure in which the muscle attachments to the patella are rearranged to alter the line of action of the quadriceps muscle. It is only carried out if prolonged conservative management fails (Insall, 1984). A distal realignment can be carried out for patella alta by repositioning the patella ligament more medially and distally (Hughston and Walsh, 1979). Selective strengthening of the vastus medialis would seem to be of value as this would advantageously affect patellar tracking (Lieb and Perry, 1968); however, this is difficult to do in practice.

References

Aglietti P., Insall J.N. and Cerulli G. (1983) Patellar pain and incongruence. I: measurement of incongruence. *Clin. Orthop.* **176**, 217–223

Amis A.A. (1989) Anterior cruciate ligament replacement. *J. Bone Joint Surg.* **71B**, 819–824

Aragona J., Parsons J.R., Alexander H. *et al.* (1981) Soft tissue attachment of a filamentous carbon-absorbable polymer tendon and ligament replacement. *Clin. Orthop.* **160**, 268–278

Barrack R.L., Skinner H.B. and Buckley S.L. (1989) Proprioception in the anterior cruciate deficient knee. *Am. J. Sports Med.* **17**, 1–6

Beck C., Drey D., Young J. *et al.* (1986) Instrumental testing of functional knee braces. *Am. J. Sports Med.* **14**, 253–256

Bishop R.E.D. and Denham R.A. (1977) A note of the ratio between tensions in the quadriceps tendon and infrapatella ligament. *Eng. Med.* **6**, 53–54

Branch T.P., Hunter R. and Donath M. (1989) Dynamic EMG analysis of anterior cruciate deficient legs with and without bracing during cutting. *Am. J. Sports Med.* **17**, 35–41

Carlson J.M. and French J. (1989) Knee orthoses for valgus protection. *Clin. Orthop.* **247**, 175–192

Clancy W.G., Nelson D.A., Reider B. *et al.* (1982) Anterior cruciate ligament reconstruction using one-third of the patella ligament, augmented by extra articular tendon transfers. *J. Bone Joint Surg.* **64A**, 352–359

Clancy W.G., Ray J.M. and Zoltan D.J. (1988) Acute tears of the anterior cruciate ligament. *J. Bone Joint Surg.* **70A**, 1483–1488

Cook F.F., Tibone J.E. and Redfern F.C. (1989) A dynamic analysis of a functional brace for anterior cruciate ligament insufficiency. *Am. J. Sports Med.* **17**, 519–524

Cox A.J. (1990) Biomechanics of the patello-femoral joint. *Clin. Biomech.* **5**, 123–130

Dahlstedt L., Dalen N. and Jonsson U. (1990) Goretex prosthetic ligament vs. Kennedy ligament augmentation device in anterior cruciate ligament reconstruction. *Acta Orthopaed. Scand.* **61**, 217–224

Fisher L.R. and McLellan D.L. (1989) Questionnaire assessment of patient satisfaction with lower limb orthoses from a district hospital. *Prosthet. Orthot. Int.* **13**, 29–35

France E.P., Paulos L.E., Jayaraman G. *et al.* (1987) The biomechanics of lateral knee bracing. Part II: Impact response of the braced knee. *Am. J. Sports Med.* **15**, 430–438

Frankel V.H. and Nordin M. (1980) *Basic Biomechanics of the Skeletal System*. Lea and Febinger, Philadelphia, pp. 115–117

Garrick J.G. and Requa R.K. (1987) Prophylactic knee bracing. *Am. J. Sports Med.* **15**, 471–476

Goodfellow J. and O'Connor J. (1978) The mechanics of the knee and prosthesis design. *J. Bone Joint Surg.* **60A**, 358–369

Hehne H.J. (1990) Biomechanics of the patellofemoral joint and its clinical relevance. *Clin. Orthop.* **258**, 73–85

Hughston J.C. and Walsh W.M. (1979) Proximal and distal reconstruction of the extensor mechanism for patellar subluxation. *Clin. Orthop.* **144**, 36–42

Indelicato P.A., Pascale M.S. and Huegel M.O. (1989) Early experience of the GORE-TEX polytetrafluoroethylene anterior cruciate ligament prosthesis. *Am. J. Sports Med.* **17**, 55–62

Insall J.N. (1984) Disorders of the patella. In: Insall J.N. (ed.), *Surgery of the Knee*. Churchill Livingstone, Edinburgh, pp. 191–260

Insall J.N., Goldberg V. and Salvati E. (1972) Recurrent dislocation and the high-riding patella. *Clin. Orthop.* **88**, 67–69

Jenkins D.H.R. and McKibbin B. (1980) The role of carbon fibre implants as tendon and ligament substitutes in clinical practice. A preliminary report. *J. Bone Joint Surg.* **62B**, 497–499

Kapandji I.A. (1970) *The Physiology of the Joints*, vol. 2. Churchill Livingstone, Edinburgh

Kennedy J.C. (ed) (1979) The Injured Adolescent Knee. Williams and Wilkins, Baltimore

Knutzen K.M., Bates B.T. and Hamill J. (1983) Electrogoniometry of post surgical knee bracing in running. *Am. J. Phys. Med.* **62**, 172–179

Knutzen K.M., Bates B.T. and Hamill J. (1984) Knee brace influences on the tibial rotation and torque patterns of the surgical limb. *J. Orthop. Sports Phys. Ther.* Sept/Oct, 116–122

Lam S.J.S. (1986) Reconstruction of the anterior cruciate ligament using the Jones procedure and its Guy's Hospital modification. *J. Bone Joint Surg.* **50A**, 1213–1224

Lieb F.J. and Perry J. (1968) Quadriceps function. An anatomical and mechanical study using amputated limbs. *J. Bone Joint Surg.* **50A**, 1535–1548

Liggins A.B. (1989) Quantitative Assessment of Knee Stabilization Orthoses. PhD Thesis, University of Salford, UK

Liggins A.B. (1989) Quantitative Assessment of Knee Stabilization Orthoses. PhD Thesis, University of Salford, UK

Liggins A.B. and Bowker P. (1991) A quantitative assessment of orthoses for stabilisation of the anterior cruciate ligament deficient knee. *Eng. Med. (Proc. I Mech. E, Part H)* **205**, 81–87

Maltry J.A., Noble P.C., Woods G.W. *et al.* (1989) External stabilisation of the anterior cruciate ligament deficient knee during rehabilition. *Am. J. Sports Med.* **17**, 550–554

Maquet P.G.J. (1984) *Biomechanics of the Knee*. Springer, Berlin

Marquette S.H. (1988) Stabilising anterior cruciate ligament injuries: biomechanical requirements of orthotic design. *Orthot. Prosthet.* **41**, 18–28

Morrison J.B. (1967) The Forces Transmitted by the Human Knee Joint during Activity. PhD Thesis, Department of Bioengineering, University of Strathclyde, Glasgow, Scotland

Morrison J.B. (1969) Function of the knee in various activities. *Biomed. Eng.* **4**, 573–579

Muller W. (1983) *The Knee. Form, Function and Ligament Reconstruction*. Springer, Berlin

Nicholas J.A. (1973) The five-one construction for anteromedial instability of the knee. *J. Bone Joint Surg.* **55A**, 899–922

Nissan M. (1980) Review of some basic assumptions in knee biomechanics. *J. Biomech.* **13**, 375–381

Nordin M. and Frankel V.H. (1980) Biomechanics of the knee. In: Frankel V.H. and Nordin M. (eds), *Basic Biomechanics of the Skeletal System*. Lea and Febiger, Philadelphia, pp. 113–148

Noyes F.R., Mooar P.A., Matthews D.S. *et al.* (1983) The symptomatic anterior cruciate-deficient knee Part I: The long-term functional disability in athletically active individuals. *J. Bone Joint Surg.* **65A**, 154–162

Odensten M., Hamberg P., Nordin M. *et al.* (1985) Surgical or conservative treatment of the acutely torn anterior cruciate ligament. *Clin. Orthop.* **198**, 87–93

Palastanga, N., Field D. and Soames R. (1989) *Anatomy and Human Movement*. Heinemann Medical Books, Oxford

Perry J. Antonelli D. and Ford W. (1975) Analysis of knee joint forces during flexed knee stance. *J. Bone Joint Surg.* **57A**, 962–967

Pratt D.J. (1990) A three dimensional electrogoniometric study of selected knee orthoses. *Clin. Biomech.* **6**, 67–72

Schutte M.J., Dabezies E.J., Zimny M.L. *et al.* (1987) Neural anatomy of the human anterior cruciate ligament. *J. Bone Joint Surg.* **69A**, 243–247

Seedholm B.B., Dowson D. and Wright V. (1974) The load-bearing function of the menisci: a preliminary study. In: Ingwersen O.S., Van Linge B., Van Rhens T.J.G. (eds), *The Knee Joint. Recent Advances in Basic Research and Clinical Aspects*. Excerpta Medica, Amsterdam, pp. 37–42

Segal P. and Jacob M. (1989) *The Knee*. Wolfe Medical, London

Seireg A. and Arvikar R.J. (1975) The prediction of

muscular load sharing and joint forces in the lower extremities during walking. *J. Biomech.* **8**, 89–102

Tietz C.C., Hermanson B.K., Kronmal R.A. *et al.* (1987) Evaluation of the use of braces to prevent injury to the knee in collegiate football players. *J. Bone Joint Surg.* **69A**, 2–9

Waugh W. (1984) Knee replacement. In: Jackson J.P. and Waugh W. (eds), *Surgery of the Knee Joint.* Chapman and Hall, London, pp. 351–391

Wojtys E.M., Loubert P.V., Sampson S.Y. *et al.* (1990) Use of a knee-brace for control of tibial translation and rotation. *J. Bone Joint Surg.* **72A**, 1323–1329

Zarins B. and Rowe C.R. (1986) Combined anterior cruciate ligament reconstruction using semitendinosus tendon and iliotibial tract. *J. Bone Joint Surg.* **66A**, 160–176

9

Knee–ankle–foot orthoses

David Condie and John Lamb

9.1 Introduction

The previous chapter has described the clinical and biomechanical considerations in the design and use of knee orthoses. Knee–ankle–foot orthoses may also be employed to treat disorders of knee function. As an introduction to the discussion of this category of orthoses, three occasions when a knee–ankle–foot orthosis (KAFO) might be employed in preference to a knee orthosis (KO) will first be defined.

Some patients may present with functional disorders which affect both the knee and the ankle. On these occasions it may be both simpler and more effective to prescribe a single KAFO rather than both a KO and an AFO.

Even for patients who present with an isolated knee disorder, there are occasions when due to the severity of the disorder the magnitude of the required controlling forces dictates the use of a KAFO in order to maximize the length of the lever arms and the limb–orthoses contact areas through which these forces are applied.

Finally in some patients with an isolated knee disorder problems may be encountered in successfully suspending a KO. On these occasions a KAFO may be prescribed, the below-knee section of this serving to overcome the suspension problem.

Two principal types of fabrication are used for KAFO manufacture:

1. A conventional metal and leather design (Figure 9.1(a)), or

2. A contemporary moulded thermoplastic design (Figure 9.1(b)).

Conventional fabrication utilizes metal side bars incorporating hinged knee joints, interconnected by curved transverse metal bands to provide structural stiffness. The inner surfaces of the bands are padded and covered with soft leather to provide a cushioned interface with the limb. The essential interconnection with the shoe is achieved either through a clevis type ankle joint (a U-shaped hinge) and shoe attachment stirrup or via spurs or pins attached to the distal ends of the side bars which engage in a matching tube inserted transversely into the shoe heel.

The metal side bars are produced in both steel for applications in which strength is required or aluminium where light weight is the more important consideration and in a range of sizes to accommodate the differing size and weight of patients and degree of loading. The most commonly used cross-sectional shape of the side bars is round edged rectangular. Although some experimental laboratory work has been carried out to measure side bar loading values (Trappitt and Berme, 1981; and Abou Ghaida *et al.*, 1987–88), at present no method exists of accurately identifying, in the clinical or workshop environment, the precise side bar design which is appropriate to any particular patient. The orthotist, in specifying the side bar design of the KAFO, therefore still decides on this empirically and from experience.

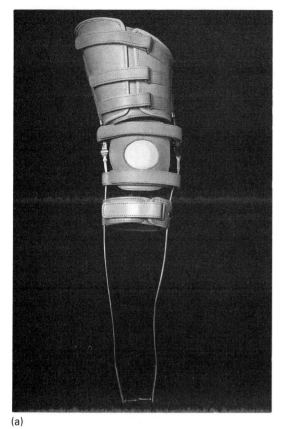

(a)

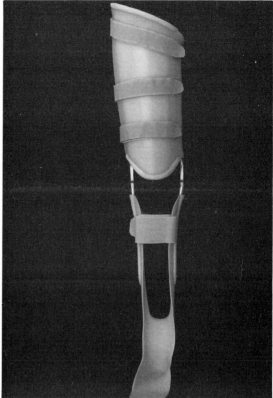

(b)

Figure 9.1 (a) Conventional metal and leather KAFO. (b) Contemporary thermoplastic KAFO

Contemporary thermoplastic construction, described originally by Yates (1968) and popularized in the UK by Tuck (1974), uses moulded plastic sections both above and below the knee, interconnected by similar side bar/knee joint components as are used in conventional fabrication. The below-knee plastic section includes a footpiece which fits inside the shoe and thus this design of orthosis, unlike conventional construction, does not require any direct attachment to the shoe.

Biomechanically the function of both types of orthosis is similar. Conventional designs apply the controlling forces through their transverse bands, while in contemporary designs this is achieved by the moulded plastic sections. In both cases the shoe forms an essential component of the orthotic mechanical system and additional control straps or pads may also be employed depending on the specific function of the orthosis.

Where a KAFO is not required to exert any

specific control over ankle or foot function it is customary to employ either a free acting ankle joint attached to the shoe as previously described, or to trim the plastic below-knee section posteriorly at ankle level in order to minimize the restriction of ankle function (Figure 9.2).

There are however specific occasions when the biomechanical function of the KAFO at the knee joint depends on the concurrent control of motion at the ankle joint. In addition, some patients with a knee disorder also exhibit impaired ankle or foot function. In both these situations it will be necessary to utilize either an appropriate design of orthotic ankle which controls ankle joint movement, or to form and trim the plastic below-knee section in such a way as to effect the necessary control of ankle or foot function.

In the next sections only the functionally significant construction features of each design of orthosis will be described.

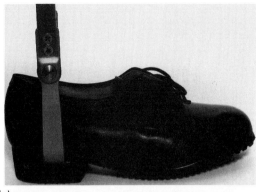

(a)

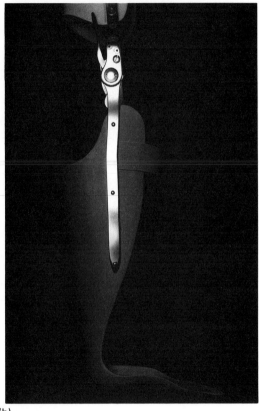

(b)

Figure 9.2 (a) Free ankle joint. (b) Thermoplastic below-knee section trimmed to minimize resistance to motion

9.2 Anatomy and biomechanics

The ankle, knee and hip joint anatomy and biomechanics relevant to the discussion of the uses of KAFOs is contained in Chapters 6, 8 and 10 respectively.

9.3 Clinical applications

Advances in medical and surgical practice over recent years have significantly reduced the numbers of patients who require the prescription of a KAFO. The biomechanical basis for the use of KAFOs is divided into three sections which relate to the nature of the principal impairment being addressed. These are:

1. Weakness of the muscles which control the knee joint (and perhaps the hip and ankle joints).
2. Upper motor neurone lesions which result in hypertonicity (spasticity) of the lower limb musculature.
3. Loss of structural integrity of the hip or knee joints.

9.3.1 Muscle weakness

Weakness of the muscles of the lower limbs, including those controlling the knee joint, will most commonly result from spinal cord damage due to trauma or congenital abnormality such as spina bifida or as a consequence of a lower motor neurone disease such as poliomyelitis. Injury to a nerve or tendon may also result in specific knee joint muscle weakness.

Orthotic treatment is directed at compensating for the muscle weakness thereby enabling a better level of physical activity. The specific treatment objectives, biomechanical requirements and appropriate orthotic designs will be described for each of the commonly encountered patterns of muscle weakness.

(a) Total lower limb weakness

Total lower limb weakness (paraplegia) such as that resulting from spinal cord damage makes it impossible for an individual to achieve and maintain an upright posture. Apart from the obvious loss of mobility, this will exclude them from many everyday activities. There are also physiological consequences of being unable to stand and, depending upon the location and extent of the spinal lesion, spinal stability may also be impaired.

The loss of sensation and diminished tissue viability which is also suffered by these patients creates the danger of pressure sores which therefore makes the avoidance of high limb–orthosis contact pressures a major priority.

For those patients whose spine is stable and who have some residual hip flexor muscle power, bilateral KAFOs may be successfully prescribed to provide knee and ankle stability. Standing balance may then be achieved by the patient hyperextending his hips, thus placing the centre of gravity of the trunk, head and upper limbs behind the hip joint axis. Mobility is achieved with the assistance of elbow crutches using either a bipedal or swing-through gait.

The force system required to provide knee and ankle stability is illustrated in Figure 9.3. This comprises two overlapping force systems R_2, R_3 and R_4 controlling the knee and R_1, R_2 and R_3 controlling the ankle. Contrary to some traditional practices, axial load relief is not a necessary requirement in this application and, given the presence of diminished sensation and tissue viability, an increase in ischial contact and loading is preferably avoided. In this situation it is desirable that the full length of the thigh should be encompassed by the orthosis

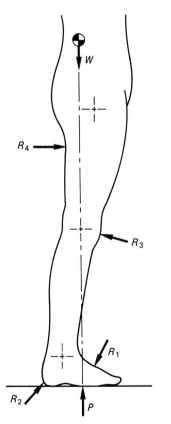

Figure 9.3 Posture adopted and orthotic force system required to achieve standing balance

since the size of the contact pressures will be minimized if the two posterior forces are as far apart and distributed over as large an area as possible.

Some variation exists in the method of application of the posteriorly directed force at the level of the knee joint. This may be achieved by using a leather knee apron positioned directly over the patella, using a single moulded infrapatellar band, or by combining the latter with a second suprapatellar force created by means of an additional strap (in conventional designs) or by modifying the construction of the above-knee section anteriorly (in contemporary designs) (see Figure 9.4).

Lehmann and Warren (1976) have demonstrated both theoretically and experimentally that where a single site of application of the posteriorly directed force is adopted this should be placed just below the knee joint line in order to minimize the shear force action upon the joint. However by using two sites of application of this force, both above and below the knee, theoretically joint shear will be completely eliminated.

This orthotic device will in addition require joints which prevent knee flexion and limit ankle dorsiflexion.

Knee joint control is achieved by using one of a range of locking joints as illustrated in Figure 9.5. These joints may be subdivided into manual or semiautomatic. Manual locks need to be manually locked and unlocked by the patient. Semiautomatic designs lock automatically when the knee is fully extended but need to be unlocked manually. Irrespective of the lock type employed, in all cases the knee joints must be locked when standing or walking and are only released to permit sitting.

In conventional designs the control of ankle joint motion is achieved by the inclusion of mechanical joints which can be adjusted to provide the required limitation of dorsiflexion. Alternatively where side bars with spurs are fitted these may be combined with rectangular sockets when no ankle movement is required or with round sockets and anterior stops when ankle plantar flexion is to be retained and dorsiflexion only prevented (Figure 9.6). It should be noted however that due to the high loadings to which the ankle joint components are subjected by this category of patient, the spurs, sockets and stops are notoriously prone to early wear, deformation and fracture.

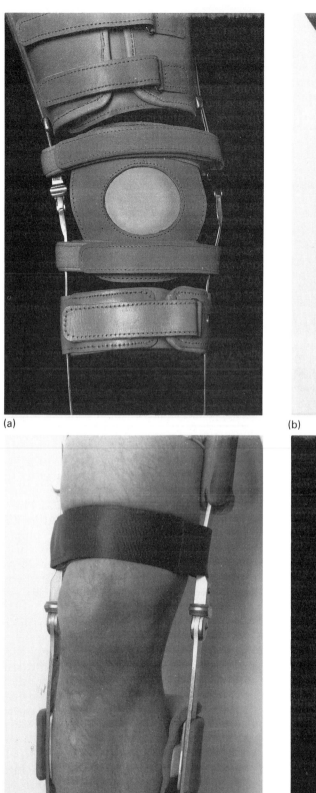
(a)

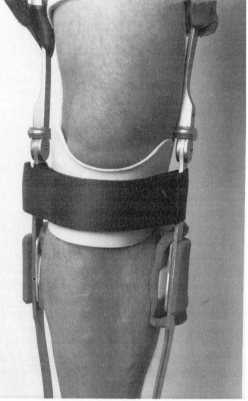
(b)

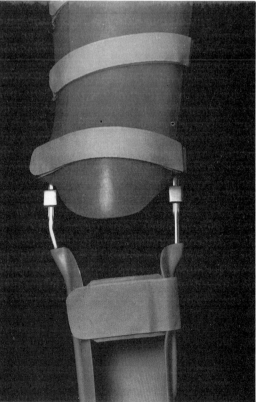
(c)

(d)

Figure 9.4 Alternative methods of providing the posteriorly directed force at the knee joint. (a) Knee apron. (b) Infrapatellar pad or strap. (c) Suprapatellar pad or strap. (d) Extended above-knee section

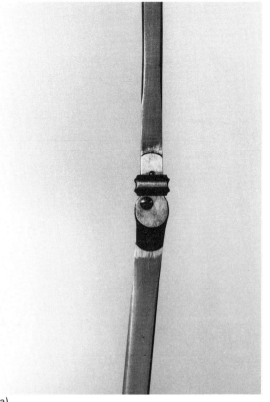

(a)

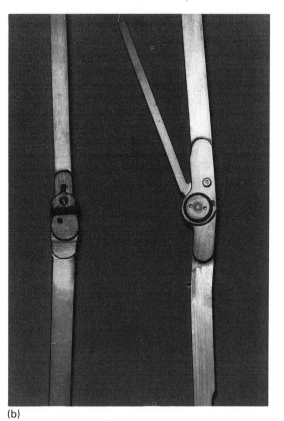

(b)

Figure 9.5 Knee lock designs. (a) Manual: ring or drop lock. (b) Automatic: ring or drop lock; bale lock

In contemporary plastic designs, the control of ankle dorsiflexion is achieved by creating a stiff ankle region within the moulded orthosis. This is achieved either by maintaining the trimline anteriorly utilizing a modified cross-sectional profile, or by employing a thicker material in the fabrication (Figure 9.7). If such a one-piece design is included in the orthosis this will inevitably result in the elimination of plantarflexion also.

Ankle movement may be permitted in contemporary designs by forming a simple overlap joint between the shank and foot pieces. Conventional metal ankle joints are also used for this purpose, while proprietary plastic and metal joints, designed specifically for use with plastic orthoses, are also available. Any one of these three methods allows a useful range of plantarflexion whilst still restricting dorsiflexion (Figure 9.8).

Several North American studies of the use of this type of orthosis have confirmed the importance of the ankle dorsiflexion limit, not only to provide stability when standing but also to significantly reduce the energy expenditure when walking with crutches (Merkel *et al.*, 1981, 1984).

Rodillo *et al.* (1988) have described an interesting use of this design of orthosis with muscular dystrophy children. They suggest that the use of such orthoses may reduce the rate of deterioration of scoliosis in these children due to the hyperlordotic posture which the orthotic device encourages.

(b) Weakness (or absence) of knee extensor power

The knee extensor muscles maintain knee stability throughout the stance phase of walking when the normal external knee moment tends to flex the knee. Total absence of knee extensor power will make normal walking impossible, although compensatory hip extension will allow an abnormal gait in many patients.

Even if the knee extensors are only weakened, the patient's gait will be insecure resulting in 'giving way' on occasions. Most patients

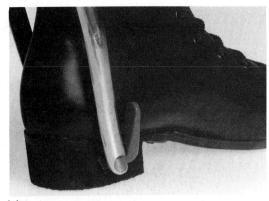

(a)

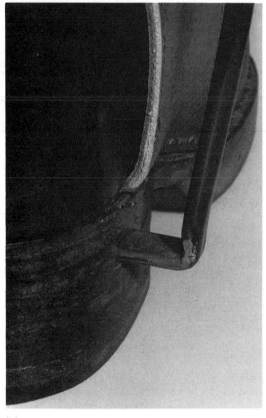

(b)

Figure 9.6 Conventional ankle joint designs which limit dorsiflexion. (a) Round spurs and sockets with anterior stops. (b) Rectangular spurs and sockets

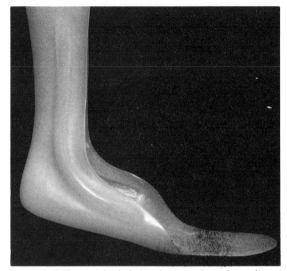

Figure 9.7 Thermoplastic below-knee section trimmed to limit dorsiflexion

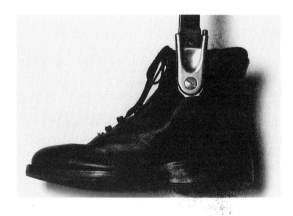

Figure 9.8 Contemporary articulated below-knee section designs which permit free plantarflexion and limit dorsiflexion

with a unilateral weakness can overcome this functional limitation by adopting compensatory gait deviations. Flexion of the trunk during the stance phase of gait will cause the ground reaction force to pass in front of the knee creating a stabilizing extension moment (Figure 9.9). Alternatively, the patient may resist flexion by manually pushing the thigh posteriorly (Figure 9.10). Both of these manoeuvres however result in a highly energy consuming and unsightly gait pattern.

Mild knee extensor weakness in the absence of a knee flexion deformity may be treated orthotically using a Floor Reaction AFO as described in Chapter 7. Severe weakness (or mild weakness in the presence of a flexion deformity) will however require the application of a KAFO, thus permitting a safer and more natural walking posture.

The force system required to resist abnormal knee flexion consists of three forces positioned as illustrated in Figure 9.11.

The same biomechanical considerations as those described for the paraplegic patient

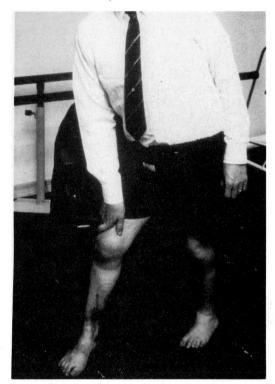

Figure 9.10 Knee stability maintained by manual pressure on the thigh

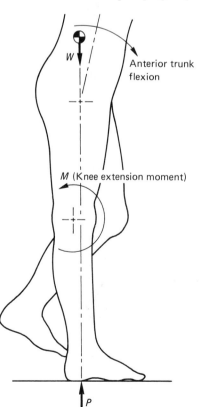

Figure 9.9 Anterior trunk flexion to achieve knee stability

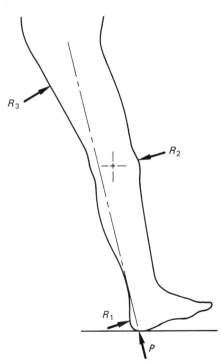

Figure 9.11 Three-force system required to prevent knee flexion

apply to the positioning of the three forces and similar variations in the method of application of the central force may be employed. The device used will also need to incorporate orthotic knee joints which provide resistance to knee flexion during the stance phase.

In those cases where knee extensor power is totally absent stability is normally achieved by employing one of the locking joint designs. Obviously this has the disadvantage of preventing knee flexion during the swing phase thus creating foot clearance problems during this part of the gait cycle. The patient will overcome this problem by circumducting the limb, hip hiking, plantarflexing the contralateral ankle and/or adopting an increased lateral sway of the trunk (Figure 9.12).

The development of the UCLA Functional Long Leg Brace was stimulated by the recognition of this problem. (Anderson and Bray, 1964). This design combines a plastic thigh shell (similar in appearance to the upper portion of a prosthetic above-knee quadrilateral socket), free knee joints with a posterior offset

and heavy duty ankle joints with adjustable dorsiflexion stops and a hydraulic damper mechanism.

Immediately after heel contact the line of action of the ground reaction force normally passes behind the anatomical knee joint axis creating a knee flexion moment which, if not resisted, will result in the leg collapsing. This tendency may be resisted by contraction of the hip extensors which will have the effect of 'pulling' the line of action forward so that it passes through or in front of the anatomical knee axis.

The Functional Long Leg Brace (FLLB) design offers an alternative mechanism for countering the knee flexion moment. Between heel strike and foot flat the effect of the force from the patient's abdomen and pelvis acting upon the anterior brim of the thigh shell creates an extension moment about the brace knee joint axis. This effect is enhanced by the posterior offset of the joint used in this design of orthosis. This moment is transmitted onto the patient's leg through the same three points

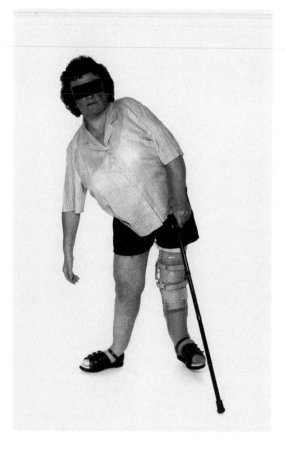

Figure 9.12 Lateral trunk sway and hip circumduction adopted to achieve foot clearance at midswing

of contact as for the conventional locked knee design of orthosis used for this group of patients.

Scott (1971) reported on a biomechanical evaluation of the FLLB, and stated that the 'combination of the partially weight bearing brim with the posteriorly offset knee joints is sufficient to stabilise a leg which was previously unstable at initial load application'.

This effect is illustrated diagrammatically in Figure 9.13 in which A_H is the component of the ground reaction force which is transmitted through the patient's leg, A_B is the component of the reaction force transmitted through the brace, and A is the resultant total support force whose line of action must pass through or in front of the anatomical knee joint axis for the knee to remain stable.

Immediately after heel contact the brace ankle joints permit free plantarflexion until foot-flat. Once rollover commences however, the resistance to dorsiflexion offered first by

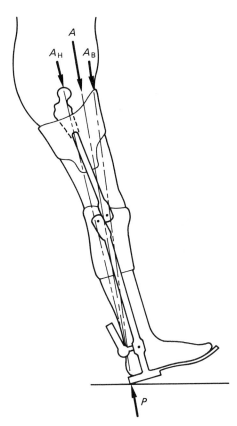

Figure 9.13 The mechanism whereby knee stability at heel contact is maintained in the functional long-leg brace

the hydraulic damper and then by the dorsiflexion stops causes the line of action of the ground reaction force to move forward, further enhancing knee stability. The orthotic requirement now is to protect the soft tissues on the posterior aspect of the knee from overstressing and damage due to the large external extension moment. This is achieved by virtue of the extension stops incorporated in the knee joints of the brace which result in a counter torque being generated between the upper section of the brace and the patient's thigh.

Regrettably this ingenious design of KAFO appears to have fallen from favour as there have been no recent reports of clinical experience of its use. Many orthotists continue to employ similar principles, utilizing both traditional and contemporary components and methods of construction with apparent success. The obvious advantage of this design of orthosis relates to the use of the free knee joints which allow the patient to flex the knee in a more normal fashion during the swing phase. Sometimes however it is necessary to employ a knee extension assist mechanism, usually an elastic cord or strap, to ensure that the knee is fully extended before heel contact. It should also be noted that this design of orthosis can only be used when a full passive range of knee extension is possible.

A variation in KAFO design for this category of impairment may be used when the patient's knee cannot be brought to full extension, either due to contracture or to bony deformity. In this situation the external knee flexion moment and the consequent orthotic contact forces required to prevent knee collapse will be significantly increased (Lehmann and Warren, 1976). This often results in intolerable pressures being generated at the limb–orthosis contact sites if the standard design of KAFO is used. The orthotic modification incorporated to deal with this situation uses an ischial weight-bearing thigh section combined with locking knee joints. During stance phase the ground reaction force is shared between the structure of the orthosis and the patient's leg. The consequent reduction in the external knee flexion moment applied to the leg results in a corresponding reduction in the magnitude of the orthosis–body counter forces required to resist this motion. Flexion of the orthosis is resisted by the locked knee joints but the associated increase in the external flexion moment applied to the orthosis requires the use of stronger and stiffer structural components.

(c) Alternative and complementary forms of treatment

Many more patients with spinal cord injuries rely upon wheelchairs for mobility than use orthoses. This is principally due to the lower energy consumption associated with wheelchair use. Wheelchair use does however have its disadvantages. At a practical level wheelchair users complain of problems of access and in particular of their restricted range of reach from the chair.

Advocates of orthotic use have drawn attention to the perceived physiological advantages of being able to stand upright. Considerations of respiratory, cardiovascular and urinary function are cited as reasons for holding this view, although there is little scientific evidence to support it. A recent study conducted in Salford (Ogilvie, 1991) did however report an apparent improvement in bone density which was attributed to orthotic use. At the present time the most practical solution for these patients would appear to be the shared use of some form of orthosis with an appropriate wheelchair.

When considering alternative treatments for patients with specific weakness of the knee extensors (in the presence of good functional hip muscles), a slightly different picture emerges and surgery does have a limited role to play in dealing with the problem of knee stability.

Knee arthrodesis, which results in a fused knee joint in a position of extension, is a well-established surgical procedure with few complications and a high success rate. The advantages of this procedure over the long-term use of an orthosis are obvious. The patient is spared the encumbrance of equipment and the time-consuming procedures involved in putting it on and taking it off. The main disadvantage of an arthrodesis is the inability to flex the knee for sitting and other activities. For this reason arthrodesis is normally only performed in those patients with a unilateral disability when a knee flexion deformity makes fitting a satisfactory orthosis difficult or when joint pain is not relieved by orthotic treatment.

9.3.2 Upper motor neurone lesions

Upper motor neurone lesions impair locomotor function through loss of the normal control of the lower limb muscles. Instead the hypertonic, more excitable muscles respond to a variety of stimuli leading to involuntary movements in a manner which is commonly referred to as 'spastic'. The pathological conditions which result in this situation include cerebral palsy, some head injuries and most commonly adult hemiplegia subsequent to a stroke or a cerebrovascular accident. The functional loss exhibited by this latter category of patients may be significantly increased by loss of sensation, proprioception and body image. Rehabilitation may be complicated by associated impairments to the patient's balance, vision and ability to communicate.

Orthotic treatment for these patients is designed to control the abnormal limb movements and thereby facilitate a more normal pattern of gait.

(a) Genu recurvatum in hemiplegia

The gait pattern of hemiplegic patients tends to be characterized by either a mass flexor or extensor response rather than the closely synchronized combination of flexion and extension required for normal function.

Individual patients exhibit widely varying abnormal patterns; however certain features arise frequently. For example, the hemiplegic patient may utilize a mass extensor response to achieve stance stability. This manoeuvre combines ankle plantarflexion and subtalar joint supination with extension of the knee (Figure 9.14(a)).

In order to avoid falling backwards, and in an attempt to achieve heel contact, the patient may flex his trunk anteriorly thereby bringing the line of action of the ground reaction force well in front of the anatomical knee joint axis, resulting in a large external knee extension moment (Figure 9.14(b)). If this pattern is not successfully corrected by physiotherapy these patients frequently develop a painful hyperextended knee, with pain felt both posteriorly due to the straining of the soft tissues normally responsible for limiting extension, and anteriorly due to impaction of the joint surfaces. A KAFO may therefore be prescribed to address these problems.

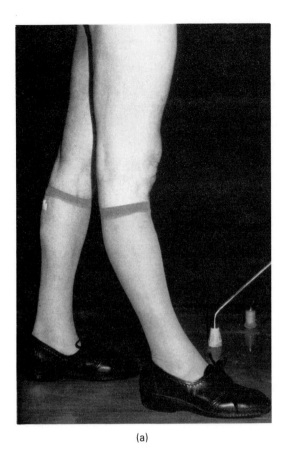

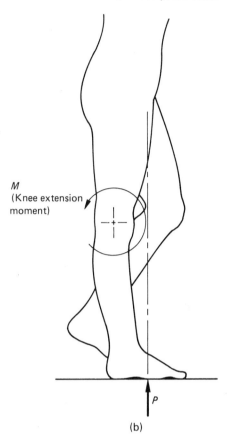

(a)

(b)

Figure 9.14 (a) Typical posture of hemiplegic patient at midstance. (b) Effect of this posture on the external knee moment

The force system necessary to achieve the required joint control is illustrated in Figure 9.15. If a conventionally fabricated design is employed this will entail the use of a posterior knee apron (Figure 9.16(a)).

If a contemporary design is utilized then the posterior surface of the below-knee section must be extended as high as possible, and the posterior surface of the above-knee section as low as possible, thus creating two complementary surfaces to provide the required anteriorly directed force (Figure 9.16(b)). Sufficient clearance must however be left between the adjacent posterior edges to allow at least 90° of knee flexion for the purposes of sitting.

The orthotic device must additionally incorporate orthotic knee joints which limit the knee extension to 175–180° while still permitting a near normal unrestricted range of knee flexion. This is achieved by using free joints with extension stops.

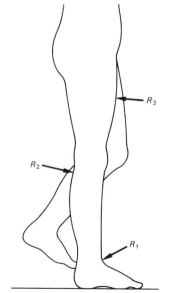

Figure 9.15 Three-force system required to prevent hyperextension of the knee

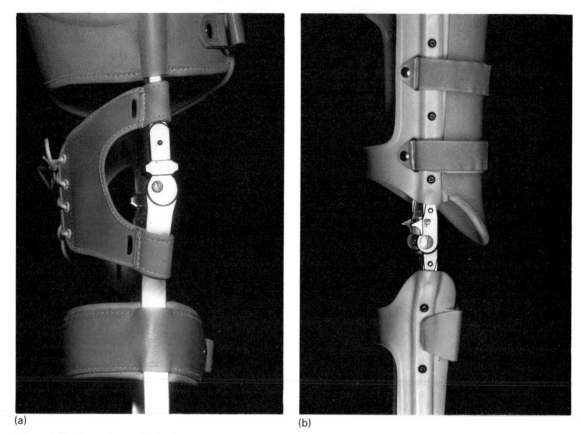

(a)   (b)

Figure 9.16 Alternative methods of providing the anteriorly directed force at the knee joint. (a) Posterior apron. (b) Extended posterior below-knee and above-knee sections of contemporary KAFO

Since spastic genu recurvatum is invariably associated with an abnormal equinovarus position of the ankle and foot, the KAFO design for this category of patient will normally include an orthotic ankle joint or the plastic below-knee section design necessary for the control of equinovarus as described in Chapter 7.

(b) Alternative and complementary forms of treatment

The management of the physical problems resulting from an upper motor neurone lesion such as a CVA will commonly entail the intensive use of therapy and drugs, and occasionally surgery. The objectives and indications for the use of these treatment methods have been discussed previously in Chapter 7.

However for the particular problem presented by a severe spastic genu recurvatum at

present (in 1992), there are no reliable practical alternatives to the use of a knee-ankle–foot orthosis.

9.3.3 Loss of structural integrity

The most common causes of impairment to the structural integrity of the knee joint are injuries to the main ligaments of the knee and joint disease, either inflammatory (rheumatoid arthritis) or degenerative (osteoarthritis). Injuries to the ligamentous structures of the knee may result in instability and on occasion pain during weight bearing. Damage to the articular surfaces of the joint will result in pain and ultimately instability or deformity due to bone loss, with associated secondary laxity of the ligaments which are as a consequence subjected to excessive loads.

The abnormal gait patterns exhibited by such patients may simply reflect the absent function of the affected tissues. For example, damage to the medial collateral ligament will result in a valgus instability of the knee joint during the stance phase of walking. In addition, patients may adopt compensatory gait deviations to obtain pain relief. For example, an asymmetric gait pattern will reduce the duration of weight bearing on the painful limb.

Many of these patients may be successfully treated orthotically using a knee orthosis as described in Chapter 8. Two groups however require a more extensive KAFO – those with severe genu recurvatum and those with severe genu varum or valgum.

Other causes of lower limb structural impairment which benefit from treatment using a KAFO include failed knee joint replacements and patients with delayed or non-union of a femoral fracture where the axial load bearing capacity of the limb is seriously compromised.

KAFOs may also have a role in the management of some hip disorders such as congenital dislocation and Perthes' disease.

The management objectives, biomechanical requirements and the means of achieving these with an orthosis will be described for each of these groups of conditions.

(a) Genu recurvatum

This condition commonly arises following injury to the posterior cruciate ligament and the posterior knee capsule (Figure 9.17). A similar situation may also arise following a prolonged period of walking with a hyperextended knee as used to achieve stability by patients with severe knee extensor weakness. In both cases, attempts to treat this condition using a simple knee orthosis are frequently unsuccessful due to the discomfort resulting from the high limb–orthosis contact forces. This problem may be overcome by using the much longer lever arms and larger limb contact areas of a KAFO to minimize these contact forces.

The force system and the orthotic structure required to treat this condition are identical to those already described in Section 9.3.2 for the treatment of spastic genu recurvatum in hemiplegia. In this instance, as ankle function is usually not impaired, free acting 'ankle joints' may be employed.

For those patients who exhibit knee extensor weakness also, the prevention of hyperextension may coincidentally prejudice knee stabil-

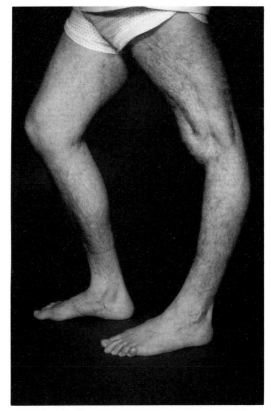

Figure 9.17 Genu recurvatum resulting from trauma to posterior soft tissues of the knee joint

ity. Any KAFO provided for such patients will therefore need to combine the features necessary to control knee extension with those necessary to maintain knee stability as described in section 9.3.1.

(b) Genu varum/valgum

During walking, the line of action of the ground reaction force passes to the medial side of the knee joint centre (Johnson *et al.*, 1990). The direct action of this force is resisted by the tibiofemoral joint surfaces, while the resulting adduction moment is resisted by both tension in the lateral collateral ligament and by the contraction of certain muscles, notably tensor fascia lata and the lateral hamstrings (Figure 9.18(a)).

Damage to the medial joint compartment, with resulting varus instability, will result in a concentration of the joint force on the damaged condyle. In addition the increased knee adduction moment will result in increased

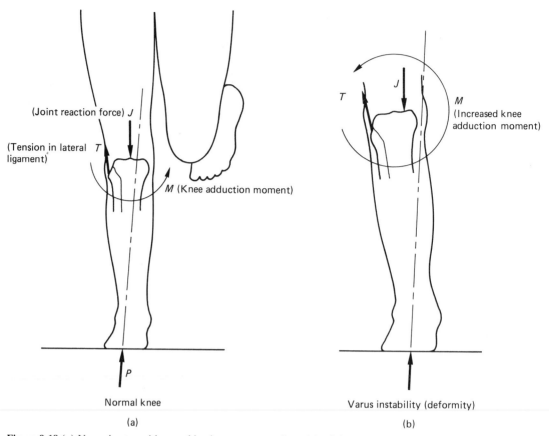

Figure 9.18 (a) Normal external knee adduction moment and resulting joint and ligament forces at midstance. (b) Increased external knee adduction moment and resulting joint and ligament forces occurring as a result of varus instability of the knee joint

tension on the lateral collateral ligament which may become overstressed (Figure 9.18(b)). Conversely damage to the lateral joint compartment will result in a concentration of pressure on this side of the joint, and, if the instability becomes severe, will result in an abduction moment about the knee joint thus placing the medial collateral ligament under stress.

Varus or valgus deformity of the knee, whether congenital in origin or acquired perhaps through trauma, will have a similar effect on the forces, the stresses at the joint surfaces and in the soft tissues.

This group of conditions illustrates very clearly the manner in which a deformity resulting from a structural impairment may create precisely the biomechanical conditions for the further deterioration of that condition. As the varus or valgus deformity or instability increases the damaging external moment will also simultaneously increase, leading to further

soft tissue damage and an even greater concentration of force at the joint surface resulting in further damage.

KAFOs may be used in all these situations to correct, as far as possible, the joint deformity and to resist any abnormal external joint moment. This will have the effect of redistributing the joint force and relieving the excessive tension in the soft tissues, thus achieving pain relief, delaying joint deterioration and permitting an improved level of patient mobility.

The force system required to achieve these objectives is illustrated in Figure 9.19. In all cases, to maximize the control exerted by the orthosis, it is recommended that the proximal and distal forces should be located as far apart as possible and the central force located as close as possible to the knee joint axis.

Once again variations exist in the method of application of the central stabilizing force. This may be achieved either by the use of a pad located at knee level on the appropriate below-

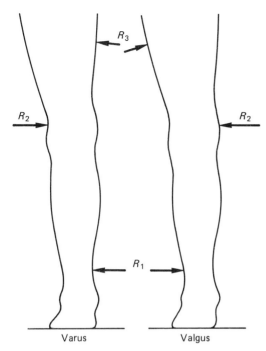

Figure 9.19 Three-force system required to control mediolateral knee instability

knee side bar, by the use of a leather knee apron wrapped around the appropriate femoral condyle and secured to the contralateral side bar, or by extending the edges of the above knee and below knee sections of the orthosis to bear against the appropriate femoral and tibial condyles (Figure 9.20).

The orthotic device will need to incorporate knee joints which resist abduction or adduction but which permit a normal range of flexion-extension when the knee range of extension is nearly normal. This may be achieved using free (posterior offset) knee joints with side bars of appropriate stiffness and strength.

A number of clinical situations may be identified which permit or require variations from this basic configuration.

First, where the alignment of the knee can be fully corrected in all planes, it may be possible in lighter weight patients to dispense with one of the knee joint/side bar assemblies without impairing the effectiveness of the orthosis as demonstrated by Nitschke (1971). (Figure 9.21).

Secondly, where it is not possible for the patient to fully extend their knee during weight

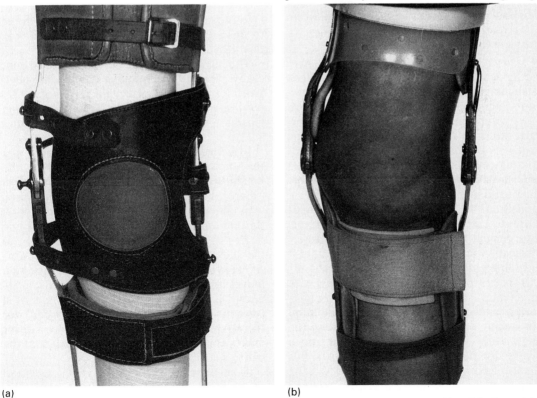

(a)   (b)

Figure 9.20 Alternative methods of providing the laterally directed force to control valgus instability of the knee. (a) Knee apron. (b) Extended above and below knee sections

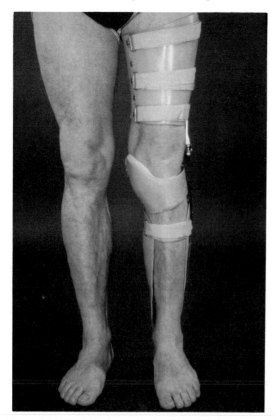

Figure 9.21 Nitschke single side bar KAFO for valgus instability of knee

bearing or to passively correct the varus/valgus malalignment fully, the resulting offset of the controlling forces, as viewed in a transverse plane, results in a couple which creates torsional stress in the orthotic device and may result in a buckling effect. This difficult problem may be alleviated by using locking knee joints and an orthotic device of increased torsional stiffness.

Finally, if the uncorrectable varus or valgus deformity exceeds approximately 10°, the orthotic contact forces required to resist further deformation may be unacceptably large resulting in intolerable pressure at the contact surfaces. The orthotic design required to deal with this situation will include an ischial weight-bearing above-knee section in combination with locking knee joints. As in the case of the patient with knee extension weakness and a knee flexion deformity (Section 9.3.1(b)), this weight-relieving orthosis functions by sharing the ground reaction force with the patient's leg. Chase (1989), in a comparative biomecha-

nical study of both ischial and non-ischial weight-bearing orthoses, demonstrated clearly that the significantly greater bending moments acting upon the ischial weight-bearing orthosis were associated with a reduction in the magnitude of the orthotic contact forces and pressures in the coronal plane.

(c) Loss of axial load bearing integrity

This form of structural impairment may be a consequence of either a joint or bony defect such as failure of a hip or knee joint replacement or a delayed or non-union of a femoral fracture. In either case the transmission of the axial force associated with normal physical activity to the limb skeleton may result in pain or axial or angular displacement, both of which may limit mobility.

A KAFO can be effectively employed to provide either partial or total relief from the axial component of the ground reaction force and hence prevent or reduce displacement and/or pain. The biomechanical requirements for such an orthosis comprise an axial load bearing area located proximal to the site of the skeletal defect and an orthotic structure capable of transmitting the ground reaction force to this area. The use of locking knee joints in this situation is therefore mandatory.

The orthortic weight-bearing area is generally created by employing either a moulded block leather thigh corset or a plastic quadrilateral shaped thigh section, these both being located under the ischial tuberosity (Figure 9.22).

Effective load relief generally requires that the orthotic structure is longer than the patient's leg, i.e. the distance from the ischial tuberosity to the bare heel. However, if used with either conventional 'free' ankle joints or a flexible plastic below-knee section, some degree of axial loading will still be applied to the skeleton when the ankle moves into dorsiflexion after midstance as the ground reaction moves forward onto the forefoot. Total continuous axial load relief requires the use of a cosmetically less acceptable 'patten end' for the KAFO which ensures that the foot never makes contact with the ground throughout the entire stance phase.

A number of investigators have reported experimental studies of the efficacy of weight-relieving KAFOs. Anderson (1977) in a study

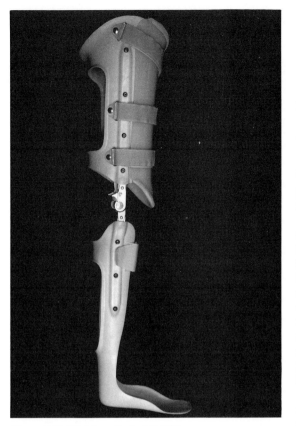

Figure 9.22 'Weight-relieving' KAFO

of static loading only, reported that using an orthosis equal in length to the patient's leg (as defined above) achieved a maximum of 50% relief of the axial load. Furthermore, it was stated that only when the orthosis was reduced to 78% of the leg length was the off-loading effect fully eliminated. Researchers at the University of Washington in a series of studies of this subject (Kirkpatrick *et al.*, 1969; Lehmann *et al.*, 1970; Lehmann and Warren, 1973) confirmed that optimum weight relief can only be obtained with the use of locked knee joints in conjunction with ankle dorsiflexion stops.

These studies also confirmed that since the unloading effect of the orthosis is achieved through a combination of the reaction of the brim of the orthosis with the tissues overlying the ischial tuberosity and the reaction of the thigh section of the orthosis with the soft tissues of the thigh, it was not possible with this design of orthosis to relieve the hip joint of all externally applied forces.

(d) Hip disorders

Congenital dislocation of the hip may exhibit up to three classical abnormalities:

1. Congenital hip dysplasia in which the acetabulum is shallow or flattened.
2. Congenital dislocation secondary to muscular or neuromuscular abnormality.
3. Congenital dislocation due to capsular laxity.

Optimum treatment is based on accurate early diagnosis, preferably during the first month of life.

Congenital hip dysplasia may require surgery to achieve effective reduction, followed by splintage for up to 6 months. Congenital dislocation of the hip due to capsular laxity is traditionally reduced manually and splinted for approximately 3 months. In both cases the objective of orthotic management is to place the femoral head in a position which allows the capsule of the joint to tighten up. This is most readily achieved by adopting a position of flexion, abduction and internal rotation of the hip.

A wide variety of orthotic designs have been developed to achieve this objective, ranging from the simple one-piece 'plastic nappy' or Stracathro (Craig) splint to the more sophisticated adjustable abduction type of device (Figure 9.23). All of these designs rely on a good fit, proximally to the pelvis or the trunk, and distally around the thigh, in providing the necessary controlling forces.

Perthes' disease (or osteochondritis of the hip) is a condition arising in childhood usually between the age of 5 and 10 years as a result of disturbance of the upper femoral epiphysis secondary to ischaemic necrosis. Initial symptoms include limping, pain and limitation of joint movements due to muscle spasm. There is considerable controversy about the treatment of Perthes' disease, but if orthotic treatment is prescribed, it is aimed at minimizing pressure on the hip joint which might cause deformation of its shape during the healing process. Such treatment may be used for as long as 4 years.

The resultant hip joint force during physical activity results from two sources. First, the direct effect of the ground reaction force transmitted to the joint surfaces and, secondly, the external hip joint moment (in both sagittal and coronal planes) which is resisted by contraction

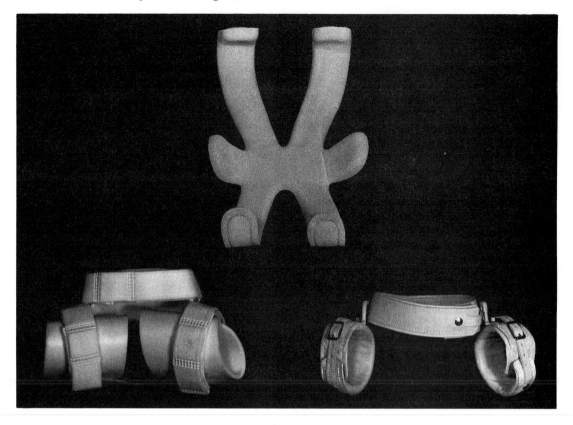

Figure 9.23 Orthoses for the management of congenital hip dysplasia

of the appropriate hip muscles. The resulting tension in these muscles causes a further increase in the hip joint resultant force. The joint pressure resulting from this force will be dependent on the area of joint contact.

In using KAFOs for the management of this condition it is necessary first to ensure that the femoral head is fully contained within the acetabulum, and secondly to provide relief of the hip joint forces arising during weight bearing.

To fulfil these orthotic objectives a weight-bearing orthotic above-knee section is required connected by rigid, normally unjointed, side bars to a patten end. The above-knee section is aligned so as to place the patient's hip joint in a position of abduction and medial rotation, ensuring maximum femoral head to acetabular congruence. Normally an outrigger is attached to the lateral side bar which maintains the leg in this position, while avoiding axial weight bearing by using a coil spring attachment (Figure 9.24).

Such an orthotic device will also inhibit contraction of the hip abduction muscles which, during normal walking, contribute significantly to the maximum joint force encountered at midstance.

Finally it should be emphasized that a number of orthopaedic surgeons disapprove of such an orthosis because its value is not proven and secondary shortening of the splinted leg due to failure to grow is a recognized complication.

(e) Alternative and complementary methods of treatment

Instability or severe deformity of the knee joint due to a loss of structural integrity can be treated surgically. In those cases of instability due to ligamentous insufficiency where the joint structure is otherwise intact, ligament replacement or augmentation procedures are appropriate. Surgery is usually followed by a carefully controlled rehabilitation period. A

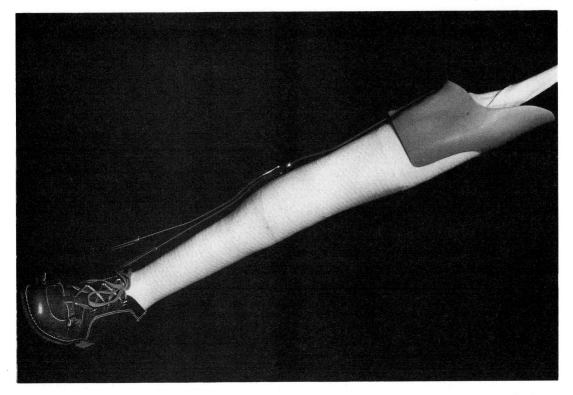

Figure 9.24 Orthosis for the management of Perthes' disease

return to contact sports is usually restricted until 1 year after surgery.

In those cases with extensive joint damage, in which pain is a feature, and when the axial load bearing capacity of the joint is seriously compromised, joint replacement may be the treatment of choice. If however there is also extensive soft tissue damage arthodesis may be the only option.

Recent advances in the materials and design of both knee joint and knee ligament replacement components have greatly increased the popularity and success of these procedures, thus dramatically reducing the numbers of patients requiring orthotic treatment.

Congenital dislocation of the hip which fails to respond to orthotic management is usually treated surgically. A wide range of procedures are employed, depending upon the particular pathology, ranging from simple adductor tenotomy to open reduction with more extensive operations such as femoral or pelvic osteotomies.

Regrettably there are as yet no proven alternative methods, surgical or otherwise, for the treatment of Perthes' disease.

9.4 Current and future developments

The design and function afforded by KAFOs has changed very little over the past 50 years. The single most notable change has been the introduction of thermoplastic materials, now used to replace leather and some of the metal components of KAFOs. This has resulted in a reduction in the weight, an improved cosmetic appearance and increased reliability of these orthoses. Additionally the improved fit attainable using these contemporary fabrication methods has increased their effectiveness. However their basic functions remain the same as their conventionally constructed predecessors.

At the present time there is little evidence of any significant development activity in the area of KAFO design. A recent review of the scientific literature (Condie, 1991) has revealed some research activity related to the analysis of the biomechanical functions of KAFOs, but no evidence of current initiatives aimed at improving KAFO function.

The reasons for this are easy to understand. The demand for KAFOs in the developed countries has unquestionably reduced during the past 10 years. The availability of an improved range of functional knee orthoses, the virtual elimination of poliomyelitis, continuing developments in pre- and post-natal screening, and in orthopaedic management especially in the field of ligament and joint replacement have all contributed to a reduction in the numbers of patients who require KAFOs.

It is obvious, however, that for a significant number of patients, KAFOs remain the preferred, if not the only possible, method of management. What therefore might be done to improve the function of the orthotic devices they receive?

The most glaring limitation of existing designs relates to the range of orthotic knee joints currently available. This is generally restricted to extension locking, limited motion and free motion joints. The biomechanical 'matching' between patient and device offered by this range of joints is particularly poor for those patients who require enhanced knee stability during stance but wish to flex their knee as normal to achieve ground clearance during swing. In the field of prosthetics a similar requirement is often provided for above-knee amputees by using one of a range of safety knees which resist flexion when loaded but are free to flex when unloaded. No reliable or suitable commercial orthotic knee joint has emerged at present which offers this function.

A further interesting development in the field of prosthetics is the ischial containment socket (ICS) which is rapidly supplanting the more traditional quadrilateral socket forms. This technique may have applications in the design of KAFOs intended to deal with a loss of structural integrity in the lower limb.

The use of KAFOs with paraplegic patients was referred to earlier in this chapter. The technique of functional electrical stimulation (FES) is well established in some parts of the world as a means of treating ankle–foot disorders in patients with upper motor neurone lesions. More recent experimental work has looked at applications of this technique for the paraplegic patient both in isolation and as part of a hybrid FES/orthotic system. Andrews and Bajd (1984) from the University of Strathclyde describe such a hybrid KAFO system designed for patients presenting with a combination of innervated and denervated muscles such as encountered in low thoracic and high lumbar lesions. A four-channel stimulator system is used in conjunction with bilateral knee orthoses incorporating locking knee joints which maintain knee extension for stance phase stability. Two channels are used to produce a contraction of the gastrocnemius muscles, causing plantarflexion of the ankle on the supporting side. The remaining two channels are employed to produce a flexion withdrawal reflex in the contralateral limb, resulting in combined ankle dorsiflexion and hip flexion thereby initiating a step. This arrangement results in a straight-leg tip-toe form of four-point gait. On the basis of this experience, it would appear reasonable to explore the practicality of applying such a hybrid approach to improving the orthotic treatment of patients with other upper motor neurone lesions, such as strokes and multiple sclerosis, in which the patient has difficulty in initiating an effective swing phase with a resulting loss of gait safety and efficiency.

In conclusion there are a number of potential avenues for the improvement of KAFO designs, but the reducing number of patients currently assessed as suitable for orthotic treatment of this type means that further development is likely to be slow in emerging.

References

Abou Ghaida H.I., Hull M.L. and Rab G.T. (1987–88) An instrumented brace for study of Legg–Calve–Perthes disease. *Biomater. Artif. Cells Artif. Organs* **15**, 719–735

Anderson E.G. (1977) The axial loading on a static knee–ankle–foot orthosis. *J. Med. Eng. Technol.* **1**, 100–102

Anderson M.H. and Bray J.H. (1964) The UCLA functional long leg brace. *Clin. Orthop.* **37**, 98–109

Andrews B.J. and Bajd T. (1984) Hybrid orthoses for paraplegics. In: *Proceedings of the 8th International Symposium on External Control of Human Extremities, Dubrovnik, Yugoslavia* (suppl.), 55–59, ETAN, Belgrade

Chase A. (1989) Biomechanical Considerations and Orthotic Prescription for Osteoarthritic Knees. Master of Philosophy Thesis, Department of Engineering, Oxford Polytechnic

Condie D.N. (1991) Lower limb orthotics. *Curr. Opin. Orthop.* **2**, 838–841

Granata C., De Lollis A., Campo G. *et al.* (1990) Analysis, design and development of a carbon fibre reinforced plastic ankle–foot orthosis prototype for myopathic patients. *J. Eng. Med.* **204H**, 91–96

Johnson F., Leitl S. and Waugh W. (1980) The distribution of load across the knee – a comparison of static and dynamic measurements. *J. Bone Joint Surg.* **62B**, 346–348

Kirkpatrick G.S., Day E.E. and Lehmann J.F. (1969) Investigation of the performance of an ischial load bearing leg brace. *Exp. Mech.* **9**, 31–35

Lehmann J.F. and Warren C.G. (1973) Ischial and patella tendon bearing braces: function, design, adjustment and training. *Bull. Prosthet. Res.* **10**, (19), 6–19

Lehmann J.F. and Warren C.G. (1976) Restraining forces in various designs of knee–ankle orthoses: their placement and effect on the anatomical knee joint. *Arch. Phys. Med. Rehabil.* **57**, 430–437

Lehmann J.F., Warren C.G., DeLateur B.J. *et al.* (1970) Biomechanical evaluation of axial loading in ischial weight-bearing braces of various designs. *Arch. Phys. Med. Rehabil.* **51**, 331–335

Merkel K.D. *et al.* (1984) Energy expenditure of paraplegic patients standing and walking with two knee– ankle–foot orthoses. *Arch. Phys. Med. Rehabil.* **65**, 121–124

Merkel K.D., Merritt J.L. and Miller N.E. (1981) Energy expenditure comparison in paraplegic patients during stance and ambulation with two types of knee–ankle–foot orthoses. *Arch. Phys. Med. Rehabil.* **62**, 513

Nitsche R.O. (1971) A single-bar above-knee orthosis. *Orthot. Prosthet.* **25**, (4), 20–25

Ogilvie C. (1991) An Investigation into the Energetic and Physical Effects of Aided Ambulation for Severely Disabled People. MD thesis, University of Leeds

Rodillo E.B., Fernandez-Bermejo E., Heckmatt J.Z. *et al.* (1988) Prevention of rapidly progressive scoliosis in Duchenne muscular dystrophy by prolongation of walking with orthoses. *J. Child Neurol.* **3**, 269–274

Scott C.M. (1971) *Functional Long Leg Brace Research.* Final Report. University of California, Prosthetics/ Orthotics Education Program, Los Angeles

Trappitt A.E. and Berme N. (1981) A transducer for the measurement of lower limb orthotic loads. *Eng. Med.* **10**, 149–153

Tuck W.H. (1974) The Stanmore cosmetic caliper. *J. Bone Joint Surg.* **56B**, 115–120

Yates G. (1968) A method for the provision of lightweight aesthetic orthopaedic appliances. *Orthopaedics* **1**, 153–162

10

Hip–knee–ankle–foot orthoses

John Stallard

10.1 Introduction

Devices which fall into the hip–knee–ankle–foot orthosis (HKAFO) category have a wide diversity of use and as a result are rich in the variety of their design. The functions for which they are used range from effective reciprocal walking, through control of limb movement, to complete immobilization of the lower limbs. First discussion will focus on some general pathological considerations and biomechanical requirements which are more widely applicable and therefore require to be dealt with separately. Next orthoses intended for paraplegic patients which are a specialized area are explored separately, and finally the orthoses which provide a more conventional control function are presented.

10.2 Pathological considerations

The principal pathological conditions for which HKAFOs are provided are complete or incomplete paraplegia. These may be traumatic or acquired in nature, or congenital lesions such as myelomeningocele. HKAFOs may also be prescribed for neurological conditions such as cerebral palsy, spinal muscular atrophy, muscular dystrophy and multiple sclerosis.

From the biomechanical point of view these pathologies present a variety of challenges. For the purposes of clarity, paraplegia is defined as a complete lesion at L1 or above, which leads to there being no motor power available at or below the hip. In the case of myelomeningocele the pathological lesions are commonly patchy with residual muscle function and attendant imbalances in the moments generated about the joints by this residual motor power. There is also an added complication that there is often uneven lateral distribution of motor control.

With the muscle weakening atrophies and dystrophies (and the now uncommon poliomyelitis), it is sometimes necessary to provide supplementary support of joints and later, as the weakness increases, full stabilization of joints where motor power has deteriorated to a stage where it is totally ineffective. The muscle dystrophies present the additional problem of good sensation, with the attendant difficulty of ensuring patient comfort as well as safe interface pressures.

In the majority of conditions which cause paraplegia at the level of the hip, the patient will have the added complication of incontinence. This presents difficulties in toileting and the accommodation of stoma bags. Some younger patients may use nappies, resulting in variable geometry in the region of one of the major orthotic support points. Whichever approach is adopted in dealing with this problem there is a need to provide a means of accommodating the clothing and appliances used within the orthotic structure. The patient must also be able to adjust his or her geometry within the orthosis and, if necessary, to discard the orthosis in order to cope with the difficulties of toileting. Self catheterization can present problems for a female patient with a hip orthosis, since it is necessary to be able to abduct the hip at least a little. In paraplegia adduction/abduction of the hip is a movement which requires to be controlled by the orthosis.

Cerebral palsy patients are rarely treated with HKAFO but they do have a role occasionally in the treatment of ataxic or athetoid conditions. A complication in providing an orthosis for this condition is the potential for triggering stretch reflexes either by surface contact or as a result of orthotic resistance. Care must always be exercised in the provision of an orthosis for such a patient and should only be supplied as part of an overall treatment plan.

10.3 Objectives of orthotic management in paraplegia

The general objective of bracing at the hip level is to permit a patient to stand or ambulate. In a few cases the requirement may be to stabilize the hips to improve sitting posture. Bearing in mind the degree of handicap associated with limited or no hip control which requires orthotic assistance, it is reasonable to question the relevance of walking or standing for such patients. Most are able to use wheelchairs very effectively and it is clearly impractical to expect that walking for the very heavily handicapped patient will approach the level of efficiency of locomotion which can be achieved using their wheelchair. Orthotic ambulation is intended to supplement the use of a wheelchair, not to replace it, with the underlying aims being:

1. To provide therapeutic benefit.
2. To improve the level of independence.

10.3.1 Therapeutic benefit from use of a HKAFO

The clinical experience of many professionals involved in the care of these patients is that ambulation does have therapeutic benefits and these have been commented on by a number of authors (Carroll, 1974; Menelaus, 1980; Rose, 1980). These perceived benefits are:

1. An improvement in bowel function.
2. An improvement in urinary drainage.
3. An improvement in peripheral circulation.
4. A reduction in osteoporosis.

Others are sceptical about these benefits and there has until recently been scant research evidence produced to support or dispel the differing views. One of the major difficulties has been the relatively small numbers of patients available for clinical trials and problems in carrying out such studies. In order to produce a control group against which comparisons may be made, patients must either be denied treatment which their clinician believes to be beneficial, or have it imposed when the belief is that it is a distraction from other treatments which are thought to be more beneficial.

Fortunately researchers are now beginning to investigate more scientifically the degree to which orthotic walking results in measurable therapeutic effects. The ethical problem of establishing a control group was solved by collaboration between two separate clinical teams in different countries who had differing views on the treatment of high level paraplegia. Mazur *et al.* (1989) compared 36 matched pairs of patients in two separate clinics, one group having received a vigorous walking treatment programme from an early age, the other having received a programme which concentrated on teaching independence in a wheelchair, but with no walking. In following up these patients between the ages of 12 and 20 they showed that the non-ambulators had twice as many fractures and five times the number of pressure sores. In addition, the ambulators proved to be more adept in a number of specific transfer tasks. To achieve these advantages the ambulant group had on average one additional hospital admission with eight additional days' hospitalization. The conclusion of the authors was that this was a small price to pay for the advantages gained.

10.3.2 Improvement in level of independence with a HKAFO

The second aim of orthotic ambulation – improvement of independence – requires careful definition. Since improved independence is not an exclusive objective of those who provide HKAFO devices, it is necessary to define it specifically in relation to ambulation. In this context independence requires patients to achieve:

1. Comparatively low energy walking. Essentially this means that patients must walk through self-motivation. If not they will discard the device when they are outside the confines of direct clinical observation and will therefore neither receive therapeutic nor any other benefit from ambulation.
2. An ability to put on and take off the orthosis without any assistance.
3. An ability to transfer from sitting to standing and vice versa when wearing the orthosis.

Each of these achievements is worth having in its own right but, unless all three can be achieved, patients will not be able to undertake of their own volition those tasks which require them to stand and walk. These include the use of working surfaces intended for the able bodied, and socializing on the same level as others who are standing.

The extent to which these two aims of ambulation can be achieved will vary depending on the degree of disability and the motivation of the patient. It is not realistic to expect every patient to achieve full independence and to ambulate in a community situation. However, the more easily and quickly the requirements of independence can be achieved, the more likely those helping individual patients will find the time to provide the necessary help. Mothers of handicapped children in particular are very busy people and cannot always spare the time to apply orthoses which are excessively time consuming to put on.

10.4 Biomechanical requirements in paraplegia

In order to achieve the objectives of orthotic management with HKAFOs when ambulation is the principal aim, it is necessary to satisfy the mechanical requirements for any form of walking, normal or handicapped (Rose, 1980). These are:

1. Stabilization of the multisegmental structure of the body.
2. Injection of propulsive forces.
3. Control of the forces used for stabilization and propulsion.

10.4.1 Stabilization of the multisegmental structure of the body

For external stabilization of a flail limb it has been shown (see Chapter 2) that each joint requires three-point fixation in the plane of movement. The factors which affect the magnitude of these forces are the degree of flexion (or extension) since this will determine the moment arm through which forces act, and the spacing between the externally applied stabilization forces. Consequently the aim in applying an HKAFO will be to hold the limbs and trunk in as good alignment as possible to minimize the moments, and to keep the stabilizing forces as far apart as possible to reduce the contact forces on the orthosis.

Orthoses which are intended to control or support the hip may do so in isolation, but more commonly they are designed to incorporate other elements which control or support the ankle and hip. When a combination of controls is required, the principles which apply in the design of AFOs and KAFOs (as described in Chapters 7 and 9) will still be relevant to those parts of the orthosis intended to control the ankle and the knee.

Although the area available for applying forces around the hip is much greater than for most other locations on the body, care must still be taken to ensure that the forces are distributed as evenly as possible in order to minimize interface pressures and reduce the risk of pressure sores. With paraplegic conditions there is particular danger because of urinary incontinence and areas of anaesthetic skin.

To provide external stabilization the vertical alignment of the centre of gravity of the body must lie within the support area of the paraplegic patient. Normal subjects have sufficient control to constantly readjust their position and thus the vertical alignment of their centre of gravity, which enables them to maintain excellent external stabilization within a very small area (Figure 10.1(a)). However, if the body is braced because the control mechanisms are absent, this facility no longer exists and a much larger support area is then required. One of the many functions of crutches is to provide that increase in support area (Figure 10.1(b)).

The means of achieving stabilization are fundamental and the same basic principles apply to all orthoses. By contrast the means of

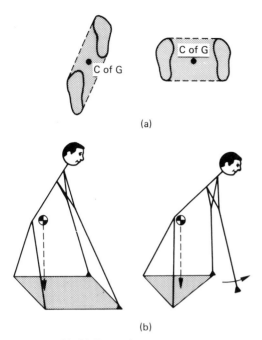

Figure 10.1 (a),(b) External support areas

achieving propulsion vary according to the design characteristics of that particular orthosis (Stallard *et al.*, 1989).

10.4.2 Propulsion and control

The precise method of ambulation offered to each individual will depend on the pathology, the biomechanical conditions which apply, the motivation and the objectives of the patient. In choosing a system it is necessary to assess each individual for all the elements which are necessary for effective walking to be achieved. The main factors to be considered are:

1. How will independence be achieved: putting on and taking off the orthosis and transferring to and from wheelchair and bed.
2. The energy cost of walking.
3. Where ambulation is to be undertaken.
4. The reliability of the orthosis from the points of view of both safety and maintenance.
5. The cost of the orthosis, including the initial hardware and training, follow-up and routine maintenance.
6. The appearance of the walking style, the orthosis, additional walking aids and the ability to disguise the use of the orthosis.

How ambulation is achieved will fundamentally affect the design of the HKAFO. Walking for paraplegic patients falls into three different categories:

1. Swing-through, swing-to or drag-to gait.
2. Swivel walking.
3. Reciprocal ambulation.

With a swing-through gait the patient uses his or her crutches or a walking aid to raise their whole body free from the ground and swing it forward. When the swing phase is restricted it is known as a swing-to gait. A further variation is to drag the feet forward along the ground, and this is sometimes known as a drag-to gait. It is not necessary (and can be a disadvantage) to have the legs separately braced because they are not called upon to move relative to each other in the swing-through, swing-to or drag-to gait. The advantage of the swing-through style is that it is relatively quick, but it has a high energy demand and is not a very stable form of walking. Because the weight of the orthosis must be lifted by the patient during each gait cycle, the lighter the orthosis the better.

In *Swivel walking* the patient causes ambulation by rocking and/or rotating the trunk to induce inertial reactions through an external frame, which imparts alternate rocking and swivelling motions to a mechanism located beneath the baseplate of the device. The details of the propulsive mechanism vary according to the individual designs of device. The advantages of this system are that it is easy to ambulate and requires no other crutches or walking aids. The orthosis – a swivel walker – allows for activities which require patients to be upright, have their hands free and provides limited mobility. However, these devices can only be used effectively on flat surfaces and provide relatively slow ambulation.

Reciprocal walking is a style of ambulation which results in the patient placing one leg in front of the other, the main propulsive forces being injected by the arms through crutches or other walking aids. The precise means by which this is done will vary according to individual designs of device. It is essential for the functioning of these orthoses that the legs are braced individually because they must move relative to one another. The advantages of this style of walking are that it is more attractive than either of the previous two methods, is quicker than swivel walking with lower energy consumption and has greater inherent stability than swing-through gait. Its disadvantages are that it requires a greater level of patient training and the structural design on the orthosis is more demanding requiring sufficient strength to avoid breakages and a mechanism to permit the reciprocal movements. This is a particular problem in the heavier patient.

10.5 Orthotic designs for paraplegia

10.5.1 Orthoses and aids for swing-through gait

(a) General considerations

In swing-through gait, ambulation is achieved by using crutches or walking frame to lift the whole body and swing it forwards. This form of locomotion is used by many groups of patients and clearly does not require HKAFOs where lower limb control at and below the hips is intact. For normal subjects research has shown that swing-through gait is, on average, 25% slower than normal walking and the heart rate is increased by 20–30 beats min^{-1} (Sankarankutty *et al.*, 1979). Clearly it is a high energy form of walking, and becomes even more so with an increase in the extent of the lower limb paralysis. When hip control is totally absent, HKAFOs are essential for this form of ambulation. In almost all cases the orthosis is designed to resist all movements of the hips, knees and frequently the ankles, and as a consequence the use of hip extension and flexion to improve the range of stride length is prevented. The HKAFO also minimizes the input of momentum, which is such an important feature of swing-through gait in normal subjects.

Few patients requiring this degree of support are effective swing-through ambulators, but these patients, with their crutches or walking frame, can mobilize over a variety of surfaces although only for a short walking distance.

The stresses which occur in HKAFOs during swing-through gait can be considerable. Vertical ground reaction forces are above those for normal walking and for two feet landings can be around 38% higher (Stallard *et al.*, 1978).

A number of devices which have been designed to allow patients to perform this type of gait are described below.

(b) Conventional HKAFO

This type of device (Figure 10.2) (Herzog and Sharrard, 1966; DHSS, 1980) uses traditional orthotic structures attached to a pelvic band to stabilize the hips, knees and ankles.

Conventional devices are usually manufactured from steel components for strength. Pelvic and thoracic bands are constructed from relatively thin metal in order to reduce the weight of the orthosis. This inevitably diminishes its structural rigidity, particularly in the lateral plane, with a consequent reduction in stability and thus an increase in the overall energy cost to the user.

In conventional devices the means of attachment are usually leather straps and buckles which are sited at chest, sacral, thigh, knee and ankle level. Having so many straps presents great difficulties for patients who wish to be independent in doffing and donning the orthosis. A further problem is the spur and

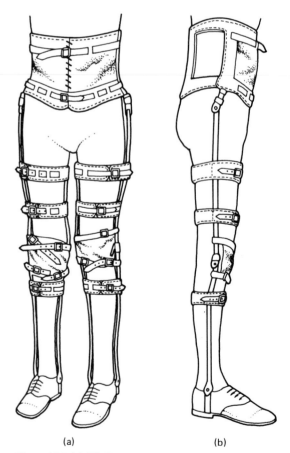

(a)   (b)

Figure 10.2 (a),(b) Conventional body brace calipers

socket location of calipers in shoes which can be very difficult to release unless the spur is exceedingly loose in the socket.

Whilst conventional HKAFOs do have a number of problems in providing a fully effective form of swing-through gait, they have the significant advantage of being readily available. In the absence of more sophisticated solutions they do allow well-motivated patients a degree of useful ambulation.

(c) Parapodium

An ingenious design, known as the Parapodium (Figure 10.3) (Motloch, 1971), typifies a more modern approach to the provision of orthotic stabilization of the hips, knees and ankles. It addresses the problems of independence, the need for rigidity, strength and ease of manufacture whilst using materials which minimize the weight of the orthosis and consequent energy cost of swing-through gait. The structure is made up of a number of modular components (a popular current trend) and

splints the lower limbs side by side. An aluminium alloy baseplate supports the feet and provides a large support area. Attached to this baseplate are brackets into which are located tubular side members which are free to rotate about the vertical axis. Joints are inserted in the vertical tubes at knee and hip level, their axes being horizontal. The side members are braced by knee-bar and sacral band assemblies through bearing brackets for the tubular side members. This arrangement allows a simple means of simultaneously locking and unlocking the hip and knee joints by rotating the side members. With the joint axes pointing forwards the joints are locked. When rotated 90° using the hinged handles on the side members, the hip and knee joint axes lie in the lateral plane and are free to hinge, thus allowing the patient to sit.

A further important feature of this design is the reduction of support points to an absolute minimum. The feet are held in position on the baseplate by a spring-loaded clamp arrangement. In addition to providing structural cross-

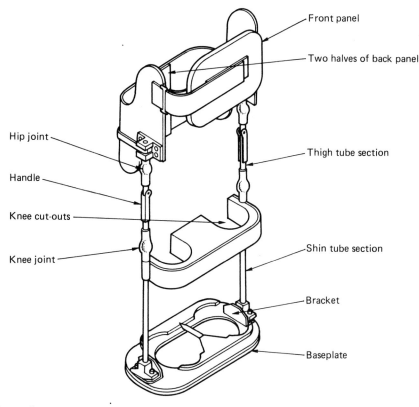

Figure 10.3 Parapodium

bracing, the knee assembly has a closed cell plastic insert which is cut to fit the patient's knees to act as a support point. Sacral band cross-bracing is shaped to pass to the rear of the patient and is plastic lined to give a sacral support point. It is also extended upwards to provide an attachment for the leather thoracic support band. This arrangement reduces the forces required to achieve complete stabilization to four (Rose and Henshaw, 1972). In addition to easing the manufacture of the kit, this minimizes the number of fastenings to be managed by the patient and therefore increases the likelihood that doffing and donning would be achieved independently. Also, as the support points are spaced as far apart as possible the stabilizing forces are reduced to the minimum necessary for each patient.

(d) Other devices

Conventional body brace and calipers and the Parapodium represent the two ends of the spectrum of devices available for swing-through gait. Variations in the design of either are clearly possible and a number are manufactured and fitted to patients. The concept of total body stabilization by means of four-point fixation which was embodied in the Parapodium has been employed in a number of other HKAFO devices and standing frames and is now widely accepted as an efficient and effective approach.

10.5.2 Swivel walking

(a) General considerations

A recognition of the high energy cost of swing-through gait led to a search for alternative forms of ambulation for patients with a total lack of hip control. Research carried out in a number of centres concentrated on mechanisms to enable paraplegic children to ambulate. Speilrein (1963) and Hall (1962) in particular described mechanisms which would result in forward motion from sideways rocking movements of the patient. These mechanisms involved swivelling components mounted on the footplates of a parapodium type of device and thus the generic term swivel walker was coined. Initially these devices achieved some success with amelic children, but their potential for providing an effective means of ambula-

tion for the growing numbers of spina bifida children was recognized by Motloch and Elliott (1966), Edbrooke (1970), and Rose and Henshaw (1972) amongst others. As their success grew a number of important variations became available.

(b) Clinical considerations

When first introduced swivel walkers were used as a primary means of ambulation for all groups of patients within the category of complete paralysis at or above the level of L1. More recent developments which have resulted in such patients achieving reciprocal walking has diminished the numbers requiring swivel walkers. Nevertheless there are three groups for whom swivel walkers are particularly suited:

1. *Very young patients.* Starting at the age of 1 year, swivel walkers can be used until sufficient upper limb coordination has developed to use crutches or walking frames. This seems to vary between 3 and 5 years.
2. *Very heavily handicapped patients.* Swivel walkers are useful for those with upper limb involvement including hemiplegia or tetraplegia up to a complete C6 level who cannot use crutches or walking frames. They can also be used for patients with significant deformity, provided they are fitted carefully. Low intelligence is not considered a contraindication (Butler *et al.*, 1982).
3. *Functional users.* Swivel walkers can be very valuable in situations in which patients with good upper limb function require only limited mobility but need to perform tasks in the upright position with free use of the hands. Cooking, woodwork, science lessons are typical examples.

Because it is such an easy device in which to ambulate it can be used by a wide age range of patients, with the old as well as the very young being able to cope with the system.

(c) Contraindications

Whilst swivel walkers can be used in all forms of paraplegia there are situations in which they are inappropriate. The main contraindications against their use are:

1. *Severe athetosis*. The strong involuntary upper limb movements associated with this condition can produce sufficient inertial reaction to overcome the inherent external stabilization afforded by the footplates of a swivel walker and cause the user to fall.
2. *Severe spinal deformity*. Swivel walkers are not intended to provide spinal support. Where spinal problems exist they should be treated with the relevant separate spinal orthosis (see Chapter 13). A spinal orthosis may be worn when using a swivel walker, but when the patient has a residual spinal deformity which cannot be comfortably supported in a swivel walker, or a deformity produces a significant displacement of the patient's centre of gravity, then the swivel mechanism cannot be evenly operated and ambulation is an unrealistic ambition.
3. *Severe hip and knee contractures*. Knee contractures in excess of 20° and hip contractures in excess of 40° cannot normally be accommodated in a swivel walker. Lesser degrees of hip flexion contracture can be accommodated if the patient has a compensatory lordosis.

(d) Swivel walker mechanics

Most swivel walker designs are based on the use of twin footplates mounted underneath a patient support structure (Figure 10.4). Stabilization of the patient is achieved through the four-point force system (as described for the Parapodium) with locations at feet, knees, hips and thorax. The footplates provide both external stabilization for the patient and a means of transmitting controlled propulsive forces so that ambulation can be achieved without the use of other aids such as crutches. When standing, the width of the support area between the inner edges of the footplates is small to facilitate easy lateral rocking, but the potential support area afforded by the inclined footplates is large which ensures good external stability.

To ambulate (Figure 10.5) the patient rocks alternately onto each footplate by making use of the inertial reaction (I) as the trunk contacts the supporting framework of the swivel walker. This in itself will not produce forward or backward motion, but three mechanisms can translate this sideways rocking into forward motion.

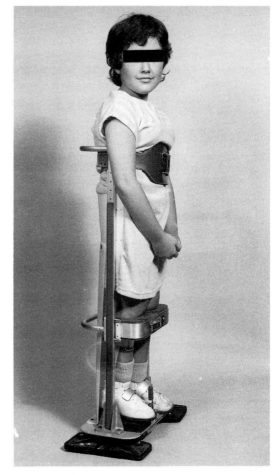

Figure 10.4 ORLAU Swivel Walker

1. *Gravitational propulsion*. The centre of mass of the system is arranged to fall slightly forward of the footplate-bearing centre so that the device is biased towards forward motion. When inclined to one side, a component of the weight, K (Figure 10.5), will cause a moment about the bearing centre tending to cause forward movement.
2. *Inertial reaction*. The inertial reaction force I used to rock onto the footplate can also produce a torque about the bearing centre, but the direction of this can be controlled by the patient so that either forward or backward motion can be selected (Figure 10.5). In the normal standing position a sideways thrust will produce a line of inertial reaction in front of the footplate-bearing centre and therefore a forward turning moment. By thrusting slightly backwards the patient can

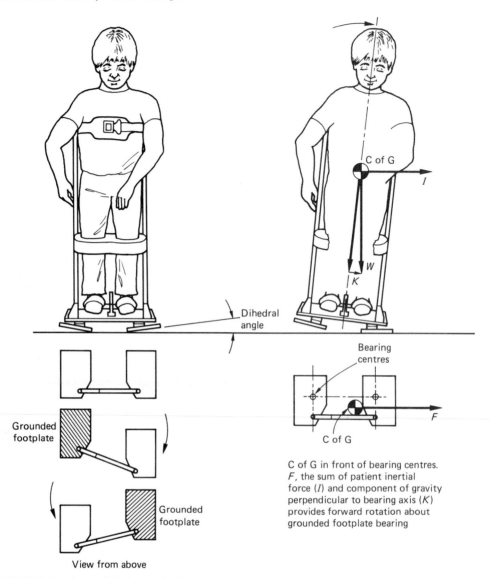

Dihedral angle

Grounded footplate

Grounded footplate

View from above

Bearing centres

C of G

C of G in front of bearing centres. *F*, the sum of patient inertial force (*I*) and component of gravity perpendicular to bearing axis (*K*) provides forward rotation about grounded footplate bearing

Figure 10.5 Swivel walker ambulation mechanics

produce an inertial reaction behind the bearing centre in order to walk backwards.
3. *Inertial torque*. More active patients also swing their arms in opposite directions and this produces an inertial torque, increasing the rotational effect produced by (2) above.

Whilst the footplates are most commonly constrained by a linking bar to move parallel to each other, an arrangement in which each footplate moves individually and is spring loaded to return to the forward alignment is possible and is sometimes preferred. There seems to be little difference in operating efficiency. Speedy operation of the spring-loaded footplates can however cause one to jam in the internally rotated position when returning to the ground and might cause a slightly unstable individual to fall.

The spacing between the footplate bearing centres does have an effect on patient ambulation performance. The closer together they are the easier it will be to rock onto alternate footplates, but there will be a consequent disadvantage – a shortening of the step length for each rocking action. Widening the bearing centres will improve step length at the cost of making it less easy to rock. Clearly there is an optimum spacing in relation to patient height. A series of tests on one child has suggested that the optimum spacing between bearing centres should be one-fifth of body height (Stallard *et al.*, 1986a).

(e) Design examples

The ORLAU Swivel Walker

This device (Figure 10.4) was developed by ORLAU (Butler *et al.*, 1982; Farmer *et al.*, 1982; Stallard *et al.*, 1986a). The design philosophy was to provide maximum independence in doffing, donning and transferring within a highly rigid structure, to maximize efficiency of ambulation, and to be so strong that it would withstand considerable maltreatment. In order to achieve this the design ideals are compromised as it is heavier, but since this only marginally affects ambulation for the patient (swivel walking requires the device only to be rocked – not lifted) it produces only a small additional inconvenience for parents or friends – not the patient.

A method of achieving independent doffing, donning and transferring was an important feature of this design. The device incorporates a chute to enable the patient to slide into the device (Stallard *et al.*, 1986a), together with easily operated fastenings.

The Salford Swivel Walker

This device (Figure 10.6) was developed at Salford University (Rose and Henshaw, 1972; Griffiths *et al.*, 1980; Rocca and Hopkins, 1978). The design philosophy was to produce as lightweight a structure as possible but with a high degree of rigidity to give efficient ambulation. Conventional straps at the knees can be adjusted for height and are lightweight. A central 'A' frame between the legs ensures secure fixation of the straps and assists the integrity of the lightweight structure. The device is lightweight, which eases handling when off the patient. As a consequence it is less robust than the ORLAU Swivel Walker and less able to withstand maltreatment.

Independence can be achieved by some patients who are able to doff and don the orthosis on the floor and then use wall bars or

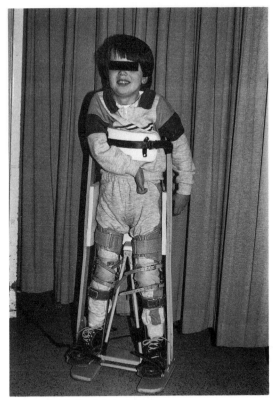

Figure 10.6 Salford Swivel Walker

other suitable apparatus to climb into the upright position.

Both these swivel walkers are comparable in performance, provided they have been correctly set up. Both incorporate features which allow minor variations in vertical alignment of the patient in order to adjust the position of the centre of gravity for best walking mechanics.

There are now a range of swivel walkers which have been designed around these well-established principles.

10.5.3 Reciprocal walking

(a) General considerations

Because of the high energy cost of swing-through gait and the restrictions inherent in swivel walking, devices have been developed which permit patients with no control of the lower limbs (primarily those with complete spinal lesions at or above L1) to ambulate reciprocally. This is a form of walking in which one leg is placed sequentially in front of the other (as in normal walking). Such a method enables patients to take body weight through the stance leg, therefore providing a potential for reducing energy cost. It is inevitable that systems of this type will require additional walking aids (e.g. crutches or walking frames) for stability and to input propulsion forces. However, when mastered, the design should enable the patient to walk over a variety of surfaces including slopes and undulations, and might permit the use of steps, etc. When successfully achieved, this style of ambulation is much closer to normal than any of the alternatives previously discussed and is perceived by many as being cosmetically much more appealing.

(b) Clinical considerations

Reciprocal walking systems demand the input of quite large forces from the upper limbs which must be carefully controlled in both direction and relative timing. It follows therefore that patients must have good upper limb strength and coordination, a reasonable degree of cardiovascular fitness and a level of intelligence which allows them to understand detailed physiotherapy instructions. A good range of hip movement on both sides is an absolute requirement. Flexion contractures of hips and knees are a disadvantage but not an absolute contraindication (depending on the system). If these are greater than 10–15° then reciprocal walking will be difficult or impossible. An increase in the patient's weight and height inevitably diminishes the efficiency of ambulation, but the ability of individual patients and orthotic systems to cope with this varies so greatly that it is impossible to set sensible limits to these. Spinal deformities can be a problem and these require individual clinical assessment. Severe scoliosis and kyphosis are contraindications to reciprocal walking.

(c) Mechanics of reciprocal walking

Reciprocal walking includes three essential features:

1. The 'swing leg' must be cleared from the ground.
2. The 'swing leg' must pivot forwards from relative hip extension to hip flexion.

3. The trunk must be progressed forwards over the stance leg from hip flexion to extension.

For normal subjects with an intact neuromuscular system this is achieved quite naturally with little apparent effort. However, where there is no control of the lower limbs, reciprocal walking demands carefully designed orthotic systems and associated patient training in order to prevent frustratingly high levels of effort for those patients who wish to adopt this form of walking.

All three elements of reciprocal walking require specific force inputs from the upper limbs (Major *et al.*, 1981), and although the exact nature of these will vary from one system to another, there are generalized principles which apply in all cases (Butler *et al.*, 1984b). These are:

1. Clearing the swing leg. This is achieved by tilting the body sideways or lifting on the relevant side, or a combination of both these. Downward and lateral forces are applied to one or both crutches (or other walking aid) for this purpose.
2. Pivoting swing leg from relative extension to flexion. This requires a forward turning moment to be generated about the swing leg hip. This can be achieved as a result of gravitational, inertial or orthotically generated mechanical forces – or a combination of these.
3. Trunk translation (hip flexion to extension) over stance leg. This occurs as a reaction to rearward forces generated in the crutches or walking aid. These may be applied unilaterally or bilaterally and require that the arm be drawn to the trunk, usually through the action of latissimus dorsi.

A typical reciprocal walking force system is shown in Figure 10.7. Control of the range of hip flexion/extension is necessary in order to limit step length. Excessive hip flexion can cause problems of external stabilization and will increase the forces required for trunk translation. In most patients there is a natural hip extension stop and, with a normal extension range, the line of the weight force of the trunk in standing passes behind the hip joint centre, giving inherent stabilization of this joint. Hip flexion deformities will lead to problems in maintaining the centre of gravity within the support area of the feet.

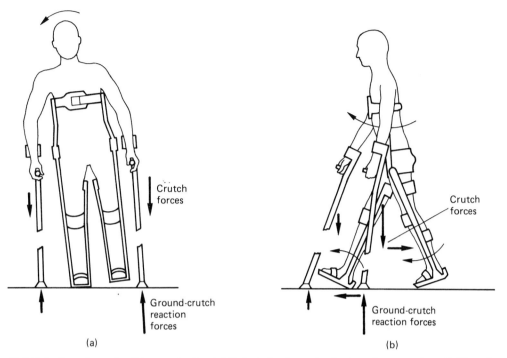

Figure 10.7 Orthotic reciprocal walking mechanics. (a) Patient clearing swing leg by using a crutch to tilt himself sideways. (b) Swing leg moving from extension to flexion under the influence of gravity and patient using latissimus dorsi to produce crutch forces to drive stance leg into extension. (Curved arrows indicate direction of rotation of body segments, straight arrows show vertical and horizontal crutch force vectors.)

(d) Design examples

There are two systems which are widely used for the provision of reciprocal walking for paraplegic patients. Both recognize that there are a number of factors which must be considered and that the final design requires a compromise of these (Stallard et al., 1979). However, whilst the fundamental principles for reciprocal walking apply in theory in both designs, there is a difference in the philosophy of compromise and this results in significant design variations.

The ORLAU ParaWalker

The compromise chosen for this system (Figure 10.8) aims for maximum efficiency of ambulation with crutches, ease of doffing, donning and transferring, and a free flowing gait style (Rose, 1979; Stallard *et al.*, 1986b; Butler and Major, 1987). In order to achieve this it provides:

1. A structure which rigidly resists adduction-abduction but which conforms for cosmetic reasons as closely as possible to the patient.

2. Limited range of low friction flexion-extension at the hips which can be overridden by an easily operated lock to permit a full range of flexion for sitting.
3. Easily operated fastening mechanisms for the support points which provide limb stabilization for the patient.
4. A high degree of mechanical safety and reliability to minimize the danger of patient injury and reduce the cost of maintenance.
5. An initial cost which does not exceed that of conventional devices supplied to patients for standing and limited mobility.

A particular advantage of the ParaWalker is the ease with which crutches may be used – elbow crutches being the most popular and efficient. The structural basis of the design ensures easy modification for growth or anatomical changes in the patient, a high degree of reliability, and a capacity for accommodating very large patients.

In order to ensure the correct prescription and service to the patient, supply of the components for this orthosis is restricted to clinical teams (doctor, orthotist, technician,

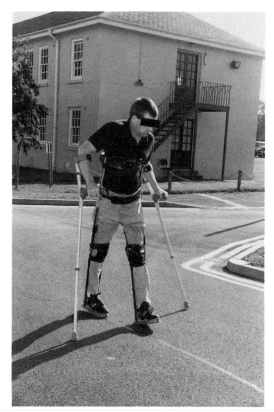

Figure 10.8 ORLAU ParaWalker

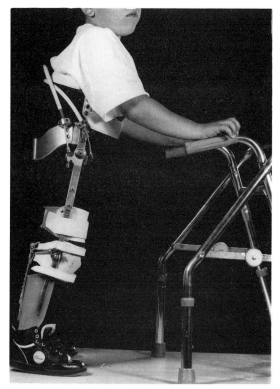

Figure 10.9 LSU Reciprocating Gait Orthosis

physiotherapist) who have received the required training.

The Louisiana State University Reciprocating Gait Orthosis (LSU-RGO)

The compromise chosen for this system (Figure 10.9) is aimed at good orthotic moulding to the patient, a stable standing posture and a lightweight construction (Douglas *et al.*, 1983; Durr-Fillauer, 1983; Yngre *et al.*, 1984; Beckman, 1987). A fundamental part of this orthosis is a system of interlinked cables joining the two hip joints (Figure 10.10) (Scrutton, 1971; Motloch, 1976). No detailed rationale has been published for the use of these cables, but it is apparent that the chosen design is based on:

1. A closely conforming polypropylene orthotic patient support structure.
2. Freely hinged metal hip joints attached to the polypropylene body brace and lower limb segments of the orthosis.

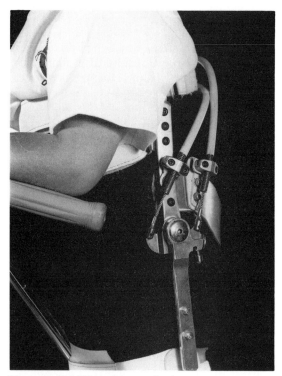

Figure 10.10 LSU hip joint mechanism

3. Twin cables linking the two hip joints to enforce relative reciprocal flexion and extension for reciprocation during walking whilst providing stable support with the hips fully extended and both feet grounded.
4. Releasable fastenings on knee joints and the interlinking cable mechanism at the hip to permit sitting.

A training programme is available which is recommended to professionals (primarily orthotists and physiotherapists) who wish to supply the orthosis. In the interests of maximizing patient opportunities for using the system this is not mandatory and components may be freely purchased from approved stockists.

The method of construction utilizes the specialist skills of professional orthotists and ensures maximum ease of fitting clothes over the device.

(e) Research results

The primary objectives of providing reciprocal walking systems are to improve the functional performance and reduce the energy cost of ambulation for paraplegic patients. During the development of such systems a number of monitoring programmes and patient reviews have been conducted, and these have all clearly identified improvements in ease of mobilization using these devices in comparison with earlier forms of walking.

(f) Patient reviews

A review of the first 27 spina bifida children supplied with an early prototype of the OR-LAU ParaWalker (Rose *et al.*, 1981) showed that there was a significant improvement in their gait assessed using the Hoffer *et al.* (1973) classification. Assessments were made 6 months after supply and compared with their performance in a variety of more conventional ambulatory orthoses assessed immediately prior to starting reciprocal walking. Following the completion of the development programme for the ParaWalker, an additional review of 52 myelomeningocele patients – all with complete lesions at or above L1 (Stallard *et al.*, 1991) – showed that the numbers of patients achieving household and community ambulatory status had increased still further to a significant degree, with 34% achieving community ambu-

latory status as compared with only 7% of the children in the earlier study. Comparison of the performances of children with spina bifida in the fully developed ORLAU ParaWalker with that of children having comparable degrees of paraplegia using conventional orthoses (Asher and Olsen, 1983), has shown that reciprocal walking gave patients an average ambulation performance in excess of 'household', whereas patients using conventional orthoses had a lower average performance in the 'therapeutic' range.

A review of the first 50 patients routinely supplied with adult ParaWalkers, all of whom had complete thoracic lesions (Moore and Stallard, 1990), showed that with an average post-supply follow-up period of 34 months, 64% were still using their device regularly. This compared favourably with 35% of a similar group of patients using more traditional orthoses with an average follow-up period of only 2 years.

Clearly from a functional point of view, there is very strong evidence to show that carefully selected and treated patients with complete spinal lesions at or above L1 do achieve very significantly better functional performance when using reciprocal walking, as compared with other styles.

(g) Relative energy cost

In addition to establishing benefits in the level of ambulation of patients using the prototype ParaWalker, Rose *et al.* (1981) also monitored changes in speed and heart rate in 14 of the 27 patients in their study. They showed that there was a mean increase in speed of 87.3% with an average decrease in heart rate of 10 beats min^{-1}. Refinement of the system has further improved efficiency, and the present average performance of routinely supplied patients in ORLAU on the basis of Physiological Cost Index (MacGregor, 1981; Butler *et al.*, 1984a) is significantly lower at 3.3 than that of the patients using the prototype system which was well in excess of 5 (Rose *et al.*, 1981; ORLAU, 1990).

Studies of the RGO (Bowker *et al.*, 1992) have shown that patients using this device have a PCI comparable with that of patients using the prototype ORLAU ParaWalker (Rose *et al.*, 1981), and that it is approximately two points lower than the same patients using conventional bilateral KAFOs for swing-through gait.

Oxygen uptake studies on both the Para-Walker (Nene and Patrick, 1989) and the RGO (Hirokawa *et al.*, 1990) show that reciprocal walking for adult patients has a very significantly lower energy cost than swing-through gait.

10.5.4 Future developments

(a) Purely mechanical systems

The main objectives of the future development of mechanical reciprocal walking systems are likely to be:

1. An improvement in lateral rigidity to further increase walking efficiency.
2. A reduction in friction of the lower limb reciprocal interlinking systems for orthoses using that design.
3. A reduction of weight to ease swing-through gait for the few patients who wish to do this and for convenience in handling the device when not worn by the patient. (The weight of the orthosis does not have a significant impact on the efficiency of reciprocal walking.)

With regard to improving lateral stiffness, this may be achieved by attention to design detail (ORLAU, 1989) and the use of newer composite materials which allow 'reshaping' after their initial construction. Whilst fundamental work is being carried out by major materials manufacturers, none has yet produced a routinely available stiff composite which is mouldable. Such a development would have important implications in many areas of orthotics.

Cables currently used on interlinked hip joint designs have high friction forces which clearly reduce walking efficiency to some degree. The use of an alternative linear bearing cable (Campbell, 1989) might partly solve this problem by reducing friction. A different approach is to eliminate the cables and use a direct lever transfer system, the fulcrum being attached to a sacral cross bracing band. This approach was first tried in the 1970s (Beyer, 1978) and has more recently been applied by Motloch (1989).

Reduction of weight can currently only be achieved at the expense of losing lateral stiffness, leading to the need for greater effort to raise the swing leg. The best hope of reducing the weight of the orthosis and retaining lateral stiffness is the use of composite materials. Those which are currently available all have some practical difficulties in their use. When newer materials eliminate these problems they are likely to impose higher costs – yet another compromise.

(b) Ambulation for bilateral lower limb deficient patients

The principles of reciprocal ambulation for paralysed patients with complete thoracic lesions should apply equally well for those with bilateral deficiency of the lower limbs. Limited experience suggests that this is the case and that such patients may be able to ambulate as successfully in a reciprocal mode with crutches (Ekus *et al.*, 1984; Meadows *et al.*, 1991). Indeed it may be easier for this group because there are greater opportunities for tuning the walking mechanics by moving the artificial limbs relative to the trunk.

(c) Functional electrical stimulation

The use of functional electrical stimulation (FES) for patients with complete paralysis of the lower limbs to help achieve reciprocal walking has been the subject of continuous research over a number of years (Petrofsky and Phillips, 1983; Kralj and Grebelnik, 1973; Petrofsky *et al.*, 1985; Marsolais and Kobetic, 1988). So far no system has gone beyond the stage of a research project and patients using pure FES have not been able to match the efficiency of walking which has been achieved with purely mechanical reciprocal walking systems. Problems with the satisfactory control of muscle contractions are likely to mean considerable delay before a system is produced which can be used as a routine clinical treatment.

An alternative approach is now receiving greater interest. FES combined with a mechanical system is widely viewed as a more practical means of improving ambulation. Systems have been developed for use with both the ORLAU ParaWalker (Patrick and McClelland, 1985) and the LSU Reciprocating Gait Orthosis (Petrofsky *et al.*, 1985). Whilst there are detailed differences in the manner in which muscle stimulation is applied, the basic philosophy of supplementing performance using an orthosis with FES applies to both. The advantages of a hybrid approach are the simplification of muscle control (patients usually providing this manually through switches) and a reduction in the number of muscles which require stimulation.

Since the major effort for walking while using reciprocating gait systems comes from the upper limbs, a prime objective of FES will be to lessen the magnitude and duration of the forces required from the upper limbs, so as to reduce fatigue in the arms. Laboratory experiments have shown that gluteal stimulation (McClelland *et al.*, 1987) can reduce the work done by the crutch forces by between 10% and 45%. This suggests there is considerable potential in this approach, which has recently been confirmed by further experimental work which has shown that overall efficiency has also resulted in the energy cost (J kg^{-1} m^{-1}) being reduced by 6–9% (Hirokawa *et al.*, 1990; Nene and Patrick, 1990).

Most experimental work on FES has been carried out using surface electrodes and external stimulators. These present practical problems for patients, the main difficulties being:

— The accurate electrode placement.
— Poor electrode adhesion over long periods.
— Significant time required to apply the system.
— The cross-stimulation of other muscles by cutaneous tracking of stimulation signals.
— The additional cost.

A viable clinical system must address all these points. Work is currently being undertaken on implantable systems but it is not yet clear whether a suitable solution which produces performance improvements at an acceptable cost will be achieved.

An additional area in which FES might provide assistance is in improving overall independence. Simple surface stimulation of the quadriceps muscles can enable paralysed patients to rise more easily from a wheelchair. Indeed systems for straightforward standing to provide ready access to high levels for paralysed patients have already been developed (Edwins *et al.*, 1988; Nash *et al.*, 1990), and these are likely to become routinely available. Adaptation of such systems for patients using mechanical orthoses is a further approach cur-

rently being investigated. The on-going problem of ensuring reliable locking of knee joints must be solved, and once solved the practical use of FES in reciprocal walking systems will become a very real option in the future.

Further work is also being carried out in a number of centres on the possibility of providing knee flexion during swing phase, and this would clearly be an exciting development.

10.6 Hip control

10.6.1 Objectives of orthotic management

In severe cases of cerebral palsy it is unrealistic to aim for independent mobility and the principal objective of providing an HKAFO is therapeutic. Commonly the treatment will be provided for patients who are severely athetoid or ataxic and in such cases additional walking aids are often needed to control aberrant upper limb and truncal movements. Anecdotal evidence has indicated that the patterned walking which such systems provide can have a real therapeutic effect, with patients advancing their ability for independent control of the limbs outwith the system. It is difficult to demonstrate conclusively that patients would not have made such advances spontaneously. However it would seem that the constraints imposed by the orthosis do not have a detrimental effect on overall control within the patient. Clearly the interrelated nature of different treatment strategies demands a team approach to ensure that the overall objectives of the treatment plan are kept firmly to the forefront.

In less severely affected cases of cerebral palsy, HKAFOs may be used to control rotational movements of the lower limb. This approach has been criticized as 'over-bracing' by some authorities, but it is the only effective orthotic solution to the problem of internal (or external) rotation of the hips, which often leads to a patient tripping over their own feet. The bracing approach requires that the knees and ankles remain freely articulated in order to preserve as much function as possible. A unilateral orthosis is often required in this situation. Quite frequently such orthoses are used to achieve rotational control until operative intervention is felt to be appropriate.

(a) Control of hip range

In conditions where motor power is available in the lower limbs, but the neuromuscular system is unable to provide the relevant controls to produce ambulation, an HKAFO can be used to impose prescribed ranges of movement upon the hips, knees and ankles. Where the degree of involvement requires a bilateral HKAFO, then usually the upper limbs and trunk are also affected and walking aids which provide additional support and control will become an essential part of the overall orthotic system.

Orthoses are used with this clinical group to achieve one of two objectives and these are:

1. As a primary orthotic device to allow patients to ambulate without constant supervision from a physiotherapist or other helper.
2. As a therapy intended to stimulate or enhance changes in neurological control which allow a patient to achieve more effective independent control of the affected limbs.

Such devices are currently in their infancy and there are few guidelines to their clinical indications. The second objective usually only follows as a byproduct of the first.

Orthoses may be used for therapeutic alignment of the hip during walking such as in Perthes' disease. With conditions of this kind, muscular power is available at the hip, and this may be tapped as a source of propulsive input. However, this must be done without disturbing the required alignment. When this is possible it may mean the use of crutches is not required.

10.6.2 Biomechanical requirements

When designing a hip orthosis consideration should be given to the pathological problem, the anatomy of the patient and the range of activities likely to be undertaken. Attention should also be given to the condition of the patient's skin in the area on which loads will be applied. The interface should be capable of transmitting the generated forces, taking account of areas of likely high pressure and sensitivity and of the characteristics of the underlying tissue.

(a) Control of hip rotation

The control of hip rotational problems necessarily requires bracing across the hip joint, and when this is the primary biomechanical problem there may be patient or parental reluctance to accept that bracing at that level is the only orthotic solution. The temptation to provide a more 'cosmetic' solution which embraces only the lower limb should be resisted since it will be ineffective.

Where the sole objective of a hip orthosis is to control rotational movements of the hip, it is theoretically not necessary to brace across the knee. However, it must be borne in mind that the leg can rotate about its longitudinal axis within a simple thigh cuff or corset. Should it not be possible to provide suitable location arrangements in the thigh area to resist rotational movements, it will be necessary to have bracing members anchored into the patient's footwear, with appropriate hinges to permit knee and ankle movements.

(b) Control of flexion-extension

Control of hip flexion-extension range can be achieved by providing a freely hinged hip joint with adjustable stops. In many cases the natural limitation of extension in the human hip joint will be adequate and only an orthotic flexion stop will be necessary.

(c) Control of hip position

In Perthes' disease (and CDH) the orthosis is often required to hold the affected hip (or hips) in a particular positional relationship between ball and socket. HKAFO devices may be prescribed which either provide a fixed relationship or a limited range for ambulation which also ensures that the required degree of abduction and/or rotation in the affected hip (or hips) is maintained.

10.6.3 Orthotic designs

(a) Control of hip range

Cerebral palsy patients who are severely athetoid or ataxic usually produce aberrant movements in abduction/adduction and rotation of the hip joint. Consequently an HKAFO provided for control purposes in this condition (as highlighted by Thompson and Patrick, 1990) will need to generate sufficient resistance in the lateral plane and about the longitudinal axis of the lower limb in order to resist these movements in individual patients. The degree of resistance required varies according to the size of the patient and the severity of their condition. In most cases the structural rigidity demanded is in excess of that which can be provided by conventional body brace–caliper structures and may need to be close to that necessary to provide efficient reciprocal walking for paraplegic patients. The flexion-extension range does not usually require to be limited, but the need for this should be assessed individually. Knee joints with a free range of flexion and extension are commonly prescribed, and knee extension assist is an additional feature which can be added. Fixed or free ankle range are features which must also be individually assessed. A walking frame which provides control of the trunk and upper limbs is usually needed for such a system if independent walking is to be achieved.

Such devices should only be prescribed within an overall treatment regime and the particular requirements of each pathological condition must be considered. It may, for example, be necessary to prevent the orthosis contacting specific areas of the patient in order to avoid triggering an unwanted muscular response. A typical system is shown in Figure 10.11.

One of the difficulties of dealing with pathological problems such as cerebral palsy which require control of the hip, is the wide range of specifications likely to be required by different patients, and judging what will be the optimum settings for any individual. For this reason, attempts have been made to design multi-adjustable systems so that they can be modified on the patient. This has been achieved for hip abduction-adduction only (Challenor, 1981) and also for a wider range of options (Farmer *et al.*, 1989), including flexion-extension.

(b) Control of hip rotation

Orthoses which are intended to control hip rotation frequently need to resist considerable torque about the longitudinal axis of the lower limbs. The structure of the orthosis must accommodate these torque demands. It must

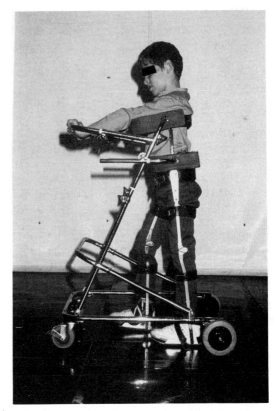

Figure 10.11 ORLAU VSO System

also produce a reaction on the patient above the hip when the control is unilateral or where there is internal rotation on one side and external rotation on the other. A structure which can rotate around the patient's trunk will not achieve the necessary reaction. Either sufficient friction must exist at the patient–orthosis interface or, preferably, bony prominences (such as the iliac crests) are used to produce a torque reaction, as discussed in Chapter 5. Where there is a similar range of internal or external rotation bilaterally, the total torque produced is balanced within the structure above the hip and rotation should not be a problem.

Theoretically it is not necessary to extend the orthosis beyond the knee in order to provide rotational control. However, it is difficult with thigh cuff arrangements to prevent the leg rotating about its longitudinal axis relative to the orthosis. Therefore, rotational control devices are commonly attached to the shoe in one way or another to increase effective rotational stability.

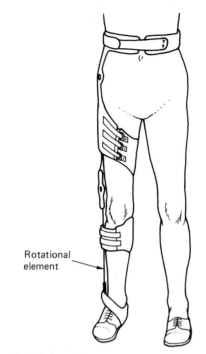

Figure 10.12 Twister Brace

One way of minimizing the 'structure' of a rotational control orthosis which is frequently used, is to employ a cable which has high torque resistance about its long axis but relatively low resistance to bending across that axis (Figure 10.12). Care must be employed with this approach because the bending which is required to permit hip and knee flexion decreases the degree of rotational control on the hip unless it is co-planar (ORLAU, 1988). The cable must be fitted to be as straight as possible with the hips and knees of the patient at their position of maximum extension in order to limit the reduction of control with the ranges used during ambulation.

(c) *Control of hip position*

When there is a clinical requirement for the ball and socket of a hip joint to be held in a particular alignment, the optimum strategy depends on a number of factors, the most important being:

— Whether there is unilateral or bilateral involvement.
— Whether some relative movement is permissible.

— Where ambulation is to be achieved.
— Whether some weight bearing through the affected hip is possible.

Complete immobilization of both hips is in many ways the simplest option. A hip spica of plaster of Paris or other suitable material may be used to fix the hips in the required position. Mobility can then be provided by a special trolley onto which the patient is placed so that they may be wheeled from one location to another. A cross-bracing bar at the distal end of the spica (commonly used to brace the orthosis) can be used as a load carrying element for the transport system. However, care must be taken to ensure that the bar and its mountings have sufficient strength to take the loads required for transportation.

When some relative hip movement is permissible, a simple hip orthosis with freely hinged hip joints, set at the required angle of abduction, may be employed (e.g. the Scottish-Rite orthosis (Figure 10.13); Lovell *et al.*, 1978). This does allow an awkward reciprocal mode of gait which is much appreciated by some patients. The stresses in such an orthosis are however bound to be large because the angle of abduction leads to high bending moments at the orthotic hip joint. This can lead to

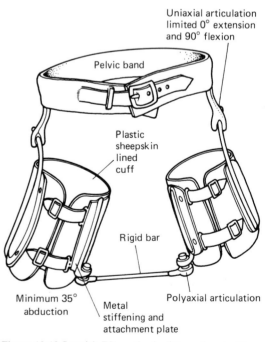

Figure 10.13 Scottish-Rite orthosis. (Reproduced with permission from Rose, 1986.)

frequent breakages and it is very difficult to achieve a high degree of mechanical reliability with such a system.

10.7 Muscular dystrophy

Swivel walkers are now commonly used for muscular dystrophy patients for whom they can prolong the walking life of the patient with both therapeutic and psychological benefit. Experience has shown that these patients have special difficulties:

1. A greater sensitivity to posture than in other groups.
2. More variability of hip and knee contractures.
3. Normal sensation in the lower limbs which can result in discomfort at the patient–orthosis interface.
4. Greater proprioceptive awareness of hip position which can lead to a wish for greater abduction.
5. General weakness, which limits the input of propulsion forces.
6. Apprehension about unsteady support and excessive step length.
7. Transfer of heavy, weak patients into the orthosis by physiotherapists and carers.

10.7.1 The ORLAU VCG Swivel Walker

A swivel walker has now been designed to accommodate these special difficulties. The ORLAU VCG Swivel Walker provides more ready adjustment of patient posture and walking mechanics so that the orthosis can be optimized for patients with the difficulties identified (Stallard *et al.*, 1992). To provide this it has the following features:

1. The facility for insertion of compensatory wedges for equinus.
2. A range of easily adjusted knee pads with sheepskin interfaces.
3. An adjustable sacral band with an Evazote lining for patient comfort.
4. A range of thoracic bands which allow the appropriate compromise between convenience and patient comfort.
5. A facility for adjusting the position of the patient support frame relative to the footplate.

6. A facility to readily adjust footplate-bearing centres.

The last two features result in much easier adjustability of the walking mechanics so that these can be optimized for patients with minimal effort. Their value is therefore not limited to patients with muscular dystrophy, but can be a useful facility for any patient who is experiencing difficulty with swivel walking.

10.8 Additional design considerations

10.8.1 Fatigue failure of materials

Cyclic loading occurs in everyday use of all types of HKAFO (Major and Stallard, 1985). Given the demanding nature of the applied loads, particularly in ambulation systems, fatigue is a likely cause of failure. Materials which have good fatigue resistance should be selected for all structural elements within such orthoses. Sudden changes of section, sharp corners and poor surface finish should be avoided in order to minimize the effect of stress raisers which might lead to the early onset of fatigue failure.

10.8.2 Structural considerations

In assessing the structural requirements of an orthosis, the degree of deformity, particularly hip flexion and adduction, is a factor which should be looked at carefully since this is likely to significantly increase the bending stresses which occur in the orthotic hip and knee joints.

Where a range of motion at the hip is necessary, the stops in the hip joint must be capable of resisting the maximum loads which can occur during any routine activity. Patient transfers frequently apply loads in excess of those experienced during walking.

Where the lower limbs are braced individually in an HKAFO (e.g. in a reciprocal walking device), the bending stresses at the orthotic hip joint will be large in routine use because of the length of the moment arm from the point of force application at the foot. These bending stresses are likely to be combined with axial loads and torque about the longitudinal axis. Not only should the mechanical strength of the joints reflect these severe demands, but the mode of failure should be ductile in nature because of the propensity of such patients to lose control and thereby produce an overload. Testing joints in accordance with an appropriate British Standard (BS2574: Part 3) will enable their characteristics to be determined, and those which have a high energy to fracture and low release of elastic energy are preferable in terms of patient safety.

10.8.3 Balanced loading

HKAFOs which brace the whole of the lower part of the body as one, the legs being splinted together rather than separately (e.g. Parapodium; Motloch, 1971), allow the potential for cross bracing the structure at the lower end. This gives the attendant advantages of increased stiffness, structural integrity and reduction of orthotic bending stresses at the level of the hip. However, when this approach is adopted, care must be taken to balance the loads through the separate limbs in order to minimize the peak stabilizing forces in each.

In cases in which a total weight-bearing function is incorporated into HKAFOs, the potential for buckling in the structures which replace the load carrying capacity of the legs must be considered, and the dynamic forces inherent in ambulation must be borne in mind since these can be considerably larger than body weight.

The range of requirements for HKAFOs is probably greater than for any other orthotic category. It is therefore incumbent upon designers of devices, and those responsible for their prescription and application, to be very clear about the objectives of treatment. The more clearly these are defined the more likely it will be that an effective prescription for an individual patient will be provided. Because the benefits of some devices in this category have been perceived as potentially spectacular, unrealistic claims have been made in the past. Whilst much can be achieved for heavily handicapped patients, it is important that the advances which have been made are kept in proportion. If they are not, newer approaches to improved patient independence may be unjustly discredited by association.

References

Asher M. and Olsen J. (1983) Factors affecting the ambulatory status of patients with spina bifida cystica. *J. Bone Joint Surg.* **65A**, 350–356

Beckman J. (1987) The Louisiana State University reciprocating gait orthosis. *Physiotherapy* **73**, 386–392

Beyer C. (1978) Personal Communication on Reciprocation Mechanisms. Breda Rehabilitation Centre, The Netherlands

Bobechko W.P., McClaurin C.A. and Motloch W.M. (1968) Toronto orthosis for Legg Perthes' disease. *Artif. Limbs* **12**, 36

Bowker P., Messenger N., Ogilvie C. *et al.* (1992). Energetics of paraplegic walking. *J. Biomech. Eng.* **14**, 344–350

British Standard (1990) Lower Limb Orthoses. Part 3. Method for the Determination of Mechanical Properties of Metal Knee Joint and Side Member Assemblies. BS 2574: Part 3

Butler P.B. and Major R.E. (1987) The ParaWalker – a rational approach to the provision of reciprocal ambulation for paraplegic patients. *Physiotherapy* **73**, 393–397

Butler P.B., Farmer I.R., Poiner R. *et al.* (1982) Use of the ORLAU Swivel Walker for the severely handicapped patient. *Physiotherapy* **68**, 324–326

Butler P., Englebrecht M., Major R.E. *et al.* (1984a) Physiological Cost Index of walking for normal children and its use as an indicator of physical handicap. *Dev. Med. Child Neurol.* **26**, 607–612

Butler P.B., Major R.E. and Patrick J.H. (1984b) The technique of reciprocal walking using the hip guidance orthosis (hgo) with crutches. *Prosthet. Orthot. Int.* **8**, 33–38

Campbell J. (1989) Reciprocating gait orthosis with linear bearing. *J. Assoc. Child. Prosthet. Orthot. Clin.* **25**, 2–5

Carroll N. (1974) The orthotic management of the spina bifida child. *Clin. Orthop.* **102**, 108–114

Challenor Y. (1981) Use of a multiply adjustable hip-control orthosis in cerebral palsy. *Inter Clin. Inform. Bull.* **17**, 1–3, 16

DHSS (1980) HKAFO. In: Rose G.K. (ed.), *Classification of Orthoses.* HMSO, London, pp. 31–37

Douglas R., Larson P., D'Ambrosia R. *et al.* (1983) The LSU Reciprocating Brace Orthosis. *Orthopaedics* **6**, 834–839

Durr-Fillauer Medical Inc. (1983) *LSU Reciprocating Brace Orthosis.* A pictorial description and application manual. Orthopaedic Division, PO Box 1678, Chattanooga, Tennessee 3740, USA

Edbrooke H. (1970) The RSI Clicking Splint. *Physiotherapy* **56**, 148–153

Edwins D.J., Taylor P.N., Crook S.E. *et al.* (1988) Practical low cost stand/sit system for mid-thoracic paraplegics. *J. Biomed. Eng.* **10**, 184–188

Ekus L., Gruger L. and Ferguson N. (1984) A reciprocation prosthesis for a patient with sacral agenesis. *Inter Clin. Inform. Bull.* **19**, 76–79

Farmer I.R., Poiner R., Rose G.K. *et al.* (1982) The adult ORLAU swivel walker – ambulation for paraplegic and tetraplegic patients. *Paraplegia* **20**, 248–254

Farmer I.R., Hodnett C., Jones N.J. *et al.* (1989) ORLAU Variable Specification Orthosis (Orthotic Device). UK Patent Application No. 8918186, filed 9 August 1989.

Griffiths J.C., Henshaw J.T., Heywood O.B. *et al.* (1980).

Clinical applications of the paraplegic swivel walker. *J. Biomed. Eng.* **2**, 250–256

Hall C.B. (1962) Ambulation of congenital bilateral lower extremity amelias and/or phocomelias. *Inter Clin. Inform. Bull.* **1**, (34)

Herzog E.G. and Sharrard W.J.W. (1966) Calipers and braces with Dundee hip lock. *Clin. Orthop.* **46**, 239

Hirokawa S., Grimm M., Le T. *et al.* (1990) Energy consumption in paraplegic ambulation using the Reciprocating Gait Orthosis and electrical stimulation of the thigh muscles. *Arch. Phys. Med. Rehabil.* **71**, 687–694

Hoffer M.M., Feiwell E., Perry R. *et al.* (1973) Functional ambulation in patients with myelomeningocele. *J. Bone Joint Surg.* **55A**, 137–148

Kralj A. and Grebelnik S. (1973) Functional electrical stimulation – a new hope for paraplegic patients? *Bull. Prosthet. Res.* 10–20, 75–102

Lovell W.W., Hopper W.C. and Purvis J.M. (1978) The Scottish–Rite Hospital Orthosis for Legg–Perthes Disease. Scientific Exhibit, Scottish Medical Meeting, Atlanta

MacGregor J. (1981) The evaluation of patient performance using long-term ambulatory monitoring technique in the domiciliary environment. *Physiotherapy* **67**, 30–33

Major R.E. and Stallard J. (1985) Fatigue and stress raisers. In: *Structures & Materials – An Introduction Based on Orthotics.* Pub. ORLAU Publishing, RJ & AH Hospital, Oswestry, pp. 27–30

Major R.E., Stallard J. and Rose G.K. (1981) The dynamics of walking using the hip guidance orthosis (hgo) with crutches. *Prosthet. Orthot. Int.* **5**, 19–22

Major R.E., Patrick J.H. and Stallard J. (1987) Exoskeletal Splint for Hip Fractures. UK Patent No. 2158226

Marsolais E.B. and Kobetic R. (1988) Development of a practical electrical stimulation system for restoring gait in the paralysed patient. *Clin. Orthop.* **233**, 65–74

Mazur J.M., Shurtleff D., Menelaus M. *et al.* (1989). Orthopaedic management of high-level spina-bifida. *J. Bone Joint Surg.* **71A**, 56–61

McClelland M., Andrews B.J., Patrick J.H. *et al.* (1987) Augmentation of the Oswestry ParaWalker Orthosis by means of surface electrical stimulation: gait analysis of three patients. *Paraplegia* **25**, 32–38

Meadows C.B., Stallard J., Wright D. *et al.* (1990) The Edinburgh–ORLAU prosthetic system to provide reciprocal locomotion in children and adults with complete transverse lower limb deficiency. *Prosthet. Orthot. Int.* **14**, 111–116

Menelaus M.B. (1980) Progress in the management of the paralytic hip in myelomeningocele. *Orthop. Clini. North Am.* **11**, 17–30

Moore P. and Stallard J. (1990) A clinical review of adult paraplegic patients with complete lesions using the ORLAU ParaWalker. *Paraplegia* **29**, 191–196

Motloch W. (1971) The Parapodium; an orthotic device for neuromuscular disorders. *Artif. Limbs* **15**, 36–47

Motloch W.M. (1976) Reciprocating gait brace. The Advance in Orthotics. In: Murdoch G. (ed.), *Device Design in Spina Bifida.* Edward Arnold, London, p. 419

Motloch W.M. (1989) Standing Brace, Parapodium and the Reciprocating Gait Orthosis. Panel Session, Spina Bifida, ISPO VI World Congress, 12–17 November, Kobe, Japan

Motloch W.M. and Elliott J. (1966) Fitting and training children with swivel walkers. *Artif. Limbs* Autumn, 27–38

Nash R.S.W., Davy M.S., Orpwood R. *et al.* (1990) Development of a wheelchair-mounted folding standing frame. *J. Biomed. Eng.* **12**, 189–192

Nene A. and Patrick J.H. (1989) Energy cost of paraplegic locomotion with the ORLAU ParaWalker. *Paraplegia* **27**, 125–132

Nene A.V. and Patrick J.H. (1990) Energy cost of paraplegic locomotion using the ParaWalker-Electrical Stimulation 'hybrid' orthosis. *Arch. Phys. Med. Rehabil.* **71**, 116–120

ORLAU (1988) Measurement of torsional stiffness of Twister Cables. *ORLAU Annu. Rep.* (14), 95–96

ORLAU (1989) ParaWalker '89 hip joint – design considerations. *ORLAU Annu. Rep.* (15), 25–29

ORLAU (1990) The PCI of ParaWalker patients. *ORLAU Annu. Rep.* (16), 41–50

Patrick J.H. and McClelland M.R. (1985) Low energy cost reciprocal walking for the adult paraplegic. *Paraplegia* **23**, 113–117

Petrofsky J.S. and Phillips C.A. (1983) Computer controlled walking in the paralysed individual. *J. Neurol. Orthop. Surg.* **4**, 153–164

Petrofsky J.S., Phillips C.A., Larson P. *et al.* (1985). Computer synthesised walking: an application of orthoses and functional electrical stimulation (FES). *J. Neurol. Orthop. Med. Surg.* **6**, 219–230

Rocca L. and Hopkins P. (1978) Swivel walkers. *Physiotherapy* **64**, 14–18

Rose G.K. (1979) The principles and practice of hip guidance articulations. *Prosthet. Orthot. Int.* **3**, 37–43

Rose G.K. (1980) Orthoses for the severely handicapped – rational or empirical choice? *Physiotherapy* **66**, 76–81

Rose G.K. (1986) Stabilising a joint or joints in a chosen position. In: *Orthotics – Principles & Practice.* William Heinemann Medical Books, London, pp. 47–49

Rose G.K. and Henshaw J.T. (1972) A swivel walker for paraplegics: medical and technical considerations. *Biomed. Eng.* **7**, 410–425

Rose G.K., Stallard J. and Sankarankutty M. (1981) Clinical evaluation of spina bifida patients using hip guidance orthosis. *Dev. Med. Child Neurol.* **23**, 30–40

Sankarankutty M., Stallard J. and Rose G.K. (1979) The relative efficiency of 'swing-through' gait on axillary, elbow and Canadian crutches compared to normal walking. *J. Biomed. Eng.* **1**, 55–57

Scrutton D. (1971) A reciprocating brace with polyplanar hip hinges used on spina bifida children. *Physiotherapy* **57**, 61–66

Speilrein R.E. (1963) An engineering approach to ambulation without the use of external power sources, of severely handicapped individuals. *J. Instit. Eng. Australia* (December)

Stallard J., Sankarankutty M. and Rose G.K. (1978) Lower-limb vertical ground reaction forces during crutch walking. *J. Med. Eng. Technol.* **2**, 201–202

Stallard J., Farmer I.R., Poiner R. *et al.* (1986a) Engineering design considerations of the ORLAU Swivel Walker. *Eng. Med.* **15**, 3–8

Stallard J., Major R.E., Poiner R. *et al.* (1986b) Engineering design considerations of the ORLAU Para-Walker and FES Hybrid System. *Eng. Med.* **15**, 123–129

Stallard J., Major R.E. and Patrick J.H. (1989) A review of the fundamental design problems of providing ambulation for paraplegic patients. *Paraplegia* **27**, 70–75

Stallard J., Major R.E. and Butler P.B. (1991) The orthotic ambulation performance of paraplegic myeolomeningocele children using the ORLAU ParaWalker treatment system. *Clin. Rehabil.* **5**, 111–114

Stallard J., Henshaw J.H., Lomas B. and Poiner R. (1992) The Orlan VCG (variable centre of gravity) swivel walker for muscular dystrophy patients. *Prosthet. Orthot. Int.*, **16**, 46–48

Thompson N. and Patrick J.H. (1990) Ambulation for cerebral palsy at ORLAU, Oswestry. *Physiotherapy* **76**, 583

Yngre D.A., Douglas R. and Roberts J.M. (1984) The reciprocating gait orthosis in myelomeningocele. *J. Paediatr. Orthop.* **4**, 304–310

11

Upper limb orthoses

David Carus, John Lamb and Garth Johnson

11.1 Introduction

The anatomy, function, control and related biomechanics of the upper limb are highly complex and interrelated. In consequence, the orthotic management of the upper limb is equally complex and specialized. This chapter provides a description of the biomechanical principles of upper limb orthotic management, using some of the common pathologies and orthoses as examples.

The orthotist is required to exercise considerable expertise when applying an upper limb orthosis to a patient. Experience has shown that there is a fine balance between improving function in one part of the upper limb and restricting function in another. The ultimate aim of the orthosis is to improve function, but the patient may consider the orthosis to be a hindrance when it is first applied, especially for those types of hand orthoses which are prescribed to be used during periods of tissue healing. The purpose of the orthosis should always be carefully explained to the patient.

It should be appreciated that the use of an upper limb orthosis in isolation will rarely achieve optimal results. These devices must be used in conjunction with an appropriate regimen of upper limb and hand therapy, which is an essential and central element of upper limb rehabilitation programmes.

11.2 Anatomy

11.2.1 Bones in the upper limb

The bones involved in movements of the 'shoulder complex' are the chest wall, scapula, clavicle and the humerus (Figure 11.1). The humerus articulates with the proximal ends of the radius and ulna at the elbow joint; the distal ends of the radius and ulna articulate with the carpus. The carpus contains eight bones which are approximately grouped into two rows; the distal row contains the trapezium, trapezoid, capitate and hamate bones and the proximal contains the scaphoid, lunate, triquetral and pisiform bones. The palm of the hand contains metacarpals for each digit. The four fingers have proximal, middle and distal phalanges whereas the thumb has only a proximal and distal phalanx – the middle phalanx was 'lost' during man's evolution (Figure 11.2). Sesamoid bones may be present at the distal interphalangeal and metacarpophalangeal joints (Kohler, 1968).

(a) Sizes of bones

Knowledge of the lengths of upper limb bones is required for the design of modular orthoses. The widely quoted anthropometric measurements made by Woodson and Conover (1964) have been summarized by Bailey (1982) and are listed in Table 11.1.

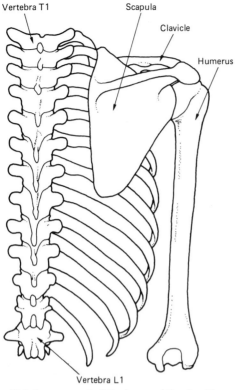

Figure 11.1 Arrangement of the bones of the shoulder

The average lengths of the finger bones are: metacarpals, 71 mm; proximal phalanges, 46 mm; middle phalanges, 28 mm; distal phalanges, 18 mm (Nordin and Frankel, 1989). The average interarticular length of the proximal phalanx of the finger bone is the sum of the lengths of the two distal phalanges, a fact which is in accordance with the mathematical Fibonacci sequence discovered in 1202 (Hoggart, 1969). The ratio of the lengths of the distal and middle phalanges and also the middle and proximal phalanges is approximately constant and has a magnitude of 0.618. Carus *et al.* (1992), however, studied the length ratios of adjacent bones for all fingers and found that this quoted ratio is inaccurate for the index and little fingers, presumably because of these fingers' roles in pinch and grasp respectively. His results are given in Table 11.2.

11.2.2 Joints of the upper limb

(a) Shoulder joint

The shoulder 'joint' is not a single joint but is rather a complex of joints between the chest wall, scapula, clavicle and humerus. The

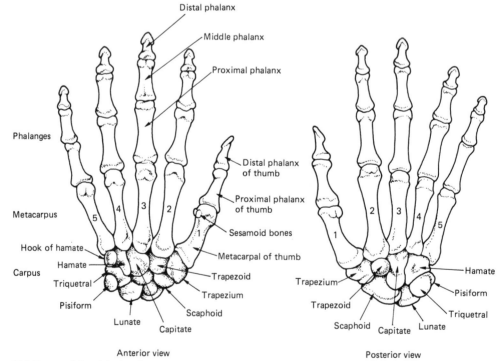

Figure 11.2 Bones of the right hand

Table 11.1 Anthropometric adult upper limb dimensions (expressed in millimetres)

| | Percentile | | | | | | | |
| | Women | | | | Men | | | |
	5th	50th	95th	SD	5th	50th	95th	SD
Hand length	170	183	201	10.2	170	191	206	9.7
Hand breadth	69	76	81	5.1	81	89	97	4.8
Hand thickness	20	25	28	2.5	30	33	36	2.0
Hand circumference	170	183	198	10.2	198	216	236	11.4
Wrist circumference	137	150	163	7.6	157	170	185	8.6
Forearm circumference (flexed)	226	249	274	15.2	259	295	330	21.6
Biceps circumference (flexed)	231	264	307	25.4	277	323	368	27.4
Shoulder to elbow length	284	310	338	15.2	338	368	399	18.5
Elbow to wrist length	211	234	257	12.7	251	287	323	21.3

Table 11.2 Ratios of interarticular lengths of finger bones between joint centres (Carus *et al.*, 1992)

	Index	Middle	Ring	Little
DP/MP	0.811	0.735	0.734	0.928
MP/PP	0.551	0.559	0.605	0.544
PP/MC	0.612	0.675	0.722	0.540

DP, distal phalange; MC, metacarpal; MP, middle phalange; PP, proximal phalange.

humeral head articulates on the glenoid socket of the scapula but its range of motion is insufficient for the large multiplanar excursions of the arm. This deficit is compensated for by additional rotation and translation between the scapula and the chest wall. The clavicle, whose role is not fully understood, represents an additional structural link allowing the application of multidirectional forces at the lateral aspect of the scapula through the acromioclavicular joint. Medially, it is attached to the sternum by the approximately spherical sternoclavicular joint. From the kinematic point of view, the acromion can move on the surface of a sphere having a radius equal to the length of the clavicle; the constraints of scapula movement are therefore determined by this movement of the acromion combined with the requirement to maintain contact with the chest wall. The end result of this structural arrangement is that the arm can transmit substantial loads to the trunk from a wide range of positions.

The available three-dimensional motion at the shoulder complex makes it difficult to define ranges of motion in the simple manner used for single axis joints. The values normally quoted are based on simple movements in the standard anatomical planes or with axial rotation of the humerus. The American Academy of Orthopedic Surgeons (AAOS); (1965) quotes ranges for these standard movements, as have Boone and Azen (1979). More recently, Johnson and colleagues (1990), using a novel technique based on an electromagnetic movement sensor (Johnson and Anderson, 1990), have also made measurements of these standard maneuvres. These data are listed in Table 11.3.

There are few available data on the forces at the glenohumeral joint and virtually none on the loading of the other articulations. Estimation of forces is made difficult by the lack of data on the function of the various muscles. However Poppen and Walker (1978), assuming that both the supraspinatus and deltoid were active, calculated a force of 0.89 times body weight for abduction of the arm to 90°. This measurement, while giving some idea of the forces acting, probably bears little relation to the forces which act during heavy manual work. While it is normal to quote lower limb joint forces during gait in terms of body weight, the varied nature of upper limb tasks probably makes such normalization inappropriate.

(b) Elbow joint

The position of the hand depends upon elbow flexion and pronation-supination of the forearm which are both commonly regarded as

Table 11.3 Ranges of motion at the shoulder complex

Movement	AAOS (1965)	Boone and Azen (1979)	Johnson et al. (1990)
Flexion	158	167	137
Extension	53	62	68
Abduction	170	184	163
Internal rotation	70	69	62

part of elbow movement. The total ranges of motion, according to the American Academy of Orthopedic Surgeons (1965) and Amis and Miller (1982), are shown in Table 11.4. Functional elbow movements have been studied by Morrey *et al.* (1981) who used a two axis electrogoniometer to measure the flexion and pronation-supination associated with some common tasks (Table 11.5).

(c) Wrist, finger and thumb joints

The wrist bones are arched to form a palmar tunnel through which pass the long finger flexor tendons. This groove is covered by the tough transverse flexor retinaculum whose function is to protect the underlying soft tissues and also to act as a pulley for the flexor tendons when the wrist is flexed. The wrist bones have minimal relative movement with respect to one another. Youm and Yoon (1979) have shown that the centres of rotation of the wrist joint are located in the capitate in the manner illustrated in Figure 11.3. The ranges of normal wrist motion, described by Bird and Stowe (1982), are given in Table 11.6.

The proximal ends of the second and third metacarpals are rigidly connected to the trapezoid and capitate. As a result, these two metacarpals and the carpal bones act as a single rigid segment. The fourth and fifth metacarpals have some limited flexion movement with respect to the hamate. The fourth metacarpal is

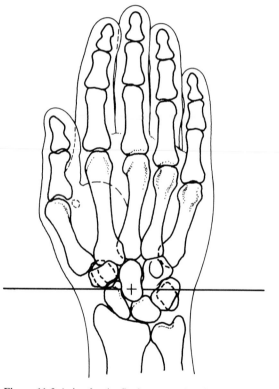

Figure 11.3 Axis of wrist flexion-extension (adapted from Youm and Yoon, 1979)

Table 11.4 Total ranges of motion at the elbow

Movement	Amis and Miller (1982)	AAOS (1965)
Flexion	142	150
Pronation	70	80–90
Supination	85	80–90

Table 11.5 Arcs of flexion (in degrees) for the performance of activities requiring elbow motion; open a door, pour from a jug, rise from a chair, read a newspaper, cut with a knife, put fork to mouth and use a telephone (Morrey *et al.*, 1981)

	Activity							
	Door	Jug	Chair	Newspaper	Knife	Fork	Glass	Telephone
Flexion range (degrees)	24–58	37–61	21–98	81–108	92–109	88–133	47–135	44–142

Table 11.6 Ranges of active motion at the wrist (Bird and Stowe, 1982)

	Age (yr)				
Movement	0–19	20–29	30–39	40–49	50–80+
Flexion	85.3	75.7	85.2	81.5	81.2
Extension	55.1	48.9	51.3	45.9	44.2
Abduction	37.1	30.5	33.4	27.1	28.8
Adduction	25.6	20.9	24.2	22.1	23.3

Table 11.7 Ranges of motion at the metacarpophalangeal joints from the neutral position

	Batmanabane and Malathi (1985)			
Movement	Index	Middle	Ring	Little
Flexion	70	90	90	95
Extension	Depends upon joint laxity			

able to flex 10–15° at the carpometacarpal joint and the fifth metacarpal can flex 20–30°. These movements are small, but are particularly important in providing maximum palm skin contact area for grasp activities.

The head of each metacarpal is unicondylar and this allows motion of the proximal phalanx in the planes of flexion-extension and abduction-adduction. The proximal phalanx can rotate about its longitudinal axis on the metacarpal head, but this movement is limited by the strong capsular ligaments. The metacarpophalangeal joint is similar in shape to a 'ball and socket'. The articular heads of the proximal and middle phalanges are bicondylar. The articular surfaces of the interphalangeal joints are congruent so they act as simple hinges and these joints can be likened to a 'tongue and groove'. Table 11.7 lists the maximum ranges of movement of the metacarpophalangeal joints according to Batmanabane and Malathi (1985). The ranges of movement of the interphalangeal joints are typically 100–110° for the proximal joint and 90° for the distal joint, according to AAOS. Wide variations in extension angles occur and these are caused by the extent of joint laxity. Measurements are from the neutral position with the fingers in the plane of the hand.

11.2.3 Musculature

The bone structure, musculature and nerve supply of the upper limb permit great dexter-ity, powerful grip, delicate precision and tactile feedback. The anatomy of the upper limb and in particular that of the wrist, hand, fingers and thumb is highly complex. A sound knowledge of the musculature is a prerequisite to satisfactory orthosis design and application.

(a) Shoulder

It is important to understand the controlling musculature of the shoulder to appreciate the relative motions of its elements. Scapulothoracic motion results from the actions of the trapezius and the rhomboids, all of which attach to the spinous processes, and serratus anterior which attaches to the anterior chest wall. Glenohumeral movements are produced by muscles at two levels. Superficially, the deltoid and the uppermost part of pectoralis major cover the glenohumeral joint and can produce abduction-adduction and flexion-extension. At the deeper level, glenohumeral motion is controlled by the 'rotator cuff' muscles all of which attach to the blade of the scapula. All of these muscles, supraspinatus, infraspinatus, subscapularis and teres minor, are attached to a strong ligamentous structure around the humeral neck. In addition to the rotator cuff, teres major attaches to the lower edge of the scapula and the shaft of the humerus. The neck of the humerus is therefore surrounded by muscles which can act in concert to produce any required movement at the glenohumeral joint.

Ultimately, any vertical loading of the shoulder must be carried by the spinal column. This is achieved by the suspension of the scapula from the cervical spine using the upper part of trapezius which acts almost medially on the clavicle in order to lift its distal end, and the levator scapulae acting vertically at the medial edge.

The scapulothoracic and glenohumeral muscle groups described above act in series; that is to say that any loading on the humerus must be reacted by both. In addition, as commonly occurs elsewhere in the musculoskeletal system, there are muscles which cross two joints (scapulothoracic and glenohumeral) to attach the humerus directly to the trunk. The majority of pectoralis major (that which attaches to the anterior chest wall) together with latissimus dorsi (attaching to spinous processes) can produce an additional adduction moment directly between the humerus and the trunk.

The result of this muscle arrangement is that the scapula can be moved independently of, but in concert with, the humerus leading to the so-called 'scapulohumeral rhythm'. This aspect of shoulder biomechanics has been studied by Poppen and Walker (1978) and Freeman and Munro (1966) who have shown that scapular rotation accompanies abduction, although other movements such as flexion have not been studied. It seems that these movements result from the need to optimize muscle use and to allow large ranges of motion without compromising the stability of a single synovial joint. This aspect is currently being examined by Pronk (1989) using a sophisticated mechanical model.

(b) Elbow

The three elbow flexors are the biceps brachii, brachialis and the brachioradialis. The biceps brachii is mostly inserted in the radial tuberosity and is the main flexor. It arises from the scapula so it also acts to stabilize the shoulder joint. The brachialis acts exclusively as an elbow flexor and is inserted in the tuberosity of the ulna. Finally, the brachioradialis acts chiefly as a flexor of the elbow but also as a supinator in extreme pronation.

The single elbow extensor is the triceps brachii. It has three muscle portions which converge into a single tendon which is inserted into the olecranon. The force exerted by the triceps is greatest when the shoulder is in flexion.

(c) Wrist and palm

Pure wrist extension is provided by the extensor carpi radialis brevis; combined flexion and adduction by the flexor carpi ulnaris; combined extension and adduction by the extensor carpi ulnaris, and combined extension and abduction is provided by the extensor carpi radialis longus. Wrist supination is provided by the supinator and bicep muscles, and pronation by the pronator quadratus and pronator teres muscles.

When the fingers are extended, the distal ends of the finger metacarpals lie in a flat plane, but they form a concave palmar arch when the fingers are flexed to grasp an object.

The palm has four compartments. The thenar and hypothenar compartments are enclosed in their own layers of fascia and each contain the short muscles for the thumb and little finger respectively. The intermediate compartment contains the long finger flexor tendons, the lumbricals and most of the blood vessels and nerves. Finally, the adductor compartment contains the adductor pollicis.

The vulnerable tendons, lumbricals, blood vessels and nerves, located in the intermediate compartment in the middle of the palm, are protected by the tough palmar aponeurosis. This is a strong fibrous sheet which is composed of strong longitudinal fibres mixed with transverse fibres which bind them together. The tissue is triangular in shape; the deep fibres in its proximal apex fuse with the flexor retinaculum, and its distal end divides into four processes, which in turn divide into two slips which fuse with the deep fascia on the back of the digits and with the strong deep transverse ligaments of the palm. The palmar aponeurosis has particular relevance in orthotic management, because it is affected by Dupuytren's disease.

(d) Fingers

Finger flexion and extension occur through the action of the extrinic muscles located in the forearm, and intrinsic muscles located in the hand. The intrinsic muscles also have a role in finger abduction and adduction. These groups of muscles are considered in turn.

Extrinsic flexor muscles

The extrinsic flexor muscles comprise the flexor digitorum sublimis and flexor digitorum profundus.

The tendon of the flexor digitorum sublimis is inserted into the finger's middle phalanx whereas the tendon of the deeper flexor digitorum profundus is inserted into the distal phalanx. The sublimis tendon is more superficial than the profundus tendon over the metacarpal and proximal half of the first phalanx. It is therefore inevitable that the two tendons must cross one another before their insertion points. This is achieved by bifurcation of the sublimis tendon in order that the profundus may pass through at the level of the metacarpophalangeal joint. The bifurcations wrap around the profundus tendon, reuniting at the proximal interphalangeal joint, proximal to the insertions into the sides of the middle phalanx.

The flexor digitorum sublimis muscle flexes the proximal interphalangeal joint and the angle of contact of the tendon with the middle phalanx increases with increasing flexion of the proximal interphalangeal joint. This muscle is a weak flexor of the metacarpophalangeal joint but only when the proximal interphalangeal joint is fully flexed.

The flexor digitorum profundus flexes the distal interphalangeal joint. However, when the proximal interphalangeal and metacarpophalangeal joints are passively flexed to 90°, the profundus tendon becomes too slack for functional use. It is also a weak flexor of the proximal interphalangeal and metacarpophalangeal joints but only when the distal interphalangeal joint is fully flexed.

Extrinsic extensor muscles

These comprise the extensor digitorum communis, the extensor indicis (for the index finger only) and the extensor digiti minimi (for the little finger only).

The tendon of the extensor digitorum communis initially develops into the extensor expansion in the region of the metacarpophalangeal joint, before insertion into the proximal phalanx to provide extension of the metacarpophalangeal joint. After the extensor expansion, the extensor digitorum communis trifurcates at the distal end of the proximal phalanx. Its middle portion develops into the median band which is inserted into the proximal end of the middle phalanx and acts as an extensor for the proximal interphalangeal joint. The two lateral bands are inserted into the proximal end of the distal phalanx and hence act as extensors for the distal interphalangeal joint. The principal role of the extensor digitorum communis is extension of the metacarpophalangeal joint which occurs in all positions of the wrist. The extensor indicis and extensor digiti minimi have deep insertions in the extensor digitorum communis tendons for the index and little fingers respectively. Their function is the same as the extensor digitorum but they have the secondary role of extending the index and little fingers individually.

Intrinsic muscles

The intrinsic muscles comprise the lumbicals whose function is both flexion and extension of finger joints, and the interossei whose function is abduction and adduction of the fingers. The little finger has intrinsic muscles in the hypothenar eminence. These are the abductor digiti minimi, flexor digiti minimi and opponens digiti minimi.

Each of the four lumbricals flexes the metacarpophalangeal joint and also extends the proximal and distal interphalangeal joints because it is inserted into the extensor tendon. There are four palmar and four dorsal interosseous muscles. The palmar interossei adduct the fingers towards the middle finger. Additionally, each flexes the metacarpophalangeal joint and extends the interphalangeal joints. The dorsal interossei abduct the fingers. The first and fourth abduct the index and ring fingers from the middle one. The second abducts the middle finger towards the index and the third adducts it towards its former position and, continuing to act, abducts it towards the ring finger. The second dorsal interosseous then restores it to its former position. Each dorsal interosseous flexes the metacarpophalangeal joint and extends the interphalangeal joints in a similar manner to the palmar interossei.

The abductor digiti minimi abducts and slightly flexes the little finger. The opponens digiti minimi draws the fifth metacarpal slightly forward and turns it towards the radial side.

Each finger, therefore, is provided with an adductor and an abductor. The index, middle and ring each have two interossei. The little has its own abductor and the fourth palmar interosseous as an adductor.

(e) Thumb

The unique function of the thumb is achieved through its four extrinsic and five intrinsic muscles.

Extrinsic muscles

These comprise the abductor pollicis longus, extensor pollicis brevis, extensor pollicis longus and flexor pollicis longus.

The abductor pollicis longus abducts the first metacarpal. It also flexes the first metacarpal due to the fact that the abductor tendon passes anteriorly to the extensor pollicis brevis and extensor pollicis longus. The extensor pollicis brevis has two roles: first, it extends the meta-carpophalangeal joint, and second it moves the first metacarpal laterally. It abducts the thumb if the wrist is stabilized by synergistic action of the flexor carpi ulnaris and particularly the extensor carpi ulnaris. If synergistic action is not provided, the extensor pollicis brevis ab-ducts the wrist. The action of the extensor pollicis longus is extension of both the proxi-mal interphalangeal and metacarpophalangeal joints. It also moves the metacarpal medially and posteriorly. The flexor pollicis longus fle-xes the interphalangeal joint and, secondarily, flexes the metacarpophalangeal joint.

Intrinsic muscles

The five intrinsic thumb muscles are divided into two groups. The lateral group comprises the flexor pollicis brevis, opponens pollicis and abductor pollicis brevis and is collectively known as the thenar eminence. The medial group comprises the two heads of the adductor pollicis. The flexor pollicis brevis flexes the metacarpophalangeal and proximal interpha-langeal joints. The opponens pollicis flexes the metacarpophalangeal joint and rotates the metacarpal medially. The abductor pollicis brevis abducts the thumb at the carpometa-carpal joint and slightly flexes the proximal phalanx. The adductor pollicis adducts the thumb's metacarpal towards the palm.

11.3 Pathology

11.3.1 Shoulder and elbow

Despite the fact that the multiple component design of the shoulder reduces the need for excessive motion, the glenohumeral joint relies largely upon the rotator cuff muscles for stabil-ity. This contrasts sharply with the knee joint, for instance, which, because of its fixed axis is able to rely upon strong ligaments to resist external loads. The result of this arrangement is that relatively minor trauma can lead to dislocation of the glenohumeral joint. This is sometimes experienced by athletes who have initially damaged the joint and subsequently suffer dislocation without a major force. Simi-larly, hemiplegic patients who can no longer control the rotator cuff muscles normally can suffer subluxation of the joint while the limb remains flaccid. Trauma to the elbow can result in flexor weakness, in which case there is a functional requirement to support the joint in a position of optimal function during the recov-ery period.

11.3.2 Wrist and hand

The upper limbs suffer a high incidence of injury such as lacerations, fractures, burns and crushing injuries. The joints of the wrists, hand and fingers are particularly susceptible to the development of contractures and deformities due to the number and close proximity of the joints and proliferation of soft tissues.

A review of 1 year's supply of upper limb orthoses in Dundee (McDougall *et al.*, 1985) revealed that the clinical indications for pres-cription were as follows:

— Traumatic injuries   61%
— Hemiplegia (typically CVA) 17%
—Relief of wrist pain   13%
— Dupuytren's contracture   9%

Within the group of traumatic injuries, the principal pathologies for prescriptions were in the following proportions:

— Tendon injuries   39%
— Joint injuries   34%
— Nerve injuries   27%

It is considered that these figures represent a typical spectrum for a European city. Varia-tions can be expected for hospitals with special-ist facilities for the treatment of patients with rheumatoid arthritis.

11.4 Biomechanical requirements and objectives of orthotic management

11.4.1 Shoulder

The purpose of the supply of shoulder orthoses for dislocation of the glenohumeral joint is to prevent subluxation in order to provide a stable structure for the transmission of loads from the upper limb to the trunk. Biomecha-nically, this can only be achieved by the appli-cation of an axial force to the humerus to provide elevation of the arm and the position-ing of the humeral head onto the glenoid.

Injuries to the brachial plexus can result in a totally flaccid limb requiring orthotic treatment for the shoulder, elbow and hand to permit passive use of the limb. The biomechanical requirement is therefore to apply supportive forces and moments to hold the arm in an elevated position. The need is to both support the weight of the limb and to assist its movement for the purposes of feeding and other simple tasks. Other patients who have flaccid limbs are those with high level spinal cord injury, in which case both limbs will almost certainly be involved. The use of external power is often indicated.

Finally, there are two occasions when there may be a need to hold the arm in a fixed abducted position. The first is immediately after surgery, in order to protect the muscle attachments around the shoulder. The second occasion is the treatment of a humeral fracture when fixed abduction maintains bone alignment. Biomechanically, this requires the mechanical support of the humerus directly onto the trunk.

11.4.2 Elbow

Weakness or the complete absence of active flexion may arise as a consequence of direct trauma to the flexor muscles or through damage to their central or peripheral nerve supplies. The patient will have varying degrees of difficulty in achieving flexion against an applied load, depending upon the extent of injury or denervation. The orthotic objectives are either to hold the elbow at a fixed angle deemed suitable to optimize function, comfort or cosmesis or else to allow motion whilst counteracting the effects of gravity.

11.4.3 Wrist, hand, fingers and thumb

The maintenance of joint mobility and prevention of deformity or contracture are the most important functions of upper limb orthoses (Muckart, 1970). The principal objectives when using an upper limb orthosis are to maintain normal joint alignment in the absence of contractures, or to return affected joints to their normal physiological positions when contractures are present. When patients have reduced muscle power or muscle imbalance, orthoses may be used to either hold joints in their position of function or to provide

assistance to dynamic motion. Orthoses may also be used to immobilize joints to provide functional stability or to prevent painful motion which may occur in osteoarthritis or rheumatoid arthritis.

The design of orthoses for the wrist and hand (including the fingers and thumb in the context of this section) is particularly difficult for three reasons. First, the lengths of finger and thumb bones are particularly short for the development of moments. This has the disadvantage that the short force lever arms about finger and thumb joints must be compensated for by proportionately greater magnitudes of applied force in order to generate the desired corrective moments. Secondly, the wrist and hand contain a large number of anatomical joints which may require orthotic management. Thirdly, orthotic prescriptions often require patients to be able to move their joints whilst orthoses are worn. These latter two factors considerably influence the biomechanical design of orthoses and are considered in turn below.

(a) Degrees of freedom

The number of degrees of freedom in the wrist and hand determines the number of force actions which should be incorporated in designs of wrist and hand orthoses. The total number of degrees of freedom is found by listing the possible movements of each bone with respect to its proximal one and summarizing them in the manner shown in Table 11.8.

Thirty degrees of freedom exist, a number which far surpasses any modern sophisticated machine. It would be unrealistic to design orthoses which are capable of exerting a moment about each joint individually and it is common practice for individual dynamic components to act upon multiple joints.

(b) Requirements for the mobilization of joints

The historical development of orthoses mirrored classical orthopaedic teaching, in that joint rest and immobilization have key roles in the management of a wide variety of disorders of the musculoskeletal system. This view is enforced by patients themselves when they experience pain when moving joints. There is, however, increasing evidence that mechanical stress and motion have beneficial effects upon

Table 11.8 Degrees of freedom in the wrist and hand

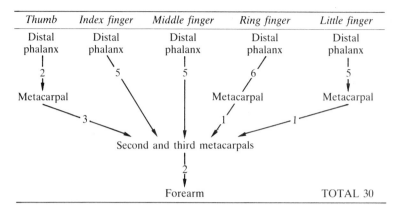

Thumb	Index finger	Middle finger	Ring finger	Little finger
Distal phalanx	Distal phalanx	Distal phalanx	Distal phalanx	Distal phalanx

the repair of bone, tendon, ligament and cartilage. Gelberman *et al.* (1982) have demonstrated that intermittent passive motion can prevent the adhesion of flexor tendon sheaths whilst tendon healing occurs. It is apparent that active mobilization can be achieved whilst an orthosis is used, provided it is structurally flexible and easily deformed by a patient's musculature. This has led to the development of 'dynamic' or 'lively' orthoses which can be elastically deformed with small values of energy.

(c) Specifications for the design of dynamic orthoses

The fundamental biomechanical principle governing the design of 'dynamic' orthoses is that energy is transferred from the orthosis to the tissues, and vice versa, when joint musculature is alternatively relaxed and contracted. The strain energy stored in the orthosis attempts to dissipate by placing the contracted joint tissues in a condition of mechanical stress. If the stiffness of the orthosis is increased, the amount of energy required to deform its shape is similarly increased. Flexible orthotic components must have low energy absorbing capacity and they are typically fabricated from elastic bands or coiled wire.

Historically, Bunnell's Weniger splint (Bunnell, 1946; Bunnell and Howard, 1950) marked the beginning of the modern evolution of dynamic hand orthoses (Figure 11.4). His orthoses were designed to exercise and mobilize joints and, at the same time, to realign joints to positions of function. His splints were enor-

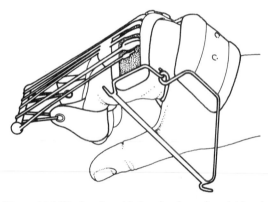

Figure 11.4 Weniger knuckle bender dynamic wrist-hand orthosis with outrigger

mously successful on young well-motivated World War Two casualties who were eager to return to civilian employment. The main disadvantage of his design is the fact that elastic bands can only exert force along their own longitudinal axes, whereas the finger tip actually follows a curve congruent with an equiangular spiral. The orthosis must include protruding rigid wires, which support the elastic bands, and which direct their lines of force. These 'outriggers', as they are named, make the orthosis conspicuous and it tended to hook onto clothes and bed covers. This problem was addressed by Moberg (1983) who commented that the problems associated with outriggers sometimes made their use impossible because of patients' negative reaction. He proposed the use of pulleys which would correctly direct the elastic bands' line of action and would also position the elastic bands in a longitudinal direction adjacent to the hand. A

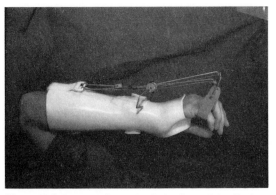

Figure 11.5 An extension orthosis for finger joint flexion contractures (for the meta carpophalangeal joints of the ring and little fingers)

minor disadvantage of this design is the high coefficient of friction between metal and elastic which necessitates the use of low friction rolling pulleys. Moberg's proposals have been widely accepted and his design is named the 'low-profile splint'. Variations of this design are in common use today (Figure 11.5).

An alternative method of applying strain energy from a dynamic orthosis is through the use of coiled wire. The advantages of using a coiled wire spring in preference to an elastic band are, first, a spring can produce both flexion and extension moments whereas elastic bands can provide tensile force only, and secondly, it is inherently smaller. The disadvantage of using coiled wire is that its axis of rotation is located at its centre so it must be carefully located adjacent to the anatomical axis of rotation.

(d) Force requirements

Ideally, an orthosis would provide a controlled moment upon each joint which requires corrective action. In practice, this is frequently impossible due to the number of degrees of freedom involved, so the design of an orthosis may have to provide correction for multiple joints with a single force input. The biomechanical principles which should be applied to the design of dynamic orthoses are explained below using the example of the 'armchair' orthosis illustrated in Figure 11.6. Strain energy, which is stored in the coil C prior to its application to the patient, produces a force F_3 in a direction approximately tangentially to the arc whose centre is at C assuming the coil's extension, CD, is not under longitudinal strain. The force vector F_3 should ideally be directed perpendicularly to the longitudinal axis of the distal phalanx in order that there is no tendency for the finger loop to slide proximally. In practice, this can only be achieved if the longitudinal axis of the distal phalanx is directed towards the coil centre. When this is not done, the finger loop must be positioned at the distal interphalangeal joint for retention. The forces F_1, F_2 and F_3, exerted by the orthosis on the hand, must be in static equilibrium. When they are resolved into their vertical and horizontal components (with respect to the proximal phalanx), then:

$$F_1 \sin \theta_1 + F_3 \sin \theta_3 = F_2$$
$$F_1 \cos \theta_1 = F_3 \cos \theta_3$$

It can be seen that all three finger joints are subjected to extension moments. Force F_3

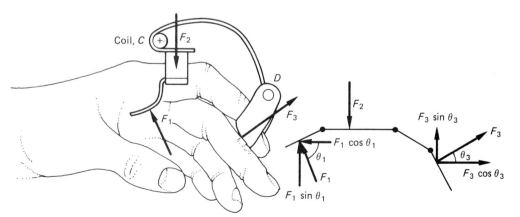

Figure 11.6 Dynamic 'armchair' finger orthosis for the extension of the interphalangeal joints

generates moments about both interphalangeal joints and independent control over each joint cannot be provided for the example shown. The magnitude of force F_3 can be altered by adjusting the coil to ensure that the force levels are tolerable to the patient. The theoretical torsional stiffness (i.e. the torque required for unit angular deformation) of a close-coiled helical spring is proportional to the modulus of elasticity of the material and the fourth power of the wire diameter, and inversely proportional to the coil diameter and the number of turns (Hearn, 1989). In algebraic terms:

$$\frac{T}{\emptyset} = \frac{E\,d^4}{64\,D\,n}$$

Hence, the stiffness of a particular coil is typically reduced by decreasing the wire gauge, increasing the coil diameter and increasing the number of turns in the coil. Care should be exercised when using this formula because coils manufactured from small gauge wire do not keep their geometrical symmetry when torsional load is increased. There is a difference between the actual torsional stiffness of coils and their theoretical values, illustrated in Figure 11.7.

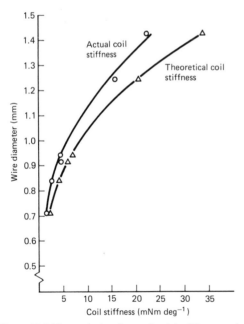

Figure 11.7 Theoretical and actual axial stiffnesses of close-coiled helical springs (Carus, 1985). The diameters of the steel coils were 7.7 mm. The results are normalized for a single turn of wire

The conditions when a dynamic orthosis could be expected to provide a satisfactory biomechanical force action are demonstrated in the following example. Figure 11.8 illustrates the structural properties of a dynamic finger orthosis which was bench tested to determine its stiffness-deformation characteristics (McDougall *et al.*, 1985). The dynamic component comprised a coiled wire, located on a rigid extension upon the hand interface component. The intersections on the force vector plot show both the magnitude and direction with which the force vector, exerted by the dynamic orthosis, acts upon the distal phalanx. For the instance shown, the orthosis would exert a force of magnitude 4 N at an inclination of 30° to the longitudinal axis of the metacarpal, used as the reference axis. When the orthosis was incorrectly prepared, however, by using a spring with greater torsional stiffness, the plot shown in Figure 11.9 was produced. It can be seen that this orthosis would be unsatisfactory because the force vector is directed in too close alignment to the longitudinal axis of the distal phalanx and the coil is too stiff, witnessed by the close proximity of the force contour lines. It would be a highly desirable goal to precisely quantify the stiffness-deformation characteristics of samples of the types of coiled wire commonly used in the manufacture of orthoses. It is believed that this has not yet been achieved, probably because of the large number of permutations. The orthotist-therapist must therefore 'feel' the stiffness-deformation characteristics of an orthosis and judge its suitability.

The force exerted by a dynamic orthosis which uses an elastic band is illustrated in Figure 11.10. Manufacturers may be able to provide stiffness data for the elastic and this can be verified in the manner described by Mildenberger *et al.* (1986). The stiffness of the elastic depends upon the magnitude of the strain energy which has to be exerted upon it to 'untangle' the polymer chains when the elastic is stretched. Its stiffness depends upon the length and cross-sectional area of the elastic and the extent of cross-link polymerization. A long elastic can be used with a low-friction pulley and an 'outrigger'. The force exerted by the elastic cord is always directed along its longitudinal axis so its line of action is affected by the position of the pulley. It is significantly easier to change the force action provided by

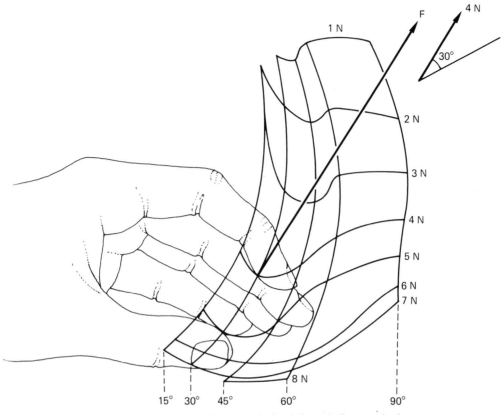

Figure 11.8 Stiffness-deformation characteristics of a correctly fitted dynamic finger orthosis

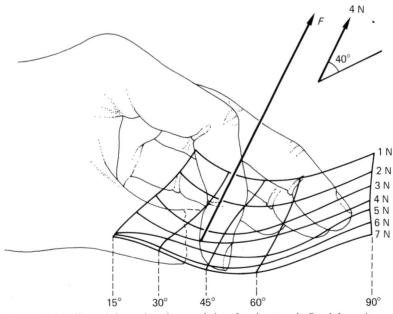

Figure 11.9 Stiffness-deformation characteristics of an incorrectly fitted dynamic finger orthosis

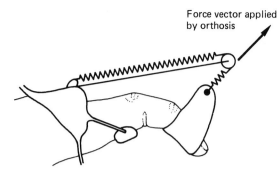

Force vector applied by orthosis

Figure 11.10 Force vector exerted by a dynamic orthosis with an elastic band

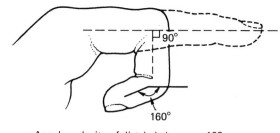

$$\frac{\text{Angular velocity of distal phalanx}}{\text{Angular velocity of middle phalanx}} = \frac{160}{90} \simeq 1.8$$

Figure 11.11 Synchronous motion of the distal and middle phalanges with respect to the proximal phalanx

this type of orthosis than that exerted by coiled wire.

The elastic cord may have a helical spring attached in series to it. The theoretical axial stiffness (i.e. the force required for unit linear extension) of an open-coiled helical spring is proportional to the fourth power of the wire diameter, and inversely proportional to the third power of the mean diameter of the coil and the number of turns;

$$\frac{W}{x} \, \alpha \, \frac{d^4 \cos(\delta)}{D^3 \, n \, [k_1 \cos^2(\delta) + k_2 \sin^2(\delta)]}$$

where k_1 and k_2 are constants and δ is the helix angle of the spring (Hearn, 1989). As before, the stiffness of a particular coil is typically reduced by decreasing the wire gauge, increasing the coil diameter and increasing the number of turns in the coil.

(e) Kinematic requirements

Orthosis design should ensure that the normal synchronous motion of the interphalangeal joints is preserved. The ratio of the average angular velocities of the distal and middle phalanges, with respect to the proximal phalanx, is approximately 1.8 because flexion of the interphalangeal joints occurs during the same time period (Figure 11.11). An idealized dynamic orthosis which would, at a particular instant, provide this ratio of angular velocities is shown in Figure 11.12. It comprises a coil G and a finger loop which is located on the distal phalanx and is illustrated by the kinematic offset, CDE. The three phalanges are denoted AB, BC and CD. The instantaneous centres of rotation I_{ij} are identified and a relative velocity

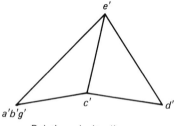

Relative velocity diagram

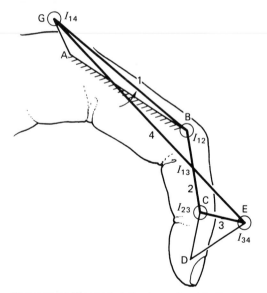

Figure 11.12 Kinematic behaviour of an idealized dynamic finger orthosis

diagram drawn. The angular velocity of the distal phalanx with respect to the proximal phalanx is given by the expression:

$$\frac{\text{velocity of E with respect to G}}{\text{distance between } I_{13} \text{ and E}}$$

$$= \frac{g'e'}{I_{13}E} = \frac{34}{20} = 1.7$$

(from scale)

and the angular velocity of the middle phalanx with respect to the proximal phalanx is given by:

$$\frac{\text{velocity of C with respect to B}}{\text{distance between C and B}}$$

$$= \frac{b'c'}{BC} = \frac{20}{22} = 0.9$$

(from scale)

The ratio of the angular velocities is 1.9, a value which is very similar to the desired value of 1.8, so this design of orthosis would ensure that the normal physiological movement of the fingers is retained for the finger joint angles shown. This design however has not been adopted for general orthotic use, presumably because the required location of components between the fingers could irritate adjacent fingers and also because the desired synchronous motion of the orthosis is not retained when the insstantaneous centre of rotation I_{13} is displaced during finger flexion and extension.

This idealized kinematic behaviour is compared with the 'armchair' orthosis illustrated in Figure 11.13. In this case, the angular velocity of the distal phalanx with respect to the proximal phalanx is:

$$\frac{\text{velocity of E with respect to G}}{\text{distance between } I_{13} \text{ and E}}$$

$$= \frac{g'e'}{I_{13}E} = \frac{35}{63} = 0.6$$

(from scale)

and the angular velocity of the middle phalanx with respect to the proximal phalanx is given by:

$$\frac{\text{velocity of C with respect to B}}{\text{distance between C and B}}$$

$$= \frac{b'c'}{BC} = \frac{32}{23} = 1.4$$

(from scale)

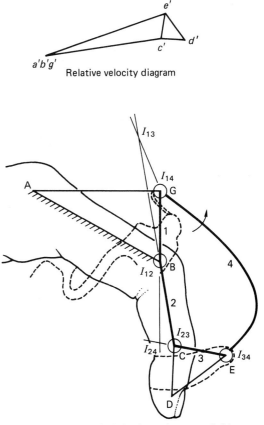

Relative velocity diagram

Figure 11.13 Kinematic behaviour of an 'armchair' dynamic finger orthosis

The ratio of the angular velocities is 0.4, a value significantly different from the desired value of 1.8. The kinematic anlaysis does appear to be disappointing but the armchair orthosis can be successfully used provided the dorsal link, GE, is able to increase in length during finger flexion to ensure synchronous interphalangeal joint motion is retained.

11.5 Description of current orthoses

References which describe the methods for fabricating upper limb orthoses include those written by Barr (1975), Malick (1978, 1979), Ellis (1981) and Rossi (1987). The essential considerations in the fabrication of upper limb orthoses are described below.

11.5.1 Materials

(a) Interface components

The principal material currently used for the construction of the interface components for upper limb orthoses is low temperature thermoplastic sheet of which a wide range is available worldwide. The majority, whilst possibly varying slightly in certain specific characteristics, all share the common feature of being mouldable between 65° and 80°C. These materials may be applied directly to the body by virtue of their low moulding temperature and they have excellent moulding characteristics. A positive cast to facilitate moulding is therefore not usually necessary. These materials generally do not possess either the strength or durability of high temperature thermoplastics, although this is usually not critical for upper limb orthoses which are required for relatively short periods of time. Orthosis construction using low temperature thermoplastics requires only a simple heat source such as a hot water bath, basic trimming tools such as knives or scissors, and suitable velcro fastening straps. Accordingly, orthoses can be quickly and relatively easily constructed from this material.

High temperature materials are also used for construction of upper limb orthoses, especially those required for long-term use. Furthermore, this material is used for the fabrication of interface modules used in some of the modular 'off-the-shelf' type orthoses systems now available. The principal advantages of using high temperature materials are that they are stronger, more rigid and durable than low temperature types. Their higher moulding temperature of 120–180°C, however, prevents the possibility of direct moulding to the patient. The moulding of these materials requires the production of a positive cast which consequently makes device fabrication both more complex and time consuming.

(c) Dynamic components

These are used to provide the required moments to the joints. The two main types of material which are used are rubber elastic and spring steel wire.

Elastic

Rubber bands or cords are widely used because they have the advantage of being readily available, cheap and easy to apply, adjust or replace. The encumberance of prominent outriggers, described by Moberg (1983), may be of little significance when these orthoses are used on motivated patients for relatively short periods of treatment in post-traumatic surgery cases. This design, however, is not usually suitable either for long-term applications or when the patient requires to use his hand for functional or occupational tasks.

Spring steel wire (piano wire)

This material is also relatively cheap and widely available. It is usually used in the form of a coil with extensions for attachment to the interface components and finger loops (Figure 11.6). The centre of the coil is normally located on, or as near as possible to, the axis of rotation of the desired joint. The coil tension can be adjusted to create the required level of flexion resistance/extension assistance. With correctly sized and shaped extensions, springs can exert arcuate force vectors which offer the potential of forming a closer biomechanical match to normal anatomical joint motion than can be achieved with orthoses which use elastic bands. Spring wire is also more controllable and versatile than elastic bands since the coils can be adjusted to provide specific functional assistance or motion control. Such springs therefore, if correctly designed and applied, offer the potential of more effective control than elastic bands. The disadvantage of using spring wire is the need to use more tools than for elastic bands. A certain degree of skill is also necessary to form the coil, shape its extension wires and to achieve a suitable and secure means of attaching them to the orthosis interface components. Finally, excessive levels of spring breakage may occur if poor quality wire is used or if the wires are incorrectly shaped.

11.5.2 Orthoses for the shoulder

(a) Glenohumeral subluxation due to muscle paralysis

The orthotic objective is to provide a proximally acting axial force on the humerus to prevent inferior subluxation. The simplest design is a sling which seeks to achieve support by a single loop around the neck with either end attached to the forearm. Cool (1989) however has demonstrated, using the free body diagram

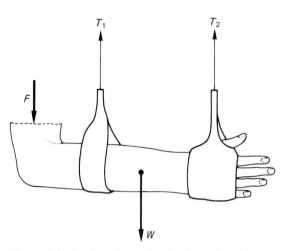

Figure 11.14 Loading of a modified collar and cuff sling for inferior subluxation of the shoulder

in Figure 11.14, that this approach cannot be successful. It can be seen in the figure that, for equilibrium of the forearm, the two tensions T_1 and T_2 cannot be equal. Since the tensions are applied at opposite ends of the same strap, their difference can only be achieved by friction around the neck which, in practice, initially leads to movement of the sling and the recurrence of subluxation. After a biomechanical analysis of the requirements, Cool proposed the design illustrated in Figure 11.15

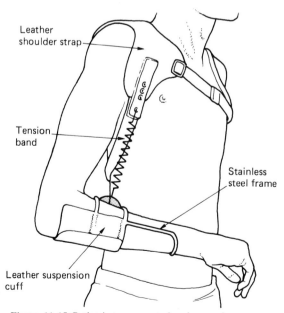

Figure 11.15 Orthosis to prevent glenohumeral subluxation. (Reproduced with permission from Cool, 1989)

where the arm is suspended from a strap attached over the injured shoulder. The lower end of the strap is attached to the proximal forearm so that the tension produces a moment sufficient to maintain it in equilibrium while supporting the humerus. This approach also avoids the problem of applying an axial force directly to the upper arm. A cuff above elbow level can only transmit axial load by friction unless there is a 'taper fit' which is likely to be prevented by large movements of soft tissue. A secure anchor is provided by a moulded cap which is held in position by a chest harness, and excessive pressure on the forearm is avoided by the use of a lightweight stainless-steel frame incorporating a plate to support the hand.

A solution favoured by the authors, and illustrated in Figure 11.16, again makes use of a rigid moulded shoulder cap attached to a condylar bearing cuff at the elbow. The cap is retained in position by straps which pass around the back of the neck (A), and over the chest (B), passing under the opposite axilla. The free body diagram in Figure 11.16 indicates how the shoulder cap is maintained in equilibrium by the applied forces.

An alternative method, used by some orthotists, is to support the arm on an orthosis attached to the trunk as shown in Figure 11.17.

(b) Brachial plexus injury

This injury is caused by traction and usually involves the spinal roots of C5 and C6. It often results from an inferior impact on the shoulder or excessive lateral displacement of the head and neck, typically as a result of a road traffic accident. The degree and permanence of the resulting paralysis depends upon the location of the lesion and also upon its severity. A typical clinical presentation is of a flail arm caused by combined denervation of wrist extensors, forearm supinators and elbow flexors. The shoulder muscles innervated by the upper trunk of the brachial plexus, namely the deltoid, supraspinatus, infraspinatus and teres minor, are also commonly involved, compromising active shoulder flexion and external rotation. The collective effect of this debilitating paralysis results in inferior displacement of the shoulder with the arm hanging limp against the trunk in a position of internal rotation and pronation.

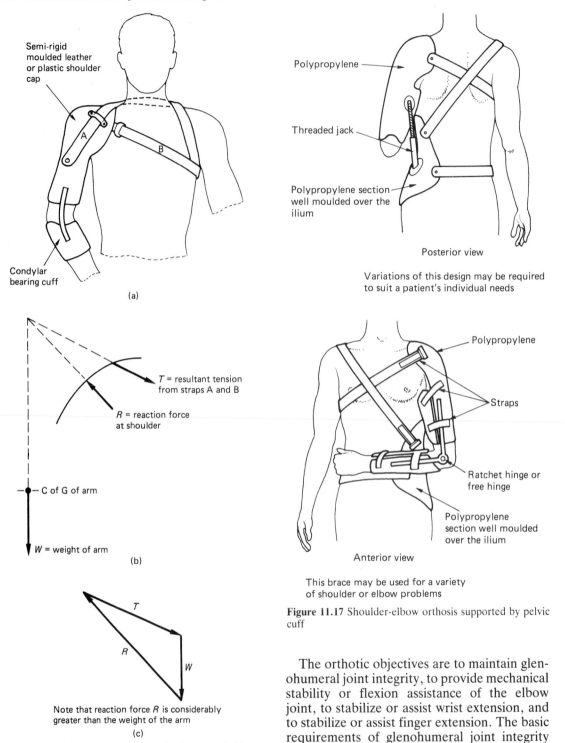

Semi-rigid moulded leather or plastic shoulder cap

A

B

Condylar bearing cuff

(a)

Polypropylene

Threaded jack

Polypropylene section well moulded over the ilium

Posterior view

Variations of this design may be required to suit a patient's individual needs

T = resultant tension from straps A and B

R = reaction force at shoulder

C of G of arm

W = weight of arm

(b)

Polypropylene

Straps

Ratchet hinge or free hinge

Polypropylene section well moulded over the ilium

Anterior view

This brace may be used for a variety of shoulder or elbow problems

Figure 11.17 Shoulder-elbow orthosis supported by pelvic cuff

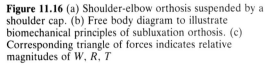

T

R

W

Note that reaction force R is considerably greater than the weight of the arm

(c)

Figure 11.16 (a) Shoulder-elbow orthosis suspended by a shoulder cap. (b) Free body diagram to illustrate biomechanical principles of subluxation orthosis. (c) Corresponding triangle of forces indicates relative magnitudes of *W, R, T*

The orthotic objectives are to maintain glenohumeral joint integrity, to provide mechanical stability or flexion assistance of the elbow joint, to stabilize or assist wrist extension, and to stabilize or assist finger extension. The basic requirements of glenohumeral joint integrity and support of the arm can usually be met by the methods described earlier for preventing subluxation (Figures 11.16, 11.17). A more extensive device, however, will be required for the collective positional control of the shoulder, elbow, wrist, hand and fingers. These orthoses are produced in several modular and bespoke designs which comprise a moulded plastic or leather shoulder cap, to which the distal components are attached. Alternatively, the device can be supported distally over the crest of the pelvis using a moulded plastic or metal shaped band, held in place by encircling straps. The structure of the orthosis is then attached to this pelvic anchor section, extended proximally to the axilla and secured to the trunk by a second lateral strap passed around the opposite axilla. The advantage of this configuration is that by not enclosing the shoulder, it reduces the likelihood of pressure problems, as well as difficulties of donning and doffing. This arrangement does not provide shoulder stability and control.

If control of the elbow is required then uniaxial ratchet type devices, which permit adjustable static positioning, are commonly used. For instance, in the case of a complete palsy of C5 and C6, there will be good hand movement but a flaccid elbow, and so an automatic locking elbow joint is provided which may be 'thrown' into different positions by a shrug of the shoulder. For wrist joint control, simple fixed or adjustable static positioning or dynamic flexion resistance/extension assistance can be used. Static positioning or dynamic assistance or resistance can be provided for the fingers. Straps are used to secure the device to the arm. If required, a removable hook or other terminal device can be operated by a cable attached at the contralateral shoulder. The Stanmore modular flail arm orthosis provides many of these facilities and uses a specially designed harness for attachment to the trunk (Figure 11.18). The weight of the arm (and orthosis) is supported by the moulded harness over the shoulder (1). In addition, because the centre of mass is frequently in front of the shoulder, there is a need to counteract the resulting moment. This reaction is provided by the lower part of the

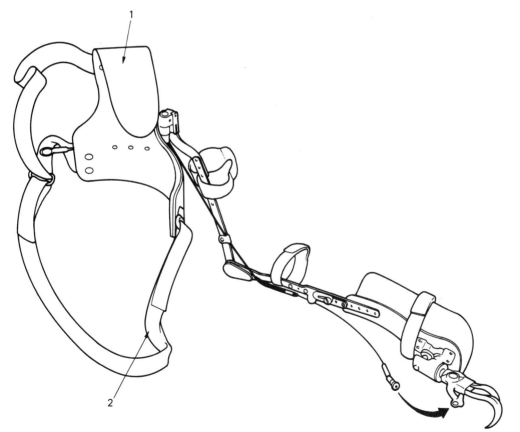

Figure 11.18 'Stanmore' modular flail arm orthosis

moulded harness which is held in position by the retaining strap (2). This orthosis has been used for a wide variety of trades and professions, including gardening, carpentry, office work and lorry driving.

(c) Functional orthosis for the flail arm

In some cases, a patient with a flail arm can gain functional benefits from mobile arm supports attached to a wheelchair or other suitable structure. These orthoses normally have four degrees of freedom. Two links in the horizontal plane permit translation and a two degree of freedom knuckle joint is used to attach a trough supporting the forearm to this linkage. The result of this arrangement is that the supported arm has three degrees of freedom in the horizontal plane and can also be rotated in a vertical plane. The orthosis must be carefully fitted to ensure that the forearm is balanced and that the hand has a functional range of motion.

11.5.3 Orthoses for the elbow

Elbow flexor weakness

The biomechanical requirements are met by a four-point force system to stabilize the elbow. The forces are applied distally on the ulnar aspect of the forearm and proximally on the posterior aspect of the humerus. A single central opposing counter force could be optimally located directly over the anterior surface of elbow joint, but this is not practical because straps applied there restrict elbow flexion and cause unacceptable pressure. In consequence, the application of anterior counter forces is usually achieved by using two separate straps located at the regions of the distal humerus and proximal forearm and situated as close to the joint axis as possible without causing impediment or discomfort during flexion. Additional proximal and distal straps are provided for the retention of the orthosis on the limb.

This condition may be treated by either dynamic or static devices. Where any degree of recovery is possible and in the absence of any other overriding pathology, then a dynamic hinged device may be used (Figure 11.19). These usually feature moulded thermoplastic cuffs at the forearm and humerus which are

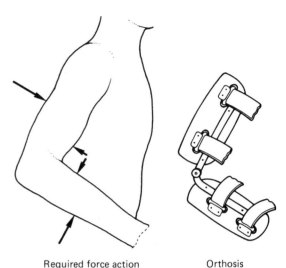

Required force action   Orthosis

Figure 11.19 Hinged elbow orthosis with free flexion and 90° extension stop

connected by one or two hinged joints. These joints may have either free motion or adjustable settings for various positions of the forearm. If no recovery is expected then simple static orthoses may be used to hold the forearm, and if required the wrist or hand, in a position of optimum function or comfort. They may also have a cosmetic role by holding the forearm in a natural flexed position thereby reinstating body symmetry.

11.5.4 Orthoses for the wrist

(a) Radial nerve palsy

Damage or transection of the radial nerve severely compromises normal wrist and hand function. A nerve lesion may result from a humeral fracture, resulting in denervation of the distal muscle group, for example the wrist extensors and extrinsic finger extensors. It may be difficult or impossible for the patient to maintain normal active wrist extension, metacarpophalangeal joint extension, wrist abduction and adduction and normal finger pinch strength. The orthotic objectives are, first, to support the wrist in an extended position, and secondly, to support the metacarpophalangeal and interphalangeal joints in functional positions to aid recovery and prevent contractures. These are usually achieved with the use of a dynamic orthosis which features separate volar forearm and hand sections, connected together

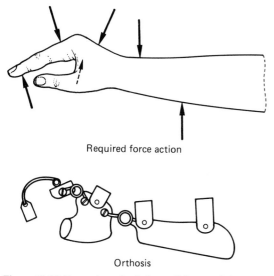

Required force action

Orthosis

Figure 11.20 Dynamic orthosis for radial nerve injury

with spring wire coils located on both sides of the wrist joint (Figure 11.20). Corrective moments about the metacarpophalangeal joints are provided with the use of a transverse dorsal bar on the proximal phalanges, connected to the hand component with wire springs. Moments about the interphalangeal joints are provided by wire springs attached at their proximal ends on the transverse dorsal bar, and at their distal ends with finger loops.

The effectiveness of this orthosis depends upon both the correct alignment of the individual orthotic components and the application of two interacting force systems. First, a wrist extension moment is achieved by the application of dorsally acting forces upon the volarly surfaces of the forearm and palm, and a volar acting force on the dorsum of the distal forearm at the region of the ulnar styloid. A second dorsal forearm strap is often added proximally to improve retention, though this is not essential for the force system. The second force system creates a flexion moment at the metacarpophalangeal joint. This is achieved by the application of volarly acting forces on the dorsum of the metacarpal and the first phalanx, the latter provided by the transverse bar. The opposing dorsally acting force is applied via the palmar section of the hand component. Extension moments about the interphalangeal joints are provided by a dorsally acting force on the distal phalanx.

(b) Wrist extensor weakness

Wrist extensor weakness results in functional deficiencies, typically weak grasp and diminished control of the hand and fingers. In the presence of this weakness, the effect of gravity tends to cause wrist flexion when the elbow is flexed. Additionally, in clinical conditions such as hemiplegia when there may be severe spasticity in the unopposed wrist flexors, severe contractures may rapidly develop.

The orthotic objective is to hold the wrist in the neutral position pending recovery, or where recovery is not possible, to hold the wrist and hand in the best functional position attainable. The biomechanical requirements are met by the application of a three-point control system to stabilize the wrist joint (Figure 11.21). The two dorsally acting forces are applied on the volar aspects, typically at the palm and mid-forearm, and the opposing dorsal counterforce is applied either over the wrist joint or immediately proximal to it. The orthotic options include both static and dynamic orthoses, the choice depending upon the precise pathology being treated, the predicted treatment outcome and the possible need to accommodate any occupational or recreational requirements. Static immobilization and support of the wrist is most easily achieved by the use of a moulded leather, or more commonly plastic, wrist-hand orthosis. This device features a volar shell with dorsal counter straps. Theoretically, only one dorsal counter strap is required but in practice additional straps are

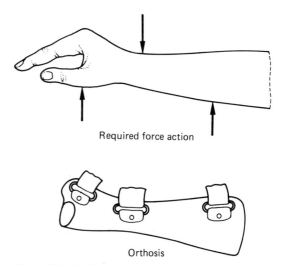

Required force action

Orthosis

Figure 11.21 Static wrist-hand orthosis

frequently added over the metacarpals and at the proximal end of the forearm section to improve attachment to the arm and improve retention. Dynamic devices most commonly feature a similar thermoplastic construction but with separate hand and forearm sections. These are coupled together by means of coiled spring wire components located on the radial and ulnar sides. The coil tensions are adjusted to counterbalance the weight of hand. Using this type of device, it is possible to maintain hand position without eliminating residual motion, or the potential for the patient to exercise the wrist joint by flexing against the resistance of the springs.

(c) The painful wrist

There are a number of conditions which cause wrist pain. Osteoarthritis results in a reduction of joint space and bone sclerosis leading to the development of osteophytes. Tenosynovitis in the tendon sheaths at the wrist joint is characterized by swelling and discomfort. Keinbock's disease (avascular necrosis of the lunate) and non-union of fractured carpal bones causes persistent pain, as does a malunion of a Colles' fracture. Static orthoses which provide compression between the thenar muscles, the dorsum of the wrist joint and the distal end of the forearm limit wrist movement and thereby alleviate pain. Static orthoses may also be prescribed prior to wrist arthrodesis surgery in order that the patient may experience the functional effects of wrist immobilization.

(d) Rheumatoid arthritis

Rheumatoid arthritis is a particularly destructive and disabling disease. It causes an ulnar drift deformity which affects all four fingers in 30% of female patients and 15% of male patients (Vaino and Oka, 1953). The deformity is caused by synovitis, the proliferation of joint membranes and an increase in joint fluids. These stretch the radial collateral ligaments and the radial hood which stabilizes the extensor tendons, leading to subluxation of the extensor tendons in the ulnar direction. Secondary contracture of the intrinsic ulnar muscles and the ulnar collateral ligament result in further ulnar drift. Ulnar drift may also be accompanied by radial deviation of the wrist which results in the typical 'zig-zag' deformity.

The pathomechanics of ulnar drift have been studied by Flatt (1971).

Orthoses may be prescribed before and after joint replacement surgery. Generally speaking, the preferred orthosis is a dynamic design which provides dorsoradially acting forces on the displaced phalanges. These devices provide gentle and continuous forces which strive to place and maintain the fingers in their normal position. Static orthoses also have a role for night-time use and are useful in relieving morning joint stiffness. They incorporate dorsal straps which exert minimal pressure upon the joints to provide correction moments during sleep. 'Posts' fixed to the volar surfaces of the orthoses can be located between the fingers to provide radially acting corrective forces.

11.5.5 Orthoses for the fingers

(a) Flexor tendon repair

The management of Zone II flexor tendon repairs remains one of the most severe rehabilitation challenges. The known risk of adhesions forming between the repaired tendon and its sheath is a strong clinical indication for early motion. Experimental studies (Matthews and Richards, 1976; Gelberman *et al.*, 1982) support the concept that the speed of healing and the strength of tendons can be improved by their mechanical environment. Hence, the purpose of an orthotic prescription is to provide relative gliding of the tendon with respect to its sheath. The most common orthosis design features a volar forearm section with an elastic band connected between it and the finger tip. The patient is encouraged to actively extend his finger against the action of the elastic band, which then returns the finger to its flexed position. This method was first described by Young and Harman (1960), and has been more recently advocated by Lister and Kleinert (Lister *et al.*, 1977). The most troublesome complication is a flexion contracture of the proximal interphalangeal joint and it is considered essential that the patient should achieve full extension of all interphalangeal finger joints during therapy.

A variety of modifications have been advocated and one of the most notable has been the use of a pulley to improve flexion of the distal interphalangeal joint and hence the excursion of the profundus tendon (Slattery and McGrouther, 1984). Figure 11.22(a) and (b)

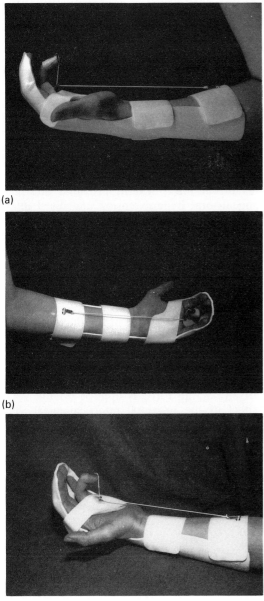

(a)

(b)

(c)

Figure 11.22 (a)–(c) Kleinert (design) orthoses with low friction pulleys

illustrates an orthosis with a low friction pulley situated on the proximal phalanx of the ring finger; Figure 11.22(c) illustrates a low friction pulley on the palm of the hand. Lin *et al.* (1989) studied the effects of incorporating a pulley to direct the line of action of the elastic band. If no pulley were used, and the elastic band provided a direct pull on the distal phalanx, the excursions of the flexor profundus

and flexor superficialis in Zone II were 10.1 and 7.8 mm respectively. When the orthosis was modified to provide a palmar pulley, under which the elastic band was passed, the excursions increased to 15 mm and 13 mm for the same tendons. Finally, if the palmar bar were retained and synergistic wrist motion was made, the corresponding tendon excursions were 19.8 and 15.2 mm respectively. In summary, the current design of an orthosis for flexor tendon repair, based upon biomechanical considerations, calls for a low profile volar elastic band, routed under a pulley, with synergistic wrist motion.

(b) Boutonnièrre deformity

This deformity is characterized by combined flexion of the proximal interphalangeal joint and hyperextension of the distal interphalangeal joint. It results from lengthening of both the middle slip of the extensor hood and the triangular retinacular ligament at the proximal interphalangeal joint. These cause palmar displacement of the lateral bands of the long extensor tendon and dorsal subluxation of the proximal phalanx. The deformity may arise either as a result of trauma, or dorsal synovitis which occurs in rheumatoid arthritis. Except for cases where the damage or deformity is slight, this condition, by its nature, is difficult to treat by the use of orthoses alone. Surgical repair is the primary method of treatment though orthoses are frequently used postoperatively.

The orthotic objectives are to hold the proximal interphalangeal joint in extension and the distal interphalangeal joint in flexion, to reduce undesirable tension in the extensor hood whilst healing takes place. This may be achieved by the application of a four-point force system (Figure 11.23). Dorsally acting forces are applied to the volar surface of the middle phalanx and at the proximal phalanx at the region adjacent to the metacarpophalangeal joint. Opposing volar counteracting forces are applied over the dorsum of the middle phalanx adjacent to the proximal interphalangeal joint, and at the distal phalanx. Orthotic options include both static and dynamic orthoses. Static devices are most widely used, particularly for immediate postoperative management and for cases for which the damage or deformity is moderate to severe. The

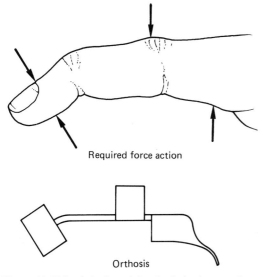

Required force action

Orthosis

Figure 11.23 Static 'safety pin' orthosis for boutonnière deformity

types of static devices include simple metal or thermoplastic volar gutters with straps over the distal phalanx and proximal interphalangeal joint regions. At a later stage in the recovery period, dynamic devices such as the Bunnell proximal interphalangeal joint extension-traction type of orthosis may be used (Figure 11.24). This consists of proximal and distal volar saddles, connected by two lengths of spring steel wire with an adjoining dorsal

velchro securing strap. The wire stiffness is sufficient to maintain passive proximal interphalangeal joint extension, yet flexible enough to also permit active flexion.

(c) Swan neck deformity

This deformity is most commonly associated with rheumatoid arthritis but may also arise as a result of ulnar neuropathy, cerebral palsy or Parkinson's disease. The appearance of the deformity is the reverse of the Boutonnière and is characterized by combined metacarpophalangeal joint flexion, proximal interphalangeal joint hyperextension and distal interphalangeal joint flexion. The condition is caused by subluxation of the lumbricals which leads to hyperextension of the proximal interphalangeal joint. This, in turn, causes tightness of the flexor digitorum profundus tendon with resulting distal interphalangeal joint flexion.

The orthotic objectives are to reduce tension in the flexor digitorum profundus tendon by holding the proximal interphalangeal joint in flexion to arrest progress of deformity. Corrective action requires the application of a four-point force system (Figure 11.25). A dorsally acting force is applied on the volar aspect of the proximal interphalangeal joint and two opposing counter forces applied at the distal end of the middle phalanx. The proximal

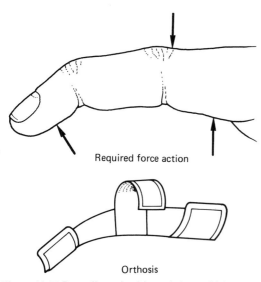

Required force action

Orthosis

Figure 11.24 Bunnell proximal interphalangeal joint extension-traction orthosis

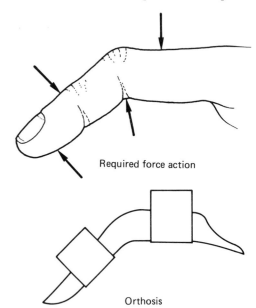

Required force action

Orthosis

Figure 11.25 Static finger orthosis for 'swan neck' deformity

interphalangeal joint is held in a straight position by a volar force on the finger tip. Static orthoses are generally used for the management of this deformity and the most common is a flexed moulded thermoplastic volar gutter with dorsal velcro securing straps. Alternatively, a moulded thermoplastic cylinder retained on the finger by its shape and intimacy of fit may be used.

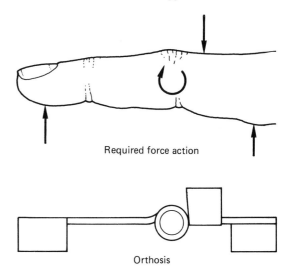

Required force action

Orthosis

Figure 11.26 Capener finger orthosis

(d) Dupuytren's contracture

This deformity most commonly involves the ring and little fingers. It is caused by progressive contracture and thickening of the longitudinal bands in the palmar fascia and results in metacarpophalangeal and proximal interphalangeal joint contractures. Surgical release of the affected tissues offers the only effective treatment for this progressive condition and the role of orthoses is therefore in postsurgical management.

The orthotic objectives are either to prevent the development of contractures which may occur during the normal soft tissue healing period, or alternatively to reduce any residual contracture which may remain postoperatively. Biomechanically, the reduction of this deformity requires the application of a three-point force system configured to create extension moments at the affected joints. Several types of orthoses are available to correct flexion of the proximal interphalangeal joint. Two of the commoner types are the Capener (Figure 11.26) and the 'armchair' (Figure 11.6), though the latter can also be used for the metacarpophalangeal joint.

The *Capener* (1967) type of orthosis features a spring wire chassis, whose side pieces are formed into a coil at the proximal interphalangeal joint. Volar saddles are located at the distal and proximal phalanges and a dorsal counter strap is located over the distal end of the proximal phalanx to effect simple three-point control. When applied to a flexed finger, the coil creates an extension moment at the PIP joint. The degree of extension assistance-flexion resistance may be adjusted either by altering the tension of the coil (by increasing or decreasing the thickness of the wire, the size or number of coils), or by bending the side pieces. The advantage of this device over the 'armchair' orthosis is that it has no dorsal projections, is less obtrusive and therefore

often more cosmetically acceptable. This design does however have some mechanical disadvantages. Its geometry and short lever arms become progressively less effective as the flexion angle increases. When used with a proximal interphalangeal flexion angle greater than 20°, the functional effect of this design is significantly compromised due to the reduced distance between the opposing force vectors.

The 'armchair' type of orthosis affects both the metacarpophalangeal and proximal interphalangeal joints. It consists of a malleable wire chassis with dorsal saddle located over the distal end of the proximal phalanx, a volar counter pad located on the palm proximal to the metacarpophalangeal joint, and a wire coil whose extension holds a finger loop which passes over the middle or distal phalanx (Figure 11.6). The spring tension exerts an extension moment on the proximal interphalangeal joint, the effect of which is to provide flexion resistance and extension assistance. Spring tension is adjusted in the same manner as described earlier. The advantage of the 'armchair' device over the Capaner type is the fact that the dorsal counter forces are further apart and this reduces the magnitudes of each of the three forces. The disadvantage of this design is that the height, length and shape of the spring, required for functional effectiveness, unavoidably causes it to protrude over the dorsum of the finger, making it more obtrusive than the Capener type. Notwithstanding this, the improved mechanical effectiveness and reduced forces exerted by the armchair orthosis compared with the Capener design render it the device of choice for the management of this condition.

11.5.6 Orthoses for the thumb

The thumb's importance for prehensile functional activities involving pinch and grasp cannot be overemphasized. It is hardly surprising, therefore, that patients may be reluctant to use orthoses which limit thumb function. In general, the number of clinical conditions which necessitate the temporary use of thumb orthoses is relatively limited, though some of the important ones are described below.

The 'game-keeper's thumb', which is a chronic metacarpophalangeal joint injury of the ulnar collateral ligament, is a painful condition which can be treated conservatively with a static opponens orthosis. The acute ulnar collateral injury is often incorrectly called a 'game-keeper's thumb'. Pichora *et al.* (1989) have reported good clinical results if the metacarpophalangeal joint is treated for 6 weeks in a removable custom-made orthosis with daily range of motion exercises. Static orthoses can also be applied for night use for patients with osteoarthritis and rheumatoid arthritis. A small number of patients with motor neurone disorders, with poor ability to provide thumb opposition, may benefit from the use of opponens orthoses for specific activities, but the majority of patients tend to reject them because they frequently interfere with sensation and function.

Dynamic orthoses are commonly prescribed for radial injuries.

11.6 Alternative and complementary treatments

Alternative and complementary treatment for patients with upper limb disorders are surgery and therapy, occasionally supplemented by functional electrical stimulation (FES). In practice, surgery and therapy can be said to be principal forms of upper limb treatment, rather than alternative and complementary. The following is an elementary description of these forms of treatment.

Surgical options involve soft tissue and bony procedures. The primary role of surgery is most commonly in the management of acute injuries, such as lacerations and fractures, though plastic surgery has a major role in the management of burns and extensive degloving injuries. Elective surgery can be performed for non-acute cases such as the lengthening of tendons to reduce contractures, or rarely, the shortening of slack tendons to improve their mechanical effect. Whenever permanent muscle denervation is present, such as may occur after irreversible nerve injury or in tetraplegia, then tendon transfer surgery may be carried out. For example, an active flexor muscle may be re-routed and attached dorsally to act as an extensor. Bony surgery, other than fracture management, is chiefly undertaken for joint fusion or replacement. Surgical fusion can eliminate painful motion or provide a position of stable function. Joint replacement surgery is now very common and joint prostheses are available for all the joints in the upper limb. Of these, metacarpophalangeal joint replacement is the commonest procedure and is typically undertaken for patients affected by rheumatoid arthritis.

The role of therapy is central in the management of the upper limb, particularly for the wrist, hand and fingers. The developments and advances in therapy treatment have resulted in the need for specialist hand therapists. Therapy is normally required for upper limb rehabilitation, irrespective of whether surgery or orthoses are employed. In the absence of surgery, the therapist endeavours to maintain joint motion, muscle power, joint control and dexterity. Postsurgery, the therapist maintains and develops joint mobility to reduce oedema, prevent contracture and to develop muscle strength. As treatment progresses, occupational therapy exercises are used to enhance function, strength, control and independence through activities of daily living (ADL) exercises supplemented by training for specific functional tasks.

A further technique used in the management of upper limb problems is functional electrical stimulation (FES), which involves the application of low voltage electrical impulses to denervated muscles to induce muscle contraction to cause joint motion. This technique involves the application of either surface or implanted electrodes to the affected muscles. Electrode signals are provided either by a table-mounted, or more commonly a patient-borne battery-powered control box. The output signal can be varied in amplitude, frequency and duration to provide the stimulus pattern best suited for the particular patient.

11.7 Current and possible future developments

An upper limb dynamic orthosis achieves its function through the transfer of energy between the orthosis and the healing or contracted tissue when muscles relax and contract. This is a *mechanically conservative system* with no external energy source. The possibility of using an external energy source to provide motion is clearly attractive whenever a patient has weakened musculature, suffers pain or lacks motivation. This has led to the development of *continuous passive motion* (CPM) machines which can be used to provide occasional, interrupted or continuous motion to affected joints.

Patients have a remarkable tolerance for CPM even in the presence of unhealed wounds. The theory which can be applied to explain this surprising fact is the 'pain gate' theory described by Melzack and Wall (1970). It is believed that CPM causes the proprioceptive receptors to provide considerable non-painful afferent input into the spinal cord ganglia. This input overwhelms the pain fibre input and thereby blocks the pain perception. Advocates of CPM report this form of treatment does not increase pain medication requirements.

The beneficial effects of CPM have been demonstrated by a variety of workers who have tested its effectiveness in different disorders. O'Driscoll *et al.* (1983) convincingly demonstrated the benefits of CPM upon joint haemarthoses; Salter *et al.*, (1981) studied its effects upon joints with septic arthritis; Gelberman *et al.* (1982) studied the effects of intermittent passive motion upon tendon healing, and Inoue *et al.* (1986) have provided strong evidence supporting the concept of early motion on ligament healing in the knee.

A convincing clinical study of the effects of CPM upon stiff finger joints was undertaken by Ketchum *et al.* (1979), who used an electrically driven hand splint to passively exercise fingers. The gains in active and passive finger joint motion achieved were compared with the results of similar stiff fingers treated by conventional means. It was shown that there was a statistically significant improvement in the mean gain of both total active and passive motion. Nowadays, the most notable commercial hand CPM machine is the Toronto Mobilimb developed by Salter and his colleagues.

Akeson *et al.* (1987) report that passive motion places in effect such fundamental cellular and tissue processes that we are probably observing only the infancy of its development. Future contributions from basic and clinical science can be expected to improve knowledge of the clinical advantages of using this type of powered orthosis.

Acknowledgements

The authors wish to thank Frau Waltraud Pinkus, head of the occupational therapy department of the Oskar-Helene-Heim Orthopaedic Hospital of the Free University of Berlin, who kindly provided the photographs used in this chapter.

References

Akeson W.H., Amiel D. and Woo S.L.-Y. (1987) Physiology and therapeutic value of passive motion. In: Helminen H., Kiviranta I., Saamanen A-M. *et al.* (eds), *Joint Loading, Biology and Health of Articular Structures*, pp. 375–394. Bristol, Wright

American Academy of Orthopedic Surgeons (1965) *Joint Motion: Method of Measuring and Recording.* American Academy of Orthopedic Surgeons, Chicago

Amis A. and Miller J. (1982) The elbow. *Clin. Rheum. Dis.* **8**, 571–594

Bailey R.W. (1982) *Human Performance Engineering: A Guide for System Designers.* Prentice-Hall, New Jersey.

Barr N.R. (1975) *The Hand: Principles and Techniques of Simple Splintmaking in Rehabilitation.* Butterworths, London.

Batmanabane M. and Malathi S. (1985). Movements at the carpometacarpal and metacarpophalangeal joints of the hand and their effect on the dimensions of the articular ends of the metacarpal bones. *Anat. Rec.* **213**, 102

Bird H. and Stowe H. (1982). The wrist. *Clin. Rheum. Dis.* **8**, 559–570

Boone D.C. and Azen S.P. (1979). Normal range of motion of joints in male subjects. *J. Bone Joint Surg.* **61A**, 756–759

Bunnell S. (1946) Active splinting of the hand. *J. Bone Joint Surg.* **28A**, 732–736

Bunnell S. and Howard L.D. Jr (1950) Additional elastic hand splints. *J. Bone Joint Surg.* **32A**, 226–228

Capener N. (1967) Lively splints. *Physiotherapy* **53**, 371–374

Carus D.A., Logan G.M., Thorpe J.R. *et al.* (1992) The technical development and clinical evaluation of a continuous passive motion system for the rehabilitation of the injured hand. In: Little E.G. (ed.), *International Conference on Experimental Biomechanics*; Limerick, Ireland, pp. 299–312. Elsevier Science Publishers BV, Amsterdam

Cool J. (1989) Biomechanics of orthoses for the subluxed shoulder. *Prosthet. Orthot. Int.* **13**, 90–96

Duncan R.M. (1989) Basic principles of splinting the hand. *Phys. Ther.* **69**, 1104–1116

Ellis M. (1981) Orthoses for the hand. In: Lamb D.W. and Kuczynski K. (eds), *The practice of hand surgery*. Blackwell Scientific Publications, Oxford, pp. 529–542

Flatt A.E. (1971) *The Pathomechanics of Ulnar Drift*; *A Biomechanical and Clinical Study*. The University of Iowa, Iowa City

Freedman L. and Munro R. (1966) Abduction of the arm in the spatula plane; scapular and glenohumeral movements. *J. Bone Joint Surg.* **48A**, 1503–1510

Gelberman R.H., Woo S.L-Y, Lothringer K. *et al.* (1982) Effects of early intermittent passive mobilization on healing canine flexor tendons. *J. Hand Surg.[Am]*, **7**, 170–175

Hearn E.J. (1989) *Mechanics of Materials*, 2nd edn. Pergamon, Oxford

Hoggart V.E. Jr (1969) *Fibonacci and Lucas Numbers*. Houghton Mifflin, Boston

Inoue M., Gomez M., Hollis V. *et al.* (1986) Medial collateral ligament healing: repair vs nonrepair. *Trans. Orthop. Res. Soc.* **11**, 78

Johnson G.R. and Anderson J.M. (1990) Measurement of three-dimensional shoulder movement by an electromagnetic sensor. *Clin. Biomech.* **5**, 123–128

Johnson G.R., Fyfe N.C.M. and Heward M. (1990) A study of the ranges of movement at the shoulder complex using an electromagnetic movement sensor. *Ann. Rheum. Dis.* **50**, 824–827

Ketchum L.D., Hibbard A. and Hassanein K.M. (1979) Follow-up report on the electrically driven hand splint. *J. Hand Surg. [Am]*, **4**, 474–481

Kohler A. (1968) *Borderlands of the Normal and Early Pathologies in Skeletal Roentgenology*, 3rd edn. Grune and Stratton, New York

Lin G-T., An K-N., Amadio P.C. *et al.* (1989) Effects of synergistic wrist motion on flexor tendon excursion in the hand. *J. Biomech.* **22**, 1048

Lister G.D., Kleinert H.E., Kutz J.E. *et al.* (1977) Primary flexor tendon repair followed by immediate controlled mobilisation. *J. Hand Surg. [Am]*, **2**, 441–451

Malick M.H. (1978) *Manual of Dynamic Hand Splinting with Thermoplastic Materials*, 2nd edn. Harmaville Rehabilitation Centre, Pittsburgh, PA

Malick M.H. (1979) *Manual of Static Hand Splinting*, 3rd edn. Harmaville Rehabilitation Centre, Pittsburgh, PA

Matthews P. and Richards H. (1976) Factors in the ad-herence of flexor tendons after repair; an experimental study in the rabbit. *J. Bone Joint Surg.* **58B**, 230–236

McDougall D.J., Carus D.A. and Jain A.S. (1985) *A Handbook of Experiences with the Application of Wrist, Hand and Finger Orthoses*. Tayside Rehabilitation Engineering Services, Dundee Limb Fitting Centre, Dundee (Mr A.S. Jain)

Melzack R. and Wall P. (1970) Psychophysiology of pain. Evolution of pain theories. *Int. Anesthesiol. Clin.* **8**, 3–34

Mildenberger L.A., Amadio P.C. and An K.N. (1986) Dynamic splinting: a systematic approach to the selection of elastic traction. *Arch. Phys. Med. Rehabil.* **67**, 241–244

Moberg E. (1983) The outrigger problem. *Scand. J. Rehabil. Med. Suppl.* **9**, 136–138

Morrey B.F., Askew L.F., An K.N. *et al.* (1981) A biomechanical study of normal functional elbow motion. *J. Bone Joint Surg.* **63A**, 872–877

Muckart R.D. (1970) Present orthotic practice in the upper extremity. In: Murdoch G. (ed.), *Prosthetic and Orthotic Practice* pp. 471–481. Edward Arnold, London

Nordin M. and Frankel V.H. (1989) *Basic Biomechanics of the Musculoskeletal System*, 2nd edn. Lea and Febiger, Philadelphia

O'Driscoll S.W., Kumaar A. and Salter R.B. (1983) The effects of continuous passive motion on the clearance of a haemarthrosis. *Clin. Orthop.* **176**, 305–311

Pichora D.R., McMurty R.Y. and Bell M.J. (1989) Gamekeeper's thumb; a prospective study of functional bracing. *J. Hand Surg. [Am]* **14**, 567–573

Poppen N.K. and Walker P.S. (1976) Normal and abnormal motion of the shoulder. *J. Bone Joint Surg.* **58A**, 195–201

Poppen N.K. and Walker P.S. (1978) Forces at the glenohumeral joint in abduction. *Clin. Orthop.* **135**, 165–170

Pronk G. (1989) A kinematic model of the shoulder girdle: a resume. *J. Med. Eng. Technol.* **13**, 119–121

Rossi J. (1987) Concepts and current trends in hand splinting. *Occup. Ther. Health Care* **4**, (3–4), 53–68

Salter R.B., Bell R.S. and Keeley F. (1981) The protective effect of continuous passive motion on living articular cartilage in acute septic arthritis; an experimental investigation in the rabbit. *Clin. Orthop.* **159**, 223–247

Slattery P.G. and McGrouther D.A. (1984) A modified Kleinert controlled mobilisation splint following flexor tendon repair. *J. Hand Surg. [Br.]* **9**, 217–218

Vaino L. and Oka M. (1953) Ulnar deviation of the fingers. *Ann. Rheum. Dis.* **12**, 122–124

Woodson W.E. and Conover D.W. (1964) *Human Engineering Guide for Equipment Designers*, 2nd edn. University of California Press

Young R.E.S. and Harman J.M. (1960) Repair of tendon injuries of the hand. *Ann. Surg.* **151**, 562–566

Youm Y. and Yoon Y.S. (1979) Analytical development in investigation of wrist kinematics. *J. Biomech.* **12**, 613–621

12

Orthoses for head and neck

Peter Convery

12.1 Introduction

Many designs of cervical orthoses are available and care must be taken to ensure that the orthotic prescription matches the patients' requirements. The aims of this chapter are to describe the functional anatomy of the cervical spine and to relate some pathological conditions to the existing range of cervical orthoses. Subsequently the two major objectives of orthotic treatment related to the functional control and stabilization of the cervical spine will be discussed.

12.2 Anatomy

The cervical spine provides support for the head whilst allowing it a degree of flexibility relative to the thorax, as well as providing protection for the spinal cord.

12.2.1 Bony elements

The first and second vertebrae are each unique and both differ from the other five cervical vertebrae. The cervical spine may be subdivided into the upper region (C1 and C2) and the lower region (C3 to C7).

The first cervical vertebrae (C1), the atlas, forms a ring with two large lateral masses whose concave superior surfaces articulate with the occipital's condyles (Figure 12.1(a)). The concave inferior surface of the lateral masses of C1 articulates with the convex supe-

rior surface of the second cervical vertebrae (C2), the axis (Figure 12.1(b)). The articulation C1/C2 is unusual in that the two vertebrae are not connected by an intervertebral disc. The odontoid process, a tooth-like peg, protrudes upwards from the body of the axis. The odontoid process fits into the ring formed by the inner surface of the anterior arch of C1, and the transverse ligament which bridges across the arch of C1. Most of the rotation of the head in the upper cervical spine occurs at the atlantoaxial joint. The spinal cord passes through the ring of the atlas and upwards through the vertebral foramen.

The C3 vertebra is similar to the remaining cervical, thoracic and lumbar vertebrae (Figure 12.2). The superior and inferior surfaces of the vertebral bodies are concave transversely and the raised lateral lips form the unciform processes. Axial loads may be transmitted through the cervical spine either through the vertebral bodies and intervertebral discs or through the two posterior facet joints, but most commonly through both. The inclination of the facet joints, at approximately 45° to the transverse plane, prevents pure lateral flexion or pure rotation. The transverse processes are grooved superiorly to allow for passage of the nerve roots. The spinous processes extend posteriorly from the posterior arch.

The vertebrae are connected viscoelastically by the intervertebral discs and ligaments. The discs permit relative motion between vertebrae and also provide assistance as a shock absorber. The discs are wedge shaped, taller

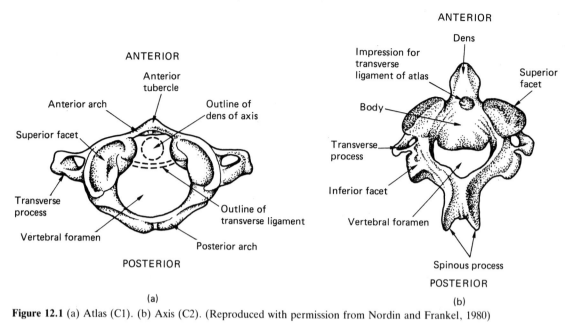

Figure 12.1 (a) Atlas (C1). (b) Axis (C2). (Reproduced with permission from Nordin and Frankel, 1980)

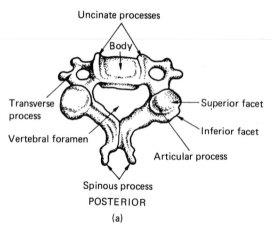

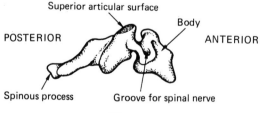

Figure 12.2 (a),(b) Typical lower cervical vertebrae. (a) Superior view. (b) Lateral view. (Reproduced with permission from Nordin and Frankel, 1980)

ventrally than dorsally, and thus contribute to the cervical lordotic curve. Flexion and extension movements of the vertebral bodies are restrained by the anterior and posterior longitudinal ligaments, whereas the ranges of movement of the transverse and spinous processes are restrained by the ligamentum nuchae, the interspinous, supraspinous, intertransverse and capsular ligaments. The transverse ligament prevents posterior translation of the odontoid within the C1 ring.

12.2.2 Muscles

The muscles in the cervical region may be grouped in terms of their location.

(a) Anterior muscles

The infrahyoid and prevertebral muscles are located anteriorly. When right and left anterior muscles act together, flexion of the head and neck occurs, and, if they act separately, lateral flexion occurs along with rotation of the head to the opposite side.

(b) Posterior muscles

Extension of the head and neck occurs when the right and left posterior cervical muscles act in unison. If the right posterior muscles act alone, the skull and neck flex laterally to the right while rotating the head to the left.

(c) *Lateral muscles*

The scalenus group, and the sternocleidomastoid muscles are positioned on the lateral aspect of the cervical region. When the right and left lateral muscles act in unison, flexion of the head and neck occurs, and if only the right muscle acts, lateral flexion of the skull and neck to the right occurs while rotating the head to the left. The levator scapulae muscle is also located laterally, and if this muscle acts on one side only and the scapula is fixed, the cervical spine will flex laterally to that side. If the levator scapulae muscles on both sides act, no movement occurs, but by so doing they help to stabilize the cervical spine.

12.3 Biomechanical considerations

The effectiveness of a cervical orthosis is dependent on the forces exerted on the patient by the orthosis. The magnitude, points of application and directions of these forces depend on:

1. The rigidity and design of the orthosis.
2. How well the orthosis is fitted.
3. The patients' attempts to move against the orthosis.

In general, forces cannot be applied by an orthosis directly on to the cervical spine due to the stiffness characteristics of the tissue surrounding the cervical spine. The forces must be applied to the stiff structures at either end of the neck, that is the head and thorax.

Motion of the neck alters the position of the centre of gravity of the head relative to the cervical spine. Shapiro *et al.* (1980) has reported that static moments about C7 due to gravity, during upright standing and sitting, are of the order of 3 Nm in extreme flexion and 1 Nm in extreme extension. The effectiveness of a cervical orthosis in immobilizing the cervical spine may be assessed from its ability to resist these moments. However, voluntary moments of 10 times those values may be applied by the patient. In addition, an accident situation such as stumbling, results in similar large moments suddenly applied involuntarily by the patient to the orthosis.

A number of researchers have studied the normal range of motion of the cervical spine. The results of a study by White and Punjabi (1990) are presented in Table 12.1. All researchers have noted that the largest sagittal motion of the cervical spine occurs between C4–C5 and C5–C6 and that this range of motion decreases with age.

Over the years, comparative studies have been undertaken to assess the performance of cervical orthoses in their ability to restrict cervical motion. The results of some of these research studies are summarized in Table 12.2.

Scientific studies of this type which attempt to compare a number of different designs of cervical orthoses are fraught with many problems. The technique adopted to measure cervical motion usually involves strapping each subject in a chair to prevent undue trunk motion, and then requesting the head to be moved in the appropriate plane. Cine-radiography may be

Table 12.1 Typical average movement values at levels in the cervical spine

Motion segment	Combined flexion-extension (°)	One-side lateral bending (°)	One-side axial rotation (°)
C0–C1	25	5	5
C1–C2	25	5	40
C2–C3	10	10	3
C3–C4	15	11	7
C4–C5	20	11	7
C5–C6	20	8	7
C6–C7	17	7	6
C7–T1	9	4	2

Table 12.2 Percentage restriction of flexion-extension motion (occip.–T1) relative to unrestrained motion

| | Type of orthosis | | | | | | | | | | |
| | Flexion-extension | | | | | Lateral bending | | | Rotation | | |
	(1)	(2)	(3)	(4)	(5)	(3)	(4)	(5)	(3)	(4)	(5)
Patients (no.)	11			7			7			7	
Normals (no.)		10	5	44	10	5	44	10	5	44	10
Collars											
Soft	23		NO	26	10	NO	8	14	NO	17	16
Thomas			75			75			75		
Camp		65									
Philadelphia	49	68		71	47		34	26		56	29
Neclock					63			43			63
Posters											
SOMI	44	89		72			34			66	
Long 2		90				90			90		
Guilford 2		90				90			90		
Four-Poster	53	94	85	79		85	54		60	73	
Cervicothoracic											
Extend. 4 Poster				87			50			82	
Yale				87			75			61	
HALO				96			96			99	

Reference: (1) Alhoff and Goldie, 1990; (2) Fisher, 1978; (3) Hartman, 1975; (4) Johnson, 1978; (5) Kaufman *et al.*, 1986.

Other researchers have used other techniques to monitor cervical motion. These alternative results may or may not be comparable with the table above.

used to detect both the cumulative cervical motion and that taking place at each intervertebral level. This procedure is repeated both with and without the orthosis being worn, to assess what percentage of restriction of movement is provided by the orthosis relative to the unrestrained motion. Johnson *et al.* (1981) have suggested that the selection and use of cervical orthoses should be based on this criterion. It must be appreciated however that all of these research results will have been influenced by whether or not the subjects assessed:

1. Required an orthosis.
2. Applied similar forces to the orthoses to achieve 'maximum' angular displacements.
3. Followed similar movement patterns.

The range of cervical motion and the forces applied to the orthosis by normal subjects may be greater than the comparable values obtained for patients who wear a cervical orthosis. Walker *et al.* (1984) determined the average maximum static force that normal subjects were able to exert with their head as:

— Anteriorly   125 N
— Posteriorly   150 N
— Laterally   170 N

Fisher (1978) placed pressure transducers between the subject and the orthosis to try to ensure that all subjects applied similar forces to the orthoses, and in order to distinguish between a slack or tight fitting orthosis. This study reported that:

1. The immobilization characteristics of the orthoses were not affected by the tightness of fit of the cervical orthosis.
2. As the subjects attempted extension of the neck the orthosis forced the proximal cervical spine into flexion but permitted extension of the distal cervical spine. Alternatively, when cervical flexion was attempted the orthosis extended the proximal cervical spine while the distal cervical spine flexed (Figure 12.3.)

This 'snaking' motion of the cervical spine has been noted by other researchers. The effectiveness of cervical orthoses in limiting the range of motion of the cervical spine is commonly presented as an assessment of relative angular movements between the occiput and T1, ignoring the intermediate relative segment angular movements. It is essential to confirm whether an orthosis encourages 'snaking' of the cervical spine. The extension in the proximal cervical spine may negate the flexion of the distal spine. If the movement of the occiput relative to T1 alone is investigated, then the results will suggest that the orthosis has apparently immobilized the cervical spine. Prescribed cervical

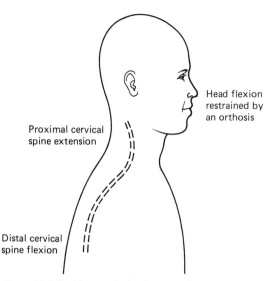

Head flexion restrained by an orthosis

Proximal cervical spine extension

Distal cervical spine flexion

Figure 12.3 Snaking cervical spine as patient attemps to flex head whilst wearing orthosis

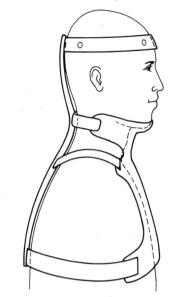

Figure 12.4 Minerva orthosis

orthoses used to stabilize an unstable neck should minimize both the 'snaking' motion and the total overall motion of the cervical spine.

This 'snaking' motion may be reduced by encapsulating the soft tissue of the neck. Some thermoplastic materials may be easily formed around the neck, thereby increasing the surface contact area and minimizing pressure levels. The orthosis may also provide an improved cosmetic appearance. The rigidity of a thermoplastic orthosis is dependent on the profile of its cross-sectional area as discussed in Chapter 2. Studies by Millington *et al.* (1987), Benzel *et al.* (1987) and Pringle (1990) suggest that a thermoplastic Minerva body jacket, as shown in Figure 12.4, is as effective as a standard halo orthosis in restricting overall cervical motion and may be more effective in reducing the 'snaking' phenomenon. This may be due to the one-piece, rear section of the thermoplastic body jacket providing total posterior contact from mid-thoracic level to the top of the head.

Cervical traction is commonly used to treat neck injuries. Traction applies a tensile force to the head stretching the soft tissues of the posterior cervical spine. The size of the intervertebral foramina is increased by traction, thereby relieving compression of the segmental nerve roots. Traction with the neck flexed provides maximum relief for nerve root compression. Figure 12.5(a) illustrates the chin strap lengthened to ensure that the line of action of the traction force passes posteriorly to the atlanto-occipital joint, whereas in Figure 12.5(b) the shortened chin strap creates traction with extension. Traction in extension can only be carried out effectively if the patient is supported on a two-level mattress as shown in Figure 12.5(b).

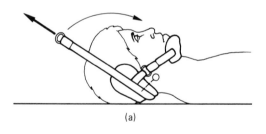

(a)

A two-level stepped mattress is required to allow extension to occur

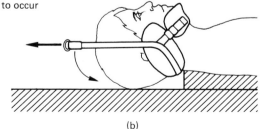

(b)

Figure 12.5 (a) Traction (flexion). (b) Traction (extension). (Reproduced with permission from Nordin and Frankel, 1980)

12.4 Description of current orthoses

Orthoses for the cervical spine can be divided into three types: collars, posters and halo/Minerva devices.

12.4.1 Collars

Collars are the simplest type of cervical orthoses and have been popularly prescribed for the treatment of a variety of cervical spine conditions. These orthoses have the advantage of low cost, ease of fabrication, convenience and good patient comfort. Although collars provide minimum motion restriction or weight transfer, they do provide warmth, psychological comfort and some support.

Collars may be subdivided into two types – soft and firm. A soft collar is a prefabricated orthosis, generally made from foam rubber and covered with a cotton stockinette, as shown in Figure 12.6. An example of a firm collar is the Philadelphia, which is fabricated in Plastazote foam and fastened with velcro-type straps at the side as shown in Figure 12.7. The Plastazote may be moulded to suit the individual patient or can be supplied prefabricated. Reinforced moulded polyethylene strips, attached to the Plastazote, provide mandible and occipital supports which extend to the upper thorax. The Yale orthosis (Figure 12.8) is similar but incorporates rivetted moulded anterior and posterior fibreglass thoracic extensions. Alternatively a firm collar may be fabricated by draping separate anterior and posterior sec-

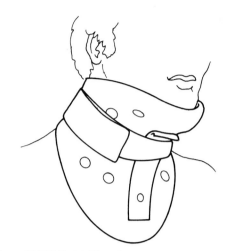

Figure 12.7 Philadelphia collar

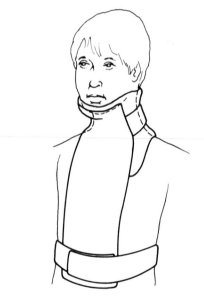

Figure 12.8 Yale orthosis

tions in a thermoplastic material, such as polyethylene, over a plaster model of the patient's neck. The two side overlaps are then fastened with velcro-type straps. Examples of prefabricated firm collars are the Thomas, Canadian and Neclock collars.

12.4.2 Posters

The poster-type orthoses are generally prefabricated and incorporate a thoracic vest to which the uprights or posts are attached. The posts extend from the vest to the occipital and

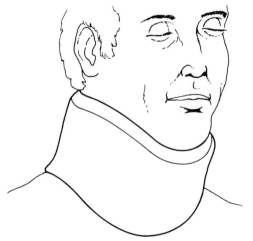

Figure 12.6 Soft collar

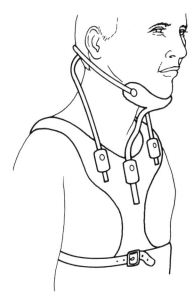

Figure 12.9 SOMI orthosis

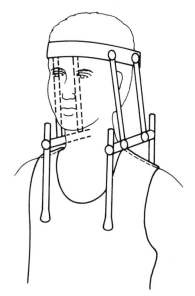

Figure 12.10 Halo orthosis

mandible areas. Examples include the four poster cervical brace and the Sterno-Occipital Mandibular Immobilizer (SOMI) brace, shown in Figure 12.9. Other examples include the two poster Guildford orthosis and the Bio-Con collar.

Cervicothoracic orthoses are of similar construction except that the vest section extends distally to provide improved contact with the trunk. These are now being increasingly used as emergency splints to protect the neck in road traffic accident victims. The Stifneck orthosis marketed in the UK by AMBU International has become particularly popular with Advanced Trauma Life Support (ATLS) teams.

12.4.3 Halo/Minerva

Additional stabilization of the head can be provided by either a halo- or Minerva-type orthosis. The halo-type orthosis is often the orthotic treatment prescribed when maximum cervical spine stabilization is required. A rigid halo ring is attached to the skull by four screws, which are applied to the outer layer of bone only. The halo is then connected by rigid uprights to a prefabricated thermoplastic vest or moulded plaster jacket, as shown in Figure 12.10. The Minerva orthosis (Figure 12.4) has a rigid one-piece posterior section extending from mid-thorax to the top of the head, to which an anterior thorax/mandible section and

a forehead strap are attached. Splinting materials which permit direct moulding onto the neck and trunk enable the Minerva orthosis to be customized for each patient. Examples of such materials are Polyform (a polyester polycaprolactone) lined with Polycushion (a closed-cell foam for padding). For long-term use the Minerva orthosis may be fabricated in a thermoplastic material moulded onto a plaster cast of the patient's neck and torso.

Whichever type of orthosis is prescribed, in all cases care needs to be taken to ensure that the cervical orthosis is fitted to the patient in the desired position. The attitude of the head in relation to the shoulders, the shape of the shoulders, and curvature of the spine all change as the patient transfers from the supine position to the sitting or standing position. Anderson *et al.* (1991) have reported that, even with a halo orthosis fitted, an average angulation of 7° and translation of 1.7 mm could still take place at the injured level, when the patient moved from the supine to the upright position.

It should be remembered that cervical orthoses have harmful as well as beneficial effects. Harmful effects include skin irritation, atrophy of muscles, ligament and joint capsule shrinkage with resulting stiffness, osteoarthritic changes due to diminished circulation to joint cartilage, and, finally, psychological disturbance of the patient. These complications are clinically highlighted by long-term use of a halo orthosis. It is therefore recommended by a number of surgeons that patients who have been using a halo orthosis for some time should be transferred to a SOMI or four-poster brace, and provided with physiotherapy treatment, before their orthotic treatment is terminated.

Finally, it is important that the patient or relative should receive clear and precise instructions as to when the orthosis should be worn, and the anticipated period of orthotic treatment.

12.5 Pathologies amenable to orthotic management: treatment objectives

There are two types of pathologies for which cervical orthoses are commonly prescribed: those requiring functional control, that is maintaining the head in a pain-free position, and those requiring postural control, that is supporting the head in a position such that progression of the cervical spine deformity is minimized.

12.5.1 Pathologies requiring functional control

The patients for whom functional control of the cervical spine is required are those suf-fering acute, subacute or chronic pain in their neck and/or arms. These will principally be patients with degenerative disorders – rheuma-toid arthritis, spondylosis and spondylitis, and those in a postoperative or post-traumatic phase. The primary treatment objective for this group of patients is to maintain the head in a pain-free position. Orthotic treatment accom-plishes this by supporting the head in the appropriate attitude and minimizing cervical movement. Thus the interface pressures be-tween the orthosis and the patient must be sufficiently large to provide functional control, but not so great that the patient experiences discomfort.

Rheumatoid arthritis (RA) is an inflamma-tory arthritis that can result in ligamentous distension and rupture, synovitis, destruction of articular cartilage, osteoporosis and erosion of bone. If 'normal' loads are applied to a cervical spine affected by chronic RA, atlan-toaxial subluxation and dislocations at the C4–C5 and C5–C6 levels may result. The atlas may also slip forward relative to the axis, permitting the odontoid process to press on, and compromise, the spinal cord. Spondylosis is a condition involving osteoarthritis of the spine, whereas spondylitis is an inflammation of the vertebrae, one form of which is ankylos-ing spondylitis which generally affects young males and results in progressive spontaneous fusion of the spine.

Table 12.3 Cervical injuries classified by Herkowitz *et al.*, 1989

Mode	Type
Hyperflexion	(a) Compression fractures of the anterior portion of the cervical vertebral bodies
	(b) Avulsion of the spinous processes
	(c) Bilateral facet dislocations if ALL posterior ligaments fail
Hyperextension	(a) Avulsion of a fragment of the anterior edge of a vertebral body or the anterior arch of C1
	(b) Compression fracture of the posterior arch of C1
	(c) Bilateral fracture of the pars interarticularis of C2, known as the 'hangman's fracture'
	(d) Odontoid fracture
	(e) Rupture of the transverse ligament
	(f) Dislocation of the atlanto-occipital joint
Axial	(a) Fractures through both the anterior and posterior arches of C1, commonly referred to as 'Jefferson fracture'
	(b) Compression fractures of the C3–C7 vertebral bodies
Flexion and rotation to right	(a) Possible left facet dislocations
Extension and rotation	(a) Possible fracture of the articular facet joints

Table 12.4 Treatment of trauma injuries

Injury	Treatment
Cervical sprains	Soft collar
Posterior arch fractures	Soft collar
Jefferson fractures	
Stable	Philadelphia orthosis
Unstable	Halo orthosis for 3 months. (If instability still exists after 3 months of halo treatment, fusion is indicated).
Transverse ligament	
Avulsion	Halo immobilization
Midsubstance tears	C1–C2 fusion
Odontoid fractures	
Avulsion of the tip	Philadelphia collar for 6 weeks
Avulsion close to C2 body (no displacement)	Halo immobilization
Avulsion close to C2 body (with displacement)	C1–C2 fusion
'Hangmans' fracture	
Stable	Philadelphia collar
Unstable	Halo orthosis for 3 months (If instability still exists then C1–C3 fusion is recommended)
Unilateral facet dislocations	Traction + halo for 3 months
Bilateral facet dislocations	Traction + fusion (Chronic subluxation occurs in over 60% of patients treated non-operatively)
Burst fractures	Operative treatment

Reference: Herkowitz *et al.*, 1989.

In the case of trauma, the treatment will vary, depending not only on the type but also on the severity of the injury. Cervical orthoses may be prescribed postoperatively to assist stabilization and permit an early hospital discharge. Orthotic treatment is recommended for soft tissue injuries; the prescribed orthosis will depend on its required function. The classification of cervical injuries by Herkowitz *et al.* (1989) is presented in Table 12.3 and his recommendations for the management of traumatic injuries are presented in Table 12.4.

Consider the case of a moving vehicle colliding with the rear of a stationary vehicle. The rapid deceleration of the moving vehicle will result in its driver being thrown forward rapidly due to inertia. If this driver is wearing a diagonal shoulder seat belt, the forward action of his body will be restrained, although his unrestrained head will pivot forward. This may result in a hyperflexion injury and possibly severe disruption of the posterior ligaments of the cervical spine. Meanwhile, the driver of the stationary vehicle may, if his head is not supported adequately by a head rest, experience a hyperextension cervical injury. A number of different mechanisms of soft tissue and bony injury to the cervical spine have been related to different trauma situations and the reader is referred to Freeman, for further details of these (1987).

The degree of immobilization perceived to be required by both postoperative and trauma patients and those with degenerative disorders will determine which of the three main types of cervical orthosis – collars, posters or halo/Minerva – is prescribed. White (1983) has emphasized that carefully documented patient assessment leads to a more rational and precise selection of orthosis. Nachemson (1987) has stated that no scientific clinical studies have demonstrated the effectiveness of orthotic treatment, although he does concede that some of the studies which have examined the restriction of cervical motion in different sorts of orthoses may be useful as prescription guides.

12.5.2 Pathologies requiring postural control

Patients may also be referred for orthotic treatment because they have excessive curvature of their cervical spine rather than neck pain. The primary objective for this group of patients is to prevent further progression of the curve by ensuring that the centre of gravity of the head is positioned such that no excessive moments are applied to the cervical spine. Good posture minimizes tissue compression or tension and other deforming forces that cause tissue dysfunction and injury. Good head posture also aligns the spine so that the joints and tissues are most flexible, and thus movement in all planes will occur most easily. Orthotic treatment can provide the posture and correct head positioning required by this category of patient. The orthosis used in any particular case should be matched to the exact stabilizing needs of the patient. Walpin (1987) has suggested that during voluntary unforced activities, the soft collar should provide sufficient limitation of cervical motion to match the clinical needs of patients with neuromuscular or osteoarticular disorders. If additional stabilization is required a four-poster or halo-type cervical orthosis may be prescribed as the adjustability of these orthoses will enable the head to be stabilized in the desired posture.

A relatively common condition requiring this approach to treatment is torticollis. This disorder involves spasm of the cervical muscles which draws the head to one side and twists the neck. A common form is congenital torticollis which follows the formation of a haematoma in the sternocleidomastoid muscle at birth. Absorption and fibrosis later occur and the muscle fails to lengthen as other neck structures grow, resulting in an increase in torticollis. Serial splinting may be necessary in order to correct the deformity.

12.6 Biomechanical function and critical assessment of orthoses

12.6.1 Collars

For a patient who flexes his head whilst wearing a firm collar, the rigidity of the stiffened anterior section of the orthosis provides the restraint to enable the neck flexion moment to be resisted by a force at the mandible together with a counter-force on the sternum of the patient as shown in Figure 12.11(a). These two resisting forces combine effectively to apply restraining extension moments about the pivot point of the cervical spine. The two forces applied to the orthosis by the mandible and sternum, shown in Figure 12.11(b), will tend to

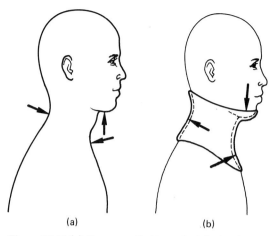

Figure 12.11 (a) Forces applied to patient flexing in a firm collar. (b) Forces applied to 'flexed' firm collar

displace the orthosis forward, away from the neck; a third force at the rear of the collar prevents this tendency. The shape of the firm collar and its limited flexibility will mean that there will often not be an intimate fit between the orthosis and the patient. Thus movement of the collar relative to the patient during use is likely to occur.

In the case of the soft collar, the flexion restraint is dependent on the compression characteristics of the soft material of the collar. If a compressive load is applied to a soft material, the resultant restraining force, R, is a function of the material stiffness (k) multiplied by the compression (d), i.e. $R = k \times d$. Thus, significant cervical flexion, with corresponding compression of the soft collar, is required before the soft material will provide a sufficient restraining force. Similarly, for a patient attempting to extend the head while restrained by a soft collar, the lack of stiffness in the collar material provides minimal resistance to extension. The extension moment is resisted by a force at the occiput and by a counter-force at the rear of the patient's spine, as shown in Figure 12.12(a). The two resisting forces effectively combine to apply restraining flexion moments about the pivot point of the cervical spine. Likewise, the two forces applied to the orthosis, as shown in Figure 12.12(b), tend to displace the orthosis posteriorly, away from the neck, and again a third force at the front of the collar prevents this tendency. If the forces generated are high, pressure on the trachea occurs causing a choking sensation and for this

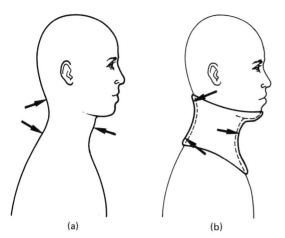

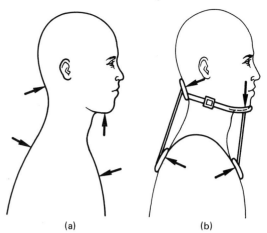

Figure 12.12 (a) Forces applied to patient extending in a soft collar. (b) Forces applied to 'extended' soft collar

Figure 12.13 (a) Forces applied to patient flexing in a four-poster orthosis. (b) Forces applied to 'flexed' four-poster orthosis

reason some collars have a central cut-out at the front. As collars seldom incorporate lateral reinforcements, they can provide little restraint to lateral bending. Their lack of rigidity, plus the possibility of rotation of the collar relative to the patient, suggests that they are unable to provide significant restraint to rotation.

12.6.2 Posters

In the four-poster or cervicothoracic orthosis, the rigidity of the uprights provides adequate restraining moments to effectively immobilize the neck. Compared with a firm collar, the greater contact of the vest section with the patient introduces longer lever arms relative to the pivot point of the cervical spine. As the patient attempts to flex the head whilst wearing the four-poster, anterior restraining forces are applied to the patient as shown in Figure 12.13(a). Likewise the two forces applied to the orthosis by the mandible and sternum (Figure 12.13(b)), tend to displace the orthosis anteriorly, away from the neck. The two posterior forces prevent this tendency for the orthosis to be 'pushed forward'. The four forces are in equilibrium. The reverse occurs if the patient attempts to extend the head while wearing the orthosis. The tendency of the orthosis to move relative to the patient during flexion or extension of the head is resisted more effectively if the sternum and scapula pads are linked under the axilla as well as over the shoulders.

In a four-poster orthosis, the uprights tend to be subjected to compressive loads along their length, and therefore may be considered to function as struts. More restraint to cervical motion is prrovided if the uprights are subjected to axial loads as opposed to bending loads applied at right angles to their length. A vertical upright subjected to a horizontal force will deflect horizontally more than the same upright will deflect vertically when subjected to a similar vertical force. The upright is more effective as a strut than as a beam. This principle is well demonstrated by the SOMI brace. If a patient wearing such an orthosis attempts to flex his head, the single anterior upright is loaded axially and therefore functions as a strut. However, if the patient attempts to extend his head, the two posterior uprights are not loaded axially; the load from the occiput acts almost at right angles to the posterior uprights (Figure 12.14). Therefore the two posterior uprights function as bending beams rather than struts. It is the flexural rigidity of the two posterior uprights which resists extension through restraining forces at the occipital pads, plus counter-forces at the sternum and scapula pads. The SOMI brace is therefore very effective in resisting head flexion but provides relatively poor resistance to head extension.

For a patient attempting to laterally bend to the right while wearing a four-poster orthosis, the contours of the mandible and occiput pads permit some movement of the head relative to

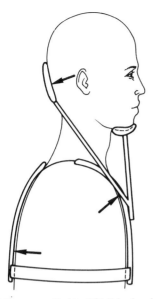

Figure 12.14 Forces applied to SOMI by head extension

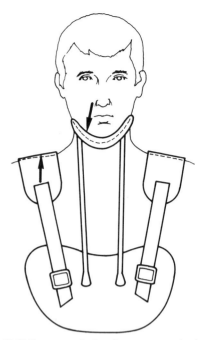

Figure 12.15 Forces applied to four-poster orthosis subjected to lateral bending of head

the orthosis, further motion is restrained by the axial forces in both the right anterior and right posterior posts, as shown in Figure 12.15. The shoulder straps prevent the sternum and scapula pads from being displaced distally. However, the lines of action of the restraining forces provided by the uprights, pass relatively close to the cervical spinal axis, and thus the moment restraining lateral bending is rather smaller than that restraining flexion.

Finally, as the patient attempts head rotation to the left, the forces applied by the head to the mandible and occipital pads result in the pads applying horizontal forces to the proximal ends of the four uprights, as shown in Figure 12.16. As the uprights are subjected to bending effects, the restraint to rotation is poor. Also, the forces applied to the uprights tend to rotate the sternum and scapula pads around the patient, a tendency which is resisted by the shear forces at the patient–orthosis interface. The fit of these pads to the patient thus largely determines the resistance to head rotation provided by the orthosis.

12.6.3 Halo/Minerva

In the case of a halo orthosis, as the patient attempts to flex his head an equal but opposite posterior restraining force is applied to the forehead by the halo ring (Figure 12.17). This restraining force has a long lever arm, acting

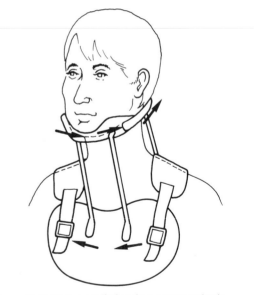

Figure 12.16 Forces applied to four-poster orthosis subjected to head rotation

well above the pivot point of the cervical spine. Thus the halo orthosis provides large restraining moments. The effectiveness of this restraining force is dependent on the rigidity of the uprights connected to the halo ring, and the fit of the halo vest/jacket to the trunk. The ten-

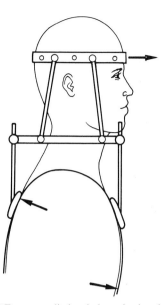

Figure 12.17 Forces applied to halo orthosis subjected to head flexion

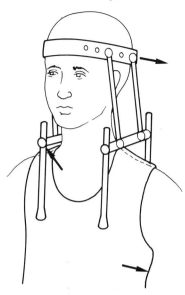

Figure 12.18 Forces applied to halo orthosis subjected to left lateral bending of the head

dency for movement of the vest relative to the patient is resisted by anterior–distal and posterior–proximal forces acting on the vest as shown.

Likewise, if the patient attempts to laterally bend the head to the left, the halo ring provides a restraining force to the right at the halo ring level, well above the pivot point of the cervical spine (Figure 12.18). The tendency for movement of the vest relative to the patient is resisted by left-distal and right shoulder forces acting on the vest.

Similarly, the uprights of a halo orthosis will be subjected to horizontal forces from the halo ring as the patient attempts to rotate his head. These horizontal forces will be transferred to the halo vest/jacket, but rotation will be resisted by the intimate fit of the vest or jacket.

Halo orthoses are often used after cervical spine fusion operations to enable early hospital discharge of a patient who previously would have been treated on traction. The forces applied to a halo orthosis as it immobilizes the cervical spine during normal daily living activities have been monitored by strain gauging the halo uprights. The halo vest is usually fitted in the supine position and the distraction is adjusted with the patient in a supine position. Koch and Nickel (1978), Walker *et al.* (1984), Lind *et al.* (1988) and Ersmark *et al.* (1988)

noted inconsistent compression/distraction forces across the neck in the seated and standing position.

Convery and Hamblen (1991) reported the results of an *in vitro* study in which a test jig was used to assess the mechanical rigidity of three types of commercial halo orthoses: the Zimmer, Fillauer, and Jerome. Repeatable three-dimensional forces and moments were applied to the 'detached' head of a model, the trunk of which was firmly fixed to the test jig. Motion of the head was measured relative to the trunk, when fitted with each orthosis. This technique ensured both repeatability and accuracy of loading conditions which are not possible with *in vivo* tests. The rigidity of the halo orthoses was found to be approximately 1 degree Nm^{-1}, with the Zimmer the most stiff and the Jerome the least stiff. The metal uprights of all three types of halo orthoses were then transferred to the same customized body jacket and the tests repeated. The rigidity of all Zimmer upright configurations was again the greatest. The study concluded that both the geometry of the uprights and the number of adjustable joints was important. The triangular configuration of the Zimmer uprights was more rigid than either the single Fillauer upright or the 'goal post' configuration of the Jerome brace. The fewer the number of adjustable joints, the greater was the rigidity of the orthosis, although reducing adjustability may limit the range of possible head positions.

12.7 Current and future developments

A testing protocol which could be used to scientifically confirm the relative functional characteristics of each design of currently used cervical orthosis would be attractive. The most effective design features could then be incorporated in future orthoses. This testing protocol should consist of two phases. First, it should include *in vitro* studies of the relative rigidity of the orthosis in shear, bending and torsion when fitted to a model whose head is detached and whose trunk is firmly fixed to a test jig. This system could be extended to employ an intact cadaveric head and trunk. Use of X-rays would confirm the degree of motion of each cervical vertebra when forces and moments are applied to the head with and without the orthoses fitted. Secondly, the protocol should involve *in vivo* clinical trials in which the forces and moments applied to the head by the orthosis are carefully monitored.

Studies should also be undertaken to investigate the possible inclusion of recent advances in materials' technology in the construction of cervical orthoses. Strong, mouldable materials are likely to permit improved functional characteristics, although patient–orthosis interface pressures would have to be carefully monitored.

12.8 Alternative and complementary treatments

Trauma cases which involve instability and/or nerve root compression should be considered for surgical treatment. White (1978) defined cervical instability at the injured level as translatory motion greater than 3 mm or angular motion greater than 11° between adjacent vertebrae. However, many surgeons continue to adopt a non-operative approach to most of these injuries.

Surgical intervention, in the case of patients with degenerative disorders is rare. Only in the case of severe subluxation, with impending neurological deficit, with or without pain, would surgical stabilization be recommended.

In all other cases involving pain, orthotic treatment would frequently be prescribed. There is no scientific evidence to suggest that orthotic treatment will halt RA progression. Pellicci *et al.* (1981), in a prospective study of the progression of RA in the cervical spines of 106 patients, has shown that the diligent use of a supportive collar did not alter the natural progression of RA.

Superficial heat or ice treatment to the neck is commonly used, although studies have not confirmed their effectiveness (Moncur and Williams, 1988). Intermittent cervical traction can be very effective in some patients with cervical spondylosis, but is not recommended for RA patients because of the potential for further damage to the joints and the risk of injury to the spinal cord. Manipulative techniques do have a place in cervical spondylosis but are contraindicated if there is any evidence of neurological loss. Physical therapy should then be restricted to gentle stretching, range of motion and isometric exercises of the neck. Transcutaneous electrical nerve stimulation may provide pain relief, although no studies have scientifically evaluated its effectiveness on the cervical spine.

For patients at risk of severe and progressive curvature of the cervical spine, surgical intervention is often employed in preference to orthotic treatment.

References

Althoff B. and Goldie I.F. (1980) Cervical collars in rheumatoid atlanto-axial subluxation: a radiographic comparison. *Ann. Rheum. Dis.* **39**, 485–489

Anderson P.A., Budorick T.E. and Salciccioli G.G. (1991) Failure of halo-vest to prevent *in-vivo* motion in patients with injured cervical spines. *Orthop. Trans.* **15**, 687

Benzel E.C., Hadden T.A. and Saulsbery C.M. (1989) A comparison of the Minerva and halo jackets for stabilization of the cervical spine. *J. Neurosurg.* **70**, 411–414

Convery P. and Hamblen D.L. (1991) Halo orthoses. *Int. J. Orthop. Trauma* **1**, 220–226

Ersmark H., Kalen R. and Lowenheim P. (1988) A methodical study of force measurements in three patients with odontoid fractures treated with a strain gauge-equipped halo-vest. *Spine* **13**, 433–435

Fisher S.V. (1978) Proper fitting of the cervical orthosis. *Arch. Phys. Med. Rehabil.* **59**, 505–507

Freeman B.L. III (1987) Fractures, dislocations and fracture-dislocations of the spine. In: Crenshaw A.H. (ed.), *Campbell's Operative Orthopaedics*, vol. 4, 7th edn. C.V. Mosby, St Louis, pp. 3109–3142.

Hartman J.T., Palumbo F. and Hill B.J. (1975) Cineradiography of the braced normal cervical spine. *Clin. Orthop. Rel. Res.* **109**, 97–102

Herkowitz H.N., Kurz L.T. and Samberg L.C. (1989) Management of cervical spine injuries. *Spine State Art Rev.* **3**, 231–241

Johnson R.M., Hart D.L., Owen J.R. *et al.* (1978) The Yale orthosis: An evaluation of its effectiveness in relating cervical motion in normal subjects and a comparison with other cervical orthoses. *Phys. Therm.* **48**, 865–871

Johnson R.M., Owen J.R., Hart D.L. *et al.* (1981) Cervical orthoses: a guide to their selection and use. *Clin. Orthop.* **154**, 34–45

Kaufman W.A., Lunsford T.R., Lunsford B.R. *et al.* (1986) Comparison of three prefabricated cervical collars. *Orthot. Prosthet.* **39**, 21–28

Koch R.A. and Nickel V.L. (1978) The halo vest: an evaluation of the motion and forces across the neck. *Spine* **3**, 103–107

Lind B., Sihlbom H. and Nordwall A. (1988) Forces and motions across the neck in patients treated with halovest. *Spine* **13**, 162–167

Millington P.J., Ellingsen J.M., Hauswirth B.E. *et al.* (1987) Thermoplastic minerva body jacket – a practical alternative to current methods of cervical spine stabilization. *Phys. Ther.* **67**, 223–225

Moncur C. and Williams H.J. (1988) Cervical spine management in patients with rheumatoid arthritis: review of the literature. *Phys. Ther.* **68**, 509–515

Nachemson A.L. (1987) Orthotic treatment for injuries and diseases of the spinal column. *Phys. Med. Rehabil.* **1**, 11–24

Pellicci P.M., Ranawat C.S., Tsairis P. *et al.* (1981) A prospective study of the progression of rheumatoid arthritis of the cervical spine. *J. Bone Joint Surg.* **63A**, 342–350

Pringle R.G. (1990) Review article: halo versus minerva – which orthosis? *Paraplegia* **28**, 281–284

Shapiro I. and Frankel V.H. (1980) Biomechanics of the cervical spine. In: Nordin M. and Frankel V.H. (eds), *Basic Biomechanics of the Musculoskeletal System*. Lea & Febiger, Philadelphia, pp. 204–224

Walker P.S., Lamser D., Hussey R.W. *et al.* (1984) Forces in the halo-vest apparatus. *Spine* **9**, 773–777

Walpin L.A. (1987) The role of orthotic devices for managing neck disorders. *Phys. Med. Rehabil.* **1**, 25–43

White A.A. (1983) Some comments on cervical orthoses. *Clin. Prosthet. Orthot.* **7**, 5–7

White A.A. and Punjabi M.M. (1990) Spinal braces: functional analysis and clinical applications. In: White A.A. and Punjabi M.M. (eds), *Clinical Biomechanics of the Spine*. J.B. Lippincott, Philadelphia, pp. 475–509

White A.A. and Punjabi M.M. (1990) Kinematics of the spine. In: White A.A. and Punjabi M.M. (eds), *Clinical Biomechanics of the Spine*. J.B. Lippincott, Philadelphia, pp. 85–125

13

Spinal orthoses

Andrew Chase, Mark Pearcy and Dan Bader

13.1 Introduction

In recent years a clearer understanding of the orthotic requirements for treating spinal disorders has evolved. This can be attributed to a number of factors; in particular the increasing involvement of bioengineers which has led to a more comprehensive knowledge of the mechanical principles applicable to the design and development of orthoses, and a departure from traditional methods of fabrication and materials which has resulted in new concepts in bracing. Many types of orthoses are employed in treating similar spinal disorders with varying opinions as to the efficacy of each orthosis for a given condition. In this chapter the objectives are to describe the functional anatomy of the spine followed by an indication of how orthoses may be applied when specific pathologies have affected the structure and/or function of the spine. This includes a statement of the clinical objectives and the biomechanical principles of some suggested orthotic systems. In analysing current management practices, a categorization of pathologies and orthotic systems emerges which can be broadly described as dynamic, postural functional and postural static. Dynamic bracing is normally associated with pathologies where correction of deformity, or at least prevention of progression, is sought; postural functional where pain relief is sought; postural static where prevention of further progression is required to preserve respiratory and other physiological functions.

13.2 Spinal anatomy

This section provides a brief review of the anatomy of the back and spine in terms of its mechanical function.

13.2.1 Bony elements

(a) Vertebral column

The vertebral column consists of the bony vertebrae connected by the intervertebral discs and ligaments (Figure 13.1).

The discs, which are capable of transmitting tensile and compressive loads, impart flexibility to the column. The longitudinal ligaments (anterior, posterior and supraspinous), having some fibres that span single levels, control the motions of individual intervertebral joints and additionally act as restraints to excessive mobility over large segments of the column. The intervertebral ligaments (ligamentum flavum, interspinous and zygapophysial joint capsules) also restrain excessive movement of intervertebral joints.

The flexibility of the vertebral column is determined to some extent by the orientation of the zygapophysial joints. In the lumbar region their facets have a sagittal component which in conjunction with the intervertebral disc acts to limit twisting of the spine to only 1° or 2°, whilst in the thoracic spine the facets are orientated more in the coronal plane so that

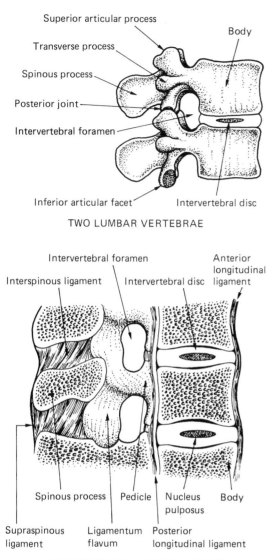

TWO LUMBAR VERTEBRAE

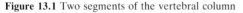

MEDIAN SAGITTAL LUMBAR SPINE

Figure 13.1 Two segments of the vertebral column

twisting is limited by the intervertebral discs and the action of the rib cage attached to the vertebrae.

(b) Rib cage

The ribs, through their attachment to the thoracic vertebrae, provide stability to this segment of the vertebral column, also limiting its mobility. However, this intimate relationship also results in rib cage deformity if the thoracic vertebral column is deformed, or vice versa.

(c) Pelvis

This bony ring is the base on which the vertebral column sits and to which it is firmly attached by the lumbosacral disc and ligaments including the iliotransverse ligaments joining the iliac wings to the transverse processes of the fifth lumbar vertebra. Disruption of the pelvis will have obvious consequences for the load bearing function of the vertebral column. The pelvis is the base on which many orthotic devices must rest and from which they obtain rotational stability.

13.2.2 Muscles

The back muscles are extremely complex, as has been described by Bogduk and Twomey (1987). Those affecting the function of the vertebral column include all the trunk muscles including the intercostal muscles and many of the limb muscles.

(a) Posterior muscles

These include all the muscles attaching to the vertebrae posteriorly. Of these, the deeper muscles may span one or two vertebrae, whilst the more superficial, more posterior muscles span several levels. In addition there are muscles which span from the pelvis to the rib cage which lie posteriorly to those attached to the vertebrae. This complexity suggests that intricate muscular control of intervertebral movements may occur and would explain some of the abnormal movements of patients with back problems.

(b) Abdominal muscles

Anteriorly the three layers of the abdominal muscles have attachments to the rib cage, to the pelvis and to the lumbar and thoracic vertebrae via the lumbodorsal fascia. They can, therefore, exert a direct action on the lumbar vertebral column. In addition they have the ability to produce an increase in intra-abdominal pressure which appears to act as a mechanism to assist extension of the spine and to relieve compressive loads produced by the contraction of the posterior muscles. Twisting movements will also be controlled by these muscles since they are the furthest removed from the axis of rotation of the vertebral column.

(c) Intercostal muscles

These muscles also have a direct action on the vertebral column due to their action on the ribs. In addition, together with the diaphragm, they can act to assist the maintenance of intra-abdominal pressure by creating an intrathoracic pressure and hence exert an extension moment on the vertebral column.

(d) Limb muscles

Some of the muscles traditionally associated with the limbs also directly affect the vertebral column. In the upper limbs, the muscles which raise the shoulder blades are directly attached to the cervical vertebrae and so affect their function, particularly when weights are held in the hands. In the lower limb, the hip muscles which act to rotate the pelvis during lifting obviously affect the vertebral column as do the psoas muscles which attach directly to the lateral aspects of the lumbar vertebrae.

13.3 General spinal biomechanics

In mechanical terms the spine can be modelled as a series of semirigid bodies, the vertebrae, separated by viscoelastic linkages, the intervertebral discs and ligaments. Attached to the spine are a collection of viscoelastic materials with varying stiffness from the stiff ribs, associated with the thoracic region, to the subcutaneous fat. These elements form part of a body cylinder, to which the spinal orthosis is attached (see Figure 5.2). The effectiveness of spinal orthoses, whether their main function is one of support, immobilization or correction or pain relief, can be assessed in biomechanical terms. The nature of the close-fitting orthosis will establish the externally applied forces which must be transmitted to the spinal column to achieve the desired therapeutic goal. The effectiveness of this force transmission will be determined by the mechanical properties, in particular the stiffness characteristics, of the intervening biological materials. Thus it is possible to apply forces more effectively through a relatively stiff material which will deform little under load, than through a low

stiffness material, which will deform to a much greater extent. This explains why, for example, spinal orthoses are more effective in holding or correcting thoracic curves, where the forces are transmitted through the ribs, than lumbar curves where the intervening soft materials are composed of muscles and viscera.

Clearly the level and duration of the externally applied loads are limited by the threshold levels associated with pain and mechanical tolerance of the soft tissues (see Chapter 5). Other limiting factors include the mechanical properties of the spinal elements. Thus a degree of elasticity will prevent total restriction of movement being achievable with a spinal orthosis. In addition, the spine in some pathologies such as osteoporosis, may not be able to tolerate a high level of loading.

The viscoelastic behaviour of the soft tissues will also result in the level of load changing over a period of time. Thus the creep phenomenon, which involves increasing deformation with time under a constant load, must also be taken into account.

Effective orthotic treatment requires an understanding of the regional kinematics of the spine in all six degrees of freedom, namely translation along each of the three coordinates and rotation about each of the three axes. Only with this knowledge can the clinician select an orthosis which will meet the specified requirements for restricting or eliminating movement. There is much information on this complex topic. However because of the inaccessibility of the spine and the complex nature of its movements, the reported results are inconsistent. The most accurate measurements *in vivo* inevitably rely upon radiography (Pearcy, 1985), although other more invasive techniques have been used, such as the insertion of Steinmann pins into the spinous processes (Gregerson and Lucas, 1967). The topic is well covered in an extensive chapter (White and Punjabi, 1990), from which a summary of the primary rotations about the three axes has been compiled in Table 13.1. These results do not take into account the accompanying or coupled rotations and translations in the other planes. For example, Pearcy (1985) has measured a translation of 2 mm in the sagittal plane during primary flexion of the upper levels of a normal lumbar spine. The kinematics of the spine will certainly change with age, with most reports indicating a reduced mobility

Table 13.1 Typical movement values at levels in the thoracic and lumbar spines

Motion segment	Combined flexion-extension (°)		One-side lateral bend (°)		One-side axial rotation (°)	
	Range	*Median*	*Range*	*Median*	*Range*	*Median*
T1–T2	3–5	4	5	5	14	9
T2–T3	3–5	4	5–7	6	4–12	8
T3–T4	2–5	4	3–7	5	5–11	8
T4–T5	2–5	4	5–6	6	5–11	8
T5–T6	3–5	4	5–6	6	5–11	8
T6–T7	2–7	5	6	6	4–11	7
T7–T8	3–8	6	3–8	6	4–11	7
T8–T9	3–8	6	4–7	6	6–7	6
T9–T10	3–8	6	4–7	6	3–5	4
T10–T11	4–14	9	3–10	7	2–3	2
T11–T12	6–20	12	4–13	9	2–3	2
T12–L1	6–20	12	5–10	8	2–3	2
L1–L2	5–16	12	3–8	6	1–3	2
L2–L3	8–18	14	3–10	6	1–3	2
L3–L4	6–17	15	4–12	8	1–3	2
L4–L5	9–21	16	3–9	6	1–3	2
L5–S1	10–24	17	2–6	3	0–2	1

with increasing age. Movements of the pathological spine are less well characterized, which probably reflects the large variations in the normal values (Table 13.1) and the unreliability of many of the measurement techniques.

The effect of lifting heavy objects is to impose substantial loads on the spine and, in particular, on the lower lumbar spine (Pearcy, 1989). The major factor contributing to these loads is contraction of the back muscles, which act on very short lever arms to provide a counterbalancing moment and hence produce large compressive forces across the intervertebral joints. However a biomechanical analysis (Figure 13.2) reveals, that to support a load of 90 kg, the forces required by the muscles would be excessive and would induce compressive stresses on the vertebrae, large enough to cause failure. There must be additional mechanisms which spare the intervertebral joints. These include the development of intra-abdominal pressure, which has been shown to increase as the weight lifted is increased (Morris *et al.*, 1961). This rise in pressure is due to contraction of the transverse and oblique abdominal muscles, whilst the recti abdomini remains quiescent. The abdominal and thoracic cavity then acts like a balloon, pushing up the diaphragm and down on the pelvic floor, thus providing an extra extensor moment (Figure 13.3). An alternative sparing mechanism on the lumbar vertebrae involves the thoracolumbar fascia and its attachment to the transverse abdominals (Graco-

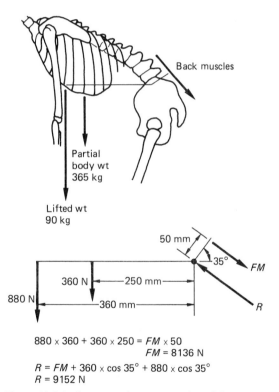

$$880 \times 360 + 360 \times 250 = FM \times 50$$
$$FM = 8136 \text{ N}$$

$$R = FM + 360 \times \cos 35° + 880 \times \cos 35°$$
$$R = 9152 \text{ N}$$

Figure 13.2 A diagrammatic representation of the estimated forces in the back during lifting

vetsky *et al.*, 1981). The action of these muscles pulling laterally on the fascia is considered to produce an extension moment on the vertebrae by virtue of the oblique direction of the fibres in the fascia. However this mechanism may

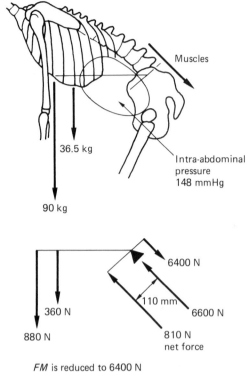

FM is reduced to 6400 N
R is reduced to 6600 N

Figure 13.3 The effects of including intra-abdominal pressure on the forces in the back during lifting

only provide extensor forces across one or two levels of the lumbar spine and the stabilizing effect of the fascia may be confined generally to a passive mechanism through its direct attachment to the vertebrae and ilia.

Balanced horizontal forces are eminently suitable for providing efficient bending moments for the correction of lateral curvature, derotation of vertebrae and immobilization of the spine. Most of the loading patterns used in practice can be shown to be mediated through a traditional three-point loading system. This system, which applies commonly to many engineering situations, involves two horizontal forces applied at either end of a spinal segment opposed by a single force acting in the opposite direction. The magnitude and position of these forces are arranged to ensure equilibrium between forces and the resulting bending moments. As it is the bending moments that produce the angular correction of the spine, by locating the middle force directly at the apex of a lateral curve, it becomes maximally efficient as a corrective force.

Some orthoses can provide support to the spine by means of compressive loading through the soft tissues, particularly in the lumbar region. These include corsets or abdominal supports, which are effective in resting and unloading the spine.

Other biomechanical mechanisms to provide stability and immobilization involve the application of tensile distraction forces, which produce a secondary resistance to lateral forces. Many spinal orthoses are based on a cage around the patient. They consist of two semicircular fixation points, one above the other, connected by a series of uprights. Each upright acts both as a splint or distractor and as a point of attachments for various accessory devices, such as localizer pads, axillary slings and abdominal pads.

13.4 Orthotic requirements for different types of pathology

13.4.1 Dynamic management

(a) Pathologies

The principal pathologies in which dynamic control of the spine is required, that is in which the correction of the deformity is sought, are:

— Idiopathic scoliosis (the most common disorder).
— Adolescent kyphosis or Scheuermann's disease.

(b) Management objectives and biomechanical requirements

In this treatment category the common objectives are to prevent the progression of the spinal curvature which, in the adolescent tends to deteriorate and to minimize structural deformity which manifests itself as soft tissue asymmetry. There is also a need to prevent high compressive stresses on the vertebrae and to improve or maintain respiratory function. In some cases the objective of the orthosis may be to maintain the degree of deformity while the patient is waiting for surgery.

The action of this group of orthoses involves three separate but interactive biomechanical principles, namely end-point control, transverse loading and curve correction. The purpose of the pelvic portion of most orthoses, for example the pelvic girdle of the Milwaukee brace, is to provide a fixed, centred reference to the base of the spine. The neck ring of the Milwaukee brace then limits the lateral sway of the neck by keeping the head and the neck centred above the pelvis. These two elements of the orthosis control the end points of the spine providing a large resistance to column buckling even when high loads are transmitted. There is a three-point loading system, applied in the transverse plane, which is also provided within these orthoses to support the spine. The purpose of these forces is to apply bending moments to the curvature of the spine in an opposite direction to the scoliotic curve and thus correct it (or at worst prevent further deterioration). These transverse loads also permit derotation of the vertebrae (Aaro *et al.*, 1981).

The same general principles apply during correction of adolescent kyphosis. In this case the three-point bending system is used to apply the maximum bending moment to correct the deformity in the sagittal plane, with no associated axial rotation.

These dynamic orthoses provide a correctional effect on the spine on a long-term basis, which involves both mechanical effects and biological adaptation.

(c) Orthoses specification

Although these orthoses are designed to prompt the wearer into maintaining a certain posture they may incorporate transverse loading systems to assist correction of deformity. The success criterion for this type of orthosis

must be acceptability on the part of the wearer. If the prompting becomes too irritating or failure to maintain the posture results in excessive pain, then compliance by the patient will be poor. The orthosis must have fairly firm attachment to the wearer to ensure constancy in the prompting action.

The Boston Thoraco-Lumbo-Sacral Orthosis (TLSO)

The Boston scoliosis bracing system has been well documented (Hall *et al.*, 1975). The brace is constructed on the basis of a straight, normal mould. The symmetry of the inner surface of the orthosis is altered by the placement of preformed pads, which make contact with chosen areas of the patient's torso. Three-dimensional dynamic correction of the spine, as indicated in Figure 13.4, is achieved using a prefabricated polypropylene module lined with polyethylene foam (Figure 13.5). The anatomical configuration of the module provides $15°$ lumbar flexion, increased anterior abdominal force, fixation at the waist and lateral torso containment. Dynamic alignment of the spine is promoted by compression pads fitted inside the module, positioned according to the degree of rotation and the apex of the curve. Additional trochanteric and anterior superior iliac spinal pads may also be required to achieve maximum correction.

The Milwaukee Cervico-Thoraco-Lumbo-Sacral Orthosis (CTLSO)

The Milwaukee CTLSO is probably the most well documented spinal brace (Blount and

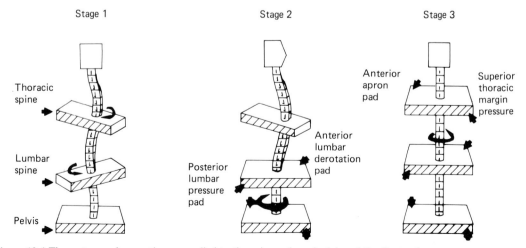

Figure 13.4 Three stages of correction as applied to the spine – the principles of the Boston brace system

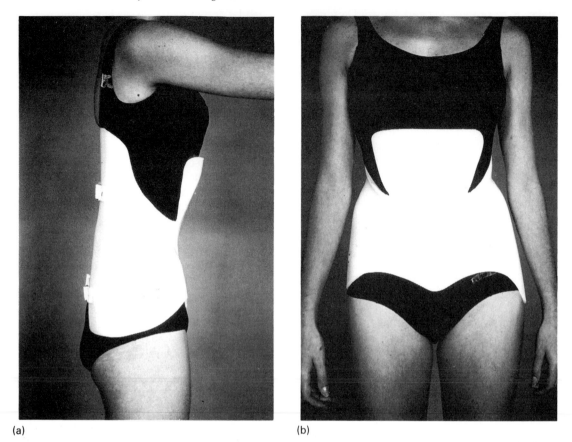

(a)   (b)

Figure 13.5 A Boston TLSO applied for a thoracolumbar idiopathic scoliosis, with apex of curve at T12/L1. (a) Lateral view; (b) anterior view

Moe, 1980) and is prescribed throughout the world. A plaster of Paris mould is produced of the subject, while maximum postural correction is maintained during the moulding process. This is achieved by applying axial traction along the length of the vertebral column and increasing the lumbar flexion. This results in a flattening of the lumbar lordosis and at the same time lateral torso forces are applied through derotation straps.

The completed orthosis comprises a moulded pelvic girdle, two adjustable posterior struts and a single anterior strut. These components extend to the occipital and mandibular level and are connected by a cervical ring. Alignment is achieved by positioning adjustable pads according to the rotation and apex of the spinal curves (Figure 13.6). Further correction may be obtained by employing axilla slings and neck ring pads.

Many orthopaedic surgeons consider the Milwaukee brace more as a 'trainer' to en-

courage the patient to adopt an improved posture rather than an orthosis. If the patient 'slouches' they become uncomfortable resting on the chin or throat support.

The Scheuermann's Thoraco-Lumbar-Sacral Orthosis (TLSO)

The mechanical objective in treating adolescent kyphosis can be achieved by employing a number of TLSO's, including the Boston, Milwaukee (Montgomery and Irwin, 1981) and the Stanmore modular system. An alternative orthosis is constructed from a rectified plaster of Paris mould of the torso and pelvis of the subject (Figure 13.7). It comprises lateral pelvic moulds, an abdominal panel, a lateroposterior thoracic panel and a sternoclavicular pad. Each panel is connected by an adjustable hinge or strut. Alignment of the spine is achieved by applying a force at the sternoclavicular and abdominal levels, which are then opposed by a

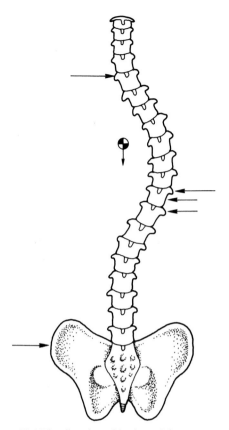

Figure 13.6 The direction of horizontal forces exerted by the Milwaukee TLSO, as viewed posteriorly

midthoracic and posterior pelvic forces. The level and direction of the midthoracic force must be determined by the apex of the kyphosis, as illustrated in Figure 13.8. A different concept has also been used in which a biofeedback audio-signal is activated by the brace user when pressure on the anterior sternal pad is increased, reminding the user to sit up and improve his posture.

(d) Critical assessment

A recent study (Chase *et al.*, 1989) involved the evaluation of the biomechanical effectiveness of the Boston brace. Interface pressure measurements were performed with the Oxford Pressure monitor at the appropriate compression pads within the brace when it was first applied, and on two further occasions within the 6-month period of brace treatment. A corresponding series of Cobb angles were also measured from standard posteroanterior radio-graphs. Results indicated initial mean corrections of 37% and 36% for thoracic and lumbar curves respectively in 14 patients with adolescent idiopathic scoliosis. However, these corrections were significantly reduced after 6 months, although it is important to note the reductions are underestimates of the initial correction, due to the dynamic nature of the initial correction, which causes progression of an unbraced curve over time. Results also indicated that the percentage correction of the curve was not determined exclusively by the mean level of force when the subjects were considered as a whole. However, in some cases, for example subjects with similar initial thoracic curves in terms of level and degree, there was a relation between applied force and curve reduction (Figure 13.9). Nevertheless, the two patients in the study with curves larger than 50° achieved little correction at any stage of treatment, despite significant levels of applied force. This confirms other findings that orthotic treatment is not effective for curves above 45°.

Scoliosis surgeons world-wide continue to use the Boston brace and consider it a valuable contribution to conservative treatment, particularly for the younger scoliosis patient.

This study has also revealed a large variation in response between patients, despite strict inclusion criteria. For seven patients who had lateral bend radiographs taken, curve flexion appeared to depend upon overall flexibility. This is illustrated in Figure 13.10. Thus subjects who had flexible spines showed large corrections, whereas subject whose radiographs indicated a relatively inflexible spine showed little improvement. It was suggested that little correction is possible unless the spine exhibits at least a 20% initial correction as measured from lateral bend radiographs. This criterion should be included when selecting suitable subjects for brace treatment.

Several studies have measured the traction forces exerted on the lateral curve by the various modified components of the Milwaukee Brace system in the management of idiopathic scoliosis. For example, Mulcahy *et al.* (1973) measured the forces through the occipital and mandibular supports for subjects in various functional positions. Results indicated average forces in the standing position of 19 N, which were shown to increase to 63 N if the patient pulled away from the thoracic pads.

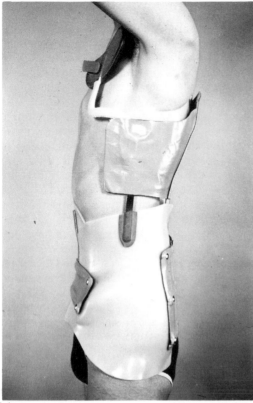

(a)

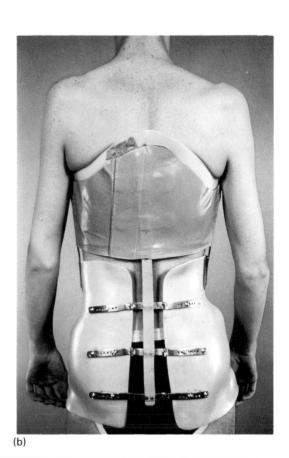

(b)

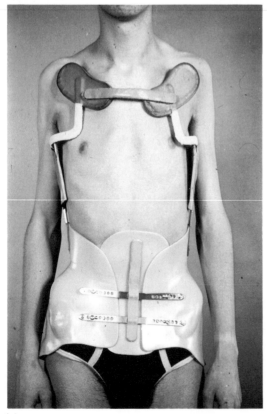

(c)

Figure 13.7 The Scheuermann TLSO: (a) lateral view indicating moulded pelvic section; (b) posterior view indicating moulded thoracic component; (c) anterior view indicating sternoclaviculum component.

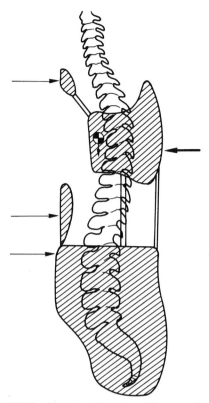

Figure 13.8 The direction of horizontal force application and distribution employed by the Scheuermann TLSO

This shows that the brace provides passive distraction when the patient moves away from the pads.

There has been a preliminary report discussing brace compliance in adolescent idiopathic scoliosis (Houghton *et al.*, 1987). These authors employed a hidden pressure switch which was activated when the patient wore the brace. Results suggested that skin condition and brace soiling produced only rough estimates of true brace compliance, which was found by measurement to be considerably less than that reported by the patient.

The medium term value of using the Milwaukee Brace for the treatment of adolescent idiopathic scoliosis is currently controversial, with some authorities providing evidence that it is of little value in the treatment of this type of scoliosis (Dickson, 1985; Edgar, 1985).

(e) Alternative and complementary treatments

In this category, the two pathologies of idiopathic scoliosis and adolescent kyphosis have been considered. Surgical intervention in these conditions has the primary objective of preventing progression or reducing the curvatures of the deformities to improve the cosmetic

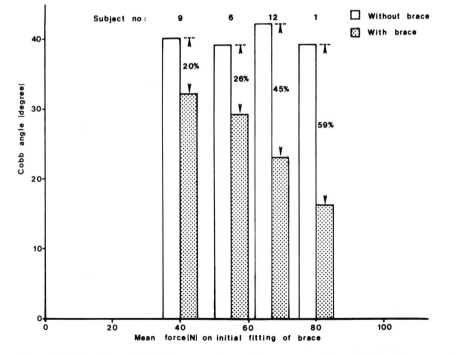

Figure 13.9 The effects of initial brace wearing on the curvature of four subjects with similar thoracic curvature. The percentage values are related to the changes in Cobb angle

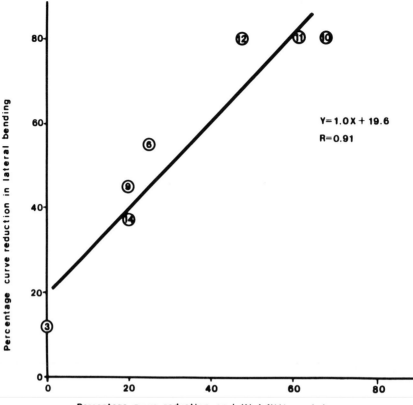

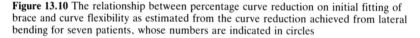

Figure 13.10 The relationship between percentage curve reduction on initial fitting of brace and curve flexibility as estimated from the curve reduction achieved from lateral bending for seven patients, whose numbers are indicated in circles

appearance of the patient. It is achieved by internal fixation of the vertebrae, approached through the anterior wall of the thorax or through the posterior aspect of the spine. A number of techniques have been employed including Harrington rods (Gaines and Leatherman, 1981), anterior spinal instrumentation (Dwyer, 1973), posterior segmental instrumentation (Griss *et al.*, 1984) and segmental wiring (Luque, 1980). Surgical techniques for adolescent kyphosis have also included the more extensive two-stage approach, which employs a kyphosis distractor and subsequent spinal fusion (Leatherman and Dickson, 1979).

Non-surgical alternative treatments include the EDF three-dimensional plaster of Paris jackets (Cotrel and Morel, 1964) and the employment of a traction-based exercise programme (Dickson and Leatherman, 1978). Preventive education also contributes to the management of adolescent spinal disorders, in particular, school screening can be employed to detect the onset of spinal and soft tissue asymmetry in those adolescents considered to be at risk (Dickson *et al.*, 1980)

13.4.2 Postural/functional management

(a) Pathologies

— Kyphosis as a result of senile osteoporosis.
— Post-operative thoracic or lumbar spinal surgery.
— Prolapsed intervertebral disc, low back pain, sciatica and ankylosing spondylitis.

(b) Management objectives and biomechanical requirements

The objective in the orthotic management of this group of pathologies is primarily to reduce deformity and also to prevent pain. This is achieved by protecting against painful movement and promoting postural realignment.

The pathologies described normally present as deformity, pain and inflammation in the thoracic, lumbar or sacral spinal segments. At the thoracic level, severe kyphosis requires a three-point force system to be applied. Anteriorly the point of application of force is at the sternoclavicular level coupled with an abdominal force. To resist these forces a posterior force is applied at the midthoracic level which is distributed over a large surface area, i.e. the body of the orthosis. Correction of deformity at the level of the thoracolumbar junction is achieved by applying anterior forces at the upper third of the sternum and at the suprapubic level, which are resisted posteriorly by a large pad in the thoracolumbar area. In the lumbosacral segment, the objective of the orthosis is normally to minimize flexion, to promote a normal upright posture and to impose forces which will increase intra-abdominal pressure.

With reference to their biomechanical objectives, this group of orthoses can be conveniently divided into two, namely, the Thoraco-Lumbo-Sacral Orthoses (TLSO) and the Lumbo-Sacral Orthoses (LSO). Within the former group, their effectiveness will be determined by the length of each moment arm from the rotational axis, and the correct alignment of the force applied through the posteriorly positioned lumbar sacral pad. This is well illustrated with the Jewett orthosis (Figure 13.11) and the thoracolumbar section of the Jones, Knight or Taylor TLSO (Figure 13.12), although the posterior force within the latter orthoses is less well defined.

The biomechanical objectives of the LSO group of orthoses are most conveniently listed as:

1. To increase the intra-abdominal pressure by exerting static lift under the diaphragm, which will diminish the loads through the lumbar lesions.
2. To place the lumbar spine in flexion and hence transfer weight bearing forwards onto the anterior part of the disc since the posterior disc is affected and thought to be causing nerve 'irritation' in many cases.

Flexion also improves the support of the disc system by diminishing translational shear forces and strengthening the effective strut mechanism. Lumbar flexion enlarges the foraminal spaces for the lumbar nerves by tightening the

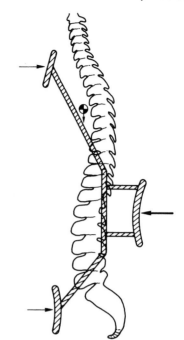

Figure 13.11 Application of three-point fixation in a Jewett brace, illustrated in the sagittal plane, when applied to flexion resistance of the thoracolumbar sacral segments

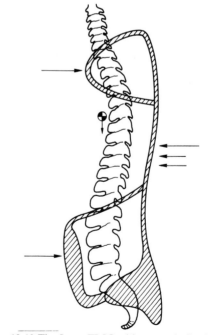

Figure 13.12 The Jones TLSO with arrows indicating the direction of horizontal force application and distribution of forces in the three-point loading system. The choice of material in the abdominal component will influence the overall mechanical integrity

posterior annulus, the longitudinal ligaments and the facet joint capsules and by separating the pedicles, which make up the roof and floor of the intervertebral foramen. This effectively improves the posterior barrier to disc protrusion.

(c) Orthoses specifications

The orthoses provide some structural support. The fit of these orthoses becomes more important as the load distribution requirement increases. The demands of functional support require a relatively rigid orthosis, which will dictate which movements the patient can perform.

Thoracolumbar flexion-hyperextension – The Jewett orthosis

This type of orthosis can be constructed from either direct measurements of the subject's torso or it can be purchased as a prefabricated orthosis. It consists of an anterolateral torso frame, to which a rotating sternal pad and a rigid suprapubic pad are attached. Posteriorly a thoracolumbar pad is connected to the frame using standard fastenings (Figure 13.11).

Thoracic kyphosis – the Jones orthosis

The Jones TLSO is a well-established orthosis for treating thoracic kyphosis (American Academy of Orthopedic Surgeons, 1975). The orthosis comprises a posterior lightweight aluminium frame which extends from the cervicothoracic level to the midsacral level. An abdominal pad is attached to the pelvic band, whilst shoulder straps are attached to the posterior frame to prevent thoracic flexion (Figure 13.12).

Lumbosacral control – the Raney flexion brace (rigid)

This plastic flexion orthosis surrounds the trunk completely (Figure 13.13), extending anteriorly from pubis to xiphisternum and posteriorly from the sacrum to the midthoracic area. The anterior abdominal shell has a deep indentation and is laced and strapped to the lumbar flexed posterior shell. It can be fabricated from an individual plaster of Paris cast or assembled from a series of modular components.

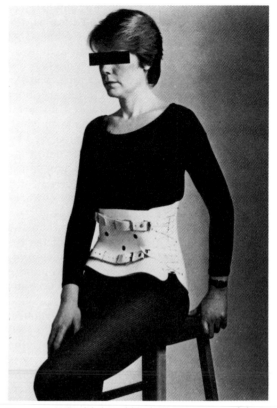

Figure 13.13 Prefabricated bivalved components of the Raney Flexion Modular Orthosis System. Note the indented abdominal cavity of the anterior component, which will effectively increase the abdominal pressure

The flexion orthosis may be prescribed for acute lumbar sprain, chronic lumbar sprain associated with postural deficits, acute sciatica with an intact annulus and recurrent back or sciatic pain postoperatively, especially for a patient with L5 root symptoms following L4 disc excision. The orthosis is demanding to wear and requires good compliance and a high tolerance of interface pressure.

Lumbosacral fabric orthoses (non-rigid)

The main component of a lumbosacral fabric orthosis is a cloth cylinder which wraps around the lower torso and pelvis and normally fastens over the anterior aspect of the torso. Ancillary components include a posterior sacral fulcrum strap, posterior rigid steels or a frame, and spirella or spring steel bones positioned at regular intervals around the cylinder. The level to which the orthosis extends, proximally and distally, is determined on an individual basis and is always a compromise between providing adequate support with a wide orthosis and allowing normal function with bending and sitting – only possible with a narrower orthosis.

(d) Critical assessment

A biomechanical analysis of the Jewett brace has been performed recently (Patwardhan *et al.*, 1990). Their analyses has indicated the effectiveness of the brace in providing the resistance to deformity, under restricted patient mobility, as long as the injury had not resulted in a loss of segmental stiffness greater than 60%.

A biomechanical investigation of a series of lumbar spinal orthoses have been reported (Grew and Deane, 1982). The authors concluded that the rigid braces are more efficient in restricting movement and that most braces produced an increase in intra-abdominal pressure. In addition the increase in temperature observed at the patient–orthosis interface can be beneficial to low back pain sufferers. In a separate study Nachemson *et al.* (1983) also measured back muscle activity, specifically the lumbar erector spinae muscles, during a range of movement tasks. The effects of lumbar spine orthoses were found to be variable, with some tasks producing a reduced myoelectric activity and others an increased activity compared to the unbraced situation.

In a recent report Willner (1990) discussed the use of a test instrument which imitates a rigid brace. This instrument could be adjusted to provide varying degrees of lordosis, abdominal support and levels of maximal dorsal support. It was found using this device that it was possible to predict whether a rigid brace would give pain relief in patients with low back pain, and it could also show how the brace might be manufactured to give optimal pain relief.

(e) Alternative and complementary treatments

The primary objective within this group of patients is to reduce pain, with the secondary aim of restoring function. Osteoporotic bone when treated surgically presents problems with fixation of the metal components into the porotic bone and frequently of an orthosis is used in the postoperative period. The literature does however suggest that two-stage segmental spinal instrumentation involving intervertebral grafting, iliac and rib grafting, followed by a second stage instrumentation can be very effective (Leatherman and Dickson, 1988). The use of drug therapy for treating back pain associated with postmenopausal osteoporosis is often worthwhile (Gordon, 1978).

Classification of the low back pain group is extremely difficult and this hampers appropriate and effective treatment. A detailed examination is required in an attempt to diagnose the site of pain and the type of lesion. Physiotherapy is an established method of symptomatic treatment and includes exercises, manipulation, electrotherapy and ergonomic advice. Drug therapy also contributes to the effective treatment of back pain and includes the use of non-steroidal anti-inflammatory drugs, muscle relaxants and pain-relieving drugs. Surgery is only appropriate when conservative measures have proved unsuccessful in relieving chronic pain or when the condition and the functional ability of the patient is profoundly impaired. Surgery is also indicated as a primary treatment in cases where there is neurological impairment of bowel or bladder control or when there is a rapid onset of progressive motor weakness.

13.4.3 Postural/static management

(a) Pathologies

— Neuromuscular disorders.
— Duchenne muscular dystrophy.
— Cerebral palsy.
— Poliomyelitis.
— Postoperative or post-traumatic management.

(b) Management objectives and biomechanical requirements

Management in this category of disorders requires the provision of support for physiological or postural benefit, or both.

In the treatment of some neuromuscular disorders, one of the primary objectives is to prevent further progression of the thoracic 'long C' scoliosis. Failure to achieve this will result in impaired pulmonary ventilation and reduced respiratory function. Postural realignment is also important when dealing with subjects who are either deficient in muscle strength or experience spastic reflexes. In both cases, orthoses will sustain postural realignment which should result in an improvement in upper limb function and head control. The objective of an orthosis for postoperative and traumatic conditions is normally to prevent movement in the region of the site of the injury or surgery.

Within this classification a division can be made in terms of the biomechanical requirements for specific patient conditions. The first group consists of Duchenne muscular dystrophy and cerebral palsy, where the objective is to apply forces in such a way as to effect an increased lumbar lordosis, tending to lock the facet joints and allow soft tissues to contract in the extended position. This is achieved during the casting process by applying occipito-mandibular traction, reducing the scoliosis and increasing the lumbar lordosis.

The second group includes subjects with poliomyelitis or those who are postoperative or post-trauma. In general terms, the objective is to compensate for neuromuscular deficiency or to prevent movement. In achieving this objective, the orthosis must apply more generalized forces by total containment of the torso and pelvis.

(c) Orthoses specification

These orthoses have to be strong to withstand the body weight of the patient. For this to be acceptable it must be supported on sections which conform well to the patient's body so that the loads are distributed over as large an area as possible.

Calot TLSO

The Calot TLSO (Figure 13.14) is an adjustable multipanel system based on the Cotrel TLSO developed at the Institut Calot, Berck-Plage in France (Young *et al.*, 1984). The

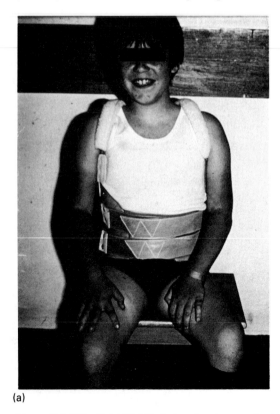

(a)

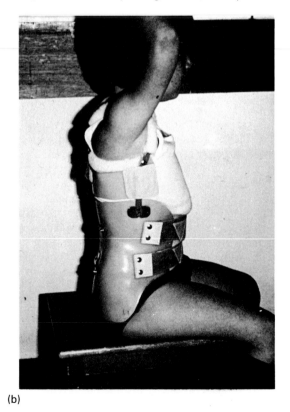

(b)

Figure 13.14 The Calot TLSO, designed to increase lumbar lordosis and optimize respiratory function. (a) anterior view; (b) Lateral view

principle of the orthosis is to promote a lumbar lordosis and, by lateral torso containment, to resist scoliotic progression. The orthosis consists of two pelvic sections, two lateral/posterior torso sections, a soft abdominal panel and shoulder straps. Each rigid section is moulded onto a rectified plaster of Paris model of the subject. All components are connected by adjustable hinges and struts.

Moulded thermoplastic or leather TLSO

In circumstances in which the primary objective of the orthosis is containment, then materials such as low density plastazote, low molecular weight polyethylene, and block leather are used to produce spinal orthoses which encase the whole of the torso and pelvis. In some instances during the casting or moulding process, corrective forces may be applied to the body. These orthoses spread the forces over the largest possible area by using the principle of total contact (Figure 13.15).

Prefabricated TLSO

A system based on the Boston Brace, named the Boston Overlap Orthosis (Figure 13.16), has been developed. It is constructed on the basis of a normal, straight torso/pelvic mould. Each module provides a 15° or 30° lumbar lordosis, is produced from polyethylene and fastens anteriorly. The module is trimmed to match the individual's size. It has the advantage of being instantly available, modular, relatively inexpensive and is very rigid.

(d) Critical assessment

Most of the experience gained with this diverse treatment group is clinically based and there are very few reports describing objective assessments of these types of orthoses. Young *et al.* (1984) compared two braces on a small group of wheelchair-bound subjects with Duchenne muscular dystrophy. Both braces produced some respiratory restriction, as measured by forced vital capacity, compared with the

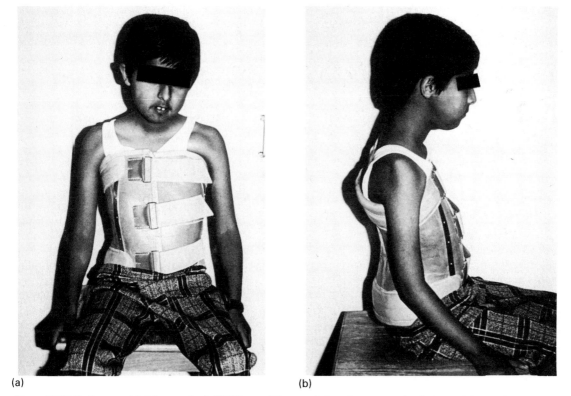

(a) (b)

Figure 13.15 Custom moulded thermoplastic TLSO, providing restriction of movement in all planes. (a) Anterior view; (b) lateral view

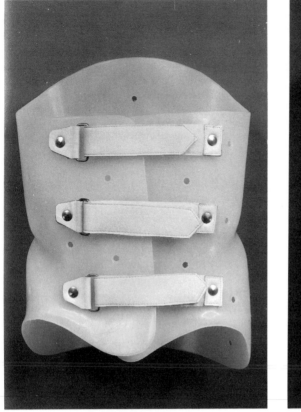

(a)

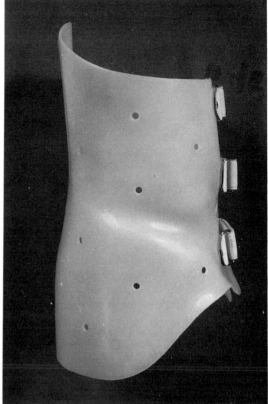

(b)

Figure 13.16 (a),(b) The Boston Overlap Modular TLSO, illustrating post-trimming and fitting. The module is preformed with a 15° or 30° lordosis

unbraced sitting position. The braces were also found to support the spine passively at an angle of lumbar lordosis similar in magnitude to that achieved when the unbraced subjects briefly produced active spinal extension.

(e) Alternative and complementary treatments

The primary objective within this group is in the preservation of function in both physical and physiological terms. Conservative treatments are the most frequently employed. Surgical intervention has been described for neuromuscular deficiencies and, in particular, Luque wiring procedures for the stabilization of patients with Duchenne muscular dystrophy (Weiman *et al.*, 1983). However risks during surgery such as sinus tachycardia, atrial and ventricular fibrillation and cardiac arrest have been well documented (Seay *et al.*, 1978). In addition, postoperative complications include

respiratory dysfunction and myoglobinuria (Boltshausen *et al.*, 1980) and may outweigh the surgical benefits.

Spinal fusion for adolescent cerebral palsy has also been recognized as having significant postoperative complications, including loss of curve correction, pressure sore formation and delayed wound healing (Lonstein and Akbarnia, 1983). More severe spinal deformities such as those observed with poliomyelitis and muscular dystrophy are more commonly managed by combining the use of spinal orthoses and custom-made seating systems (see Chapter 14).

13.5 Current and future developments

It is clear that more comparative studies need to be undertaken of an objective biomechanical nature into the efficacy of spinal orthoses in terms of correction, physical functional changes and physiological benefits. Compliance by the patient in the use of the orthosis should also be thoroughly investigated, particularly in the present economic climate in health care. Further work on the effect of orthotic treatment on long-term correction and the subsequent prevention of surgery is also needed. Many centres worldwide have considered the development of modular systems and components, which can accommodate subject growth and change in spinal shape. The potential role of prefabricated modular systems and their effectiveness both in mechanical and clinical terms should be examined. Studies should also evaluate the performance of lightweight materials which can be manufactured easily at low cost, provide good cosmesis and which improve compatability with soft tissues. Composite materials, which generally exhibit good mechanical characteristics, may be ideally suited to spinal orthosis applications.

In specific terms, thoracic and thoracolumbar control orthoses should be studied to determine the magnitude of the force produced at the soft tissue–orthosis interface at the three points of loading.

The use of internal and external electrical stimulation in conjunction with orthotic prescription should also be evaluated in relation to the management of neuromuscular spinal disorders, idiopathic scoliosis and low back pain.

References

Aaro S., Bustrom R. and Dahlborn M. (1981) The derotating effect of the Boston brace: a comparison between computer tomography and a conventional method. *Spine* **6**, 477–482

American Academy of Orthopedic Surgeons (eds) (1975) Biomechanical principles and application. In: *Atlas of Orthotics* C.V. Mosby, St Louis, pp. 354–356

Blount W.P. and Moe J.H. (1980) *The Milwaukee Brace*. Baltimore, Williams and Wilkins, pp. 119–140

Bogduk N. and Twomey L.T. (eds) (1987) *Clinical Anatomy of the Lumbar Spine*. Churchill Livingstone, Edinburgh

Boltshauser E., Steinmann B., Meyer A. *et al.* (1980) Anaesthesia induced rhabdomyolysis in Duchenne muscular dystrophy. *Br. J. Anaesth.* **52**, 559

Chase A.P., Bader D.L. and Houghton G.R. (1989) The biomechanical effectiveness of the Boston brace in the management of adolescent idiopathic scoliosis. *Spine* **14**, 636–642

Cobb J.R. (1948) Outline for the study of scoliosis. *Am. Orthop. Surg. Lect.* **5**, 261–275

Cotrel Y. and Morel G. (1964) La technique de L'E.D.F. dans la correction des scolioses. *Rev. Chir. Orthop.* **50**, 59–75

Dickson R.A. (1985) Conservative treatment for idiopathic scoliosis. *J. Bone Joint Surg.* **67B**, 176–181

Dickson R.A. and Leatherman K.D. (1978) Cotrel traction exercises, casting in the treatment of idiopathic scoliosis, *Acta Orthop. Scan.* **49**, 46–48

Dickson R.A., Stamper P., Sharp A.M. *et al.* (1980) School screening for scoliosis: cohort study of clinical course. *Br. Med. J.* **281**, 265–267

Dwyer A.F. (1973) Experience of anterior correction of scoliosis. *Clin. Orthop. Rel. Res.* **93**, 191–214

Edgar M.A. (1985) To brace or not to brace. Editorial. *J. Bone Joint Surg.* **67B**, 173–174

Gaines R.W. and Leatherman K.D. (1981) Benefits of the Harrington compression system in lumbar and thoracolumbar idiopathic scoliosis in adolescents and adults. *Spine* **6**, 483–488

Gordon G.S. (1978) Drug treatment of osteoporosis. *Ann. Rev. Pharmacol. Toxicol.* **18**, 253–268

Griss P., Harms J. and Zielke K. (1984) Ventral derotation spondylodesis. In: Dickson R.A. and Bradford D.S. (eds), *Management of Spinal Disorders*. Butterworths, London, pp. 193–236

Gracovetsky S., Farfan H.F. and Lamy C. (1981) The mechanism of the lumbar spine. *Spine* **6**, 249–262

Gregerson G.G. and Lucas D.B. (1967) An *in vivo* study of axial rotation of the human thoracolumbar spine. *J. Bone Joint Surg.* **49A**, 247–262

Grew N.D. and Deane G. (1982) The physical effect of lumbar spinal supports. *Prosthet. Orthot. Int.* **6**, 79–87

Hall J.E., Miller M.E., Schumann W. *et al.* (1975) A refined concept in the orthotic management of scoliosis. *Orthot. Prosthet.* **4**, 7–13

Houghton G.R., McInerney A. and Tew A. (1987) Brace compliance in adolescent idiopathic scoliosis. *J. Bone Joint Surg.* **69B**, 852

Leatherman K.D. and Dickson R.A. (1979) Two stage corrective surgery for congenital deformities of the spine. *J. Bone Joint Surg.* **61B**, 324–328

Leatherman K.D. and Dickson R.A. (eds) (1988) *The Management of Spinal Deformities*. Butterworth Scientific, Guildford, pp. 374–376

Lonstein J.E. and Akbarnia B.A. (1983) Operative treatment of spinal deformities in patients with cerebral palsy or mental retardation. *J. Bone Joint Surg.* **65A**, 43–55

Luque E.R. (1980) Segmental spinal instrumentation: a method of rigid internal fixation of the spine to induce arthrodesis. *Orthop. Trans.* **4**, 381

Montgomery S. and Irwin W. (1981) Scheuermann's kyphosis – long term results of Milwaukee brace treatment. *Spine* **6**, 5–8

Morris J.M., Lucas D.B. and Bresler B. (1961) Role of trunk in the stability of the spine. *J. Bone Joint Surg.* **43A**, 327–351

Mulcahy T., Galante J., DeWald R. *et al.* (1973) A

follow-up study of forces acting on the Milwaukee brace on patients undergoing treatment for idiopathic scoliosis. *Clin. Orthop.* **93**, 53–68

Nachemson A., Schultz A.B. and Andersson G.B.J. (1983) Mechanical effectiveness of lumbar spine orthoses. *Scand. J. Rehabil. Med. Suppl.* **9**, 139–143

Patwardhan A.G., Li S., Gavin T. *et al.* (1990) Orthotic stabilization of throracolumbar injuries – a biomechanical analysis of the Jewett hyperextension orthosis. *Spine* **15**, 654–661

Pearcy M.J. (1985) Stereo radiography of lumbar spine motion. *Acta Orthop Scand. Suppl.* **212**, 1–45

Pearcy M.J. (1989) Biomechanics of the spine. *Curr. Orthop.* **3**, 96–100

Raney F.L. (1969) *The Royalite Flexion Jacket.* Spinal Orthotics, Committee on Prosthetic Research and Development, National Academy of Sciences.

Seay A.R., Ziter F.A. and Thompson J.A. (1978) Cardiac arrest during induction of anaesthesia in Duchenne muscular dystrophy. *J. Pediatr.* **93**, 88–90

Weiman R.L., Gibson D.A. and Moseley C.F. (1983) Surgical stabilisation of the spine in Duchenne muscular dystrophy. *Spine* **8**, 776–780

White A.A. and Punjabi M.M. (1990) Kinematics of the spine. In: White A.A. and Punjabi M.M. (eds), *Clinical Biomechanics of the Spine.* Philadelphia: J.B. Lippincott, Philadelphia, pp. 85–125

Willner S.W. (1990) Test instrument for predicting the effect of rigid braces in cases with low back pain. *Prosthet. Orthot. Int.* **14**, 22–26

Young A., Johnson D., O'Gorman E. *et al.* (1984) A new spinal brace for use in Duchenne muscular dystrophy. *Dev. Med. Child Neurol.* **26**, 808–813

14

Seating

Geoff Bardsley

14.1 Introduction

Seating has tended in the past to be one of the more neglected aids for disabled people. Recent years, however, have seen an upsurge in interest in the subject which has resulted in major improvements in both seating systems and the services for their provision.

Is 'seating' relevant to orthotics? As the two areas share many common philosophies, particularly in their application of external structures to support the body, many orthotic principles are directly applicable to seating. This is reflected in the considerable involvement of orthotists in the prescription of seating, sometimes to the extent of providing complete seating services.

In contrast with orthotics, the study of seating is still in its infancy and consequently the knowledge and skills relating to the subject have yet to develop from an 'art-form' into a science-based subject. This chapter summarizes the 'state of the art' and its biomechanical background as practised at present.

Introductory sections describe the disabled population requiring seating, their problems in sitting and their subsequent needs. This leads to a discussion of anatomical and mechanical considerations of the process of sitting. The biomechanical support provided by a seat is described in terms of the various supportive elements which may be incorporated into a seat. Seating systems and associated devices which can provide this support are discussed subsequently. The final sections summarize the elements required in a service to provide seating and touches on current trends in research and development.

14.1.1 Population requiring seating

In the past, the need for seating has been grossly underestimated. Before embarking on a detailed discussion of seating, it is useful to gain an overall appreciation of the size of the disabled population which requires special seating provision.

In 1980, a survey was conducted in the Dundee District to determine the needs and characteristics of disabled people whose seating requirements demanded special solutions (TRES, 1981). A surprisingly large number of people, totalling 1000, were identified as having inadequate seating leading to an estimate of 200,000 people requiring special seating in the UK. The survey was not constrained to wheelchair users and in fact revealed that there are large numbers of people who are still able to walk but have significant seating problems.

The results of the survey are shown in Figure 14.1. They are subdivided to show the different pathologies in this group. The elderly dominated the results with their associated pathologies of osteoarthritis, stroke, rheumatoid arthritis or through simply being frail. Cerebral palsy accounted for the next largest group and exhibited some of the most severe problems. A group of pathologies including spinal cord injury, rheumatoid arthritis (not elderly), muscular dystrophy (with associated myopathies),

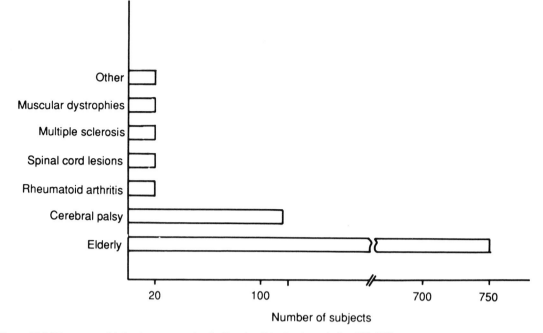

Figure 14.1 Diagnoses with inadequate seating in Dundee District (population 200 000)

and multiple sclerosis were all found to have a similar prevalence of around 0.1 per 1000. In addition, a range of assorted pathologies of a lower prevalence was identified. These included osteogenesis imperfecta, back pain, arthrogryposis, Friedreich's ataxia and lower limb amputation.

This survey concentrated on people whose seating at the time was inadequate and consequently did not include people whose seating needs had been adequately met. It could be argued that a wheelchair is a special seat and that all wheelchair users should be included in the numbers requiring special seating. This raises the total in Dundee to 2250 which, scaled appropriately, leads to an estimate of 450 000 disabled people in the UK requiring special seating.

14.2 Seating problems and needs of the disabled

The ideal seated posture fulfils the two main objectives of providing maximum body support whilst promoting a useful functional posture. These objectives frequently conflict with each other resulting in a compromise which is re-flected in seat design. For example, high activity seats tend to give upright postures with limited trunk support as this may impede function. Alternatively, low activity seats such as armchairs for relaxation tend to give a more reclined posture with extensive support to maximize comfort, but do limit reach and other functions.

The above comments apply equally to both able-bodied and disabled people. The introduction of disabilities to an individual increases his or her requirements of their seating. Inevitably such people spend much more time seated and consequently are much more sensitive to the suitability of their seating. Their ability to maintain a stable posture may be impaired and may require support provided by the seat. Clearly, the extent of support required is dependent upon the individual's sitting ability and the activities to be performed from the seated position.

The means by which a seat provides this mechanical support is constrained by the user's physical characteristics of size and shape. Further constraints may be applied from physiological (and sometimes psychological) characteristics resulting from their pathology. It is essential that the seat does not compromise their medical and physiological status and does not inhibit any potential for development or recovery.

Seating problems arise in the disabled population when their pathology impairs the mechanisms for achieving the postural objectives described above. At the same time, their disability may set different postural objectives which require specific solutions. The following section summarizes seating problems and the resulting needs of the disabled and relates them to the pathologies which cause the problems in the first place.

14.2.1 Stability

A primary concern of virtually all seating for disabled people is the promotion of postural stability. Many pathologies impair the ability of the individual to maintain a stable posture. A seat is required to compensate for this instability by providing additional support. The extent and configuration of this support is dictated by the extent of this instability in conjunction with postural needs. The support needs to be carefully matched to the individual's needs. Insufficient support will result in poor or asymmetrical postures which prevent function and may also encourage the development of deformities (Scrutton, 1991). On the other hand, excessive support may impede function by obstructing movement. It may also encourage dependence on support and discourage the development of the individual's full potential sitting ability. This applies particularly to cerebral palsy children who are developing muscle power and control.

Different pathologies may limit stability in three main ways, to various degrees and affecting different body segments.

(a) Hypertonia

The increased muscle tone characteristic of spastic cerebral palsy and stroke can prevent postural stability by the tendency for joints to be forced in to extreme positions. The extensor spasm pattern is frequently seen in cerebral palsy where all limbs are forced into extension. Alternatively, different stimuli can produce a flexor pattern. Both are posturally disturbing and can be triggered by a variety of stimuli such as noise, movement, position in space, head orientation, heat, discomfort, etc.

Positioning can have a major effect on problems of tone, especially in pathologies such as cerebral palsy. One solution frequently used for those with cerebral palsy is to flex the hips beyond 90°. This position has been found to inhibit muscle tone and diminish extensor spasm. Alternative approaches, however, have taken the reverse view and have allowed the hips to extend whilst supporting the body via the knees and chest (Pope *et al.*, 1988; Bridger *et al.*, 1989).

(b) Paresis

Muscle weakness obviously limits the individual's strength to maintain his posture, and is characteristic of all the myopathies, particularly muscular dystrophy. It is also evident in many other pathologies as a result of muscle atrophy as seen in multiple sclerosis, spastic cerebral palsy, stroke, etc. Clearly, seating requires to be much more supportive to compensate for this loss of stabilizing muscle power. Positioning can be crucial for these patients to minimize the demands on their musculature by promoting balanced postures. The centre of gravity of the head and trunk need to be positioned as close as possible to the mid-line, i.e. vertically above the midpoint between the ischial tuberosities.

(c) Dyskinesia

Constant movements such as those seen in athetosis can be highly disturbing to postural stability. They are also found in certain types of cerebral palsy and Friedreich's ataxia. They can be extreme to the extent of producing insoluble problems. Such constant movement, however, has the advantage of discouraging the development of deformities. Seating may be required to control this movement and, where possible, inhibit it. Positioning can assist in this process in a similar manner to the hypertonic individual. Alternatively, the seat may simply contain this movement and ensure that more appropriate postures are resumed when movements subside.

14.2.2 Physical characteristics

The physical characteristics of the disabled relevant to seating are primarily size and shape, as these influence the location and the contouring of the supporting surfaces. This 'dimensional matching' of seat to user is much more critical for the disabled than for able-bodied people because they are much more dependent upon support from the seat.

(a) Size

The disabled population exhibit the full range of body sizes from baby to fully grown adult. A disabled person, spending most of his time in sedentary activity, is not likely to load his skeleton to the same extent as an able-bodied person. Bone development is impaired and results in smaller body size (Bleck, 1987). Also, a large number of disabilities are associated with ageing which produces osteoporosis and a subsequent reduction in stature from loss of spinal height and increased kyphosis (Tortora and Anagnostakos, 1984). Emaciation may also occur in the disabled population including cerebral palsy and in the degenerative conditions such as muscular dystrophy, multiple sclerosis and the elderly. This readily leads to an increased susceptibility to discomfort and pressure sores from the high pressures around unprotected bony prominences.

More usually, disabled people tend to have different proportional sizes of their body segments. Leg-length development is sensitive to loading and consequently is often impaired in congenital conditions such as spina bifida. Cerebral palsy patients also have impaired development for similar reasons. Conversely some of their body segments are excessively and continuously loaded through reflex activity, resulting in comparative overdevelopment of that segment. Some conditions such as traumatic or elective amputation, thalidomide, genetic disorders, etc. can result in total absence or major size reductions in body segments.

Obesity is common in the disabled population, probably because a normal food intake may be maintained whilst their energy requirements are reduced by their disability. This imbalance results in a build up of fat. The elderly, those with spina bifida and some degenerative conditions such as muscular dystrophy can also exhibit obesity. In addition a range of hormonal or psychological problems can result in obesity with subsequent disability in otherwise normal people.

Obese people can present major difficulties for seating through difficulties in transferring from seat to seat and from providing support through highly mobile fatty tissues. They remain susceptible to pressure sores but little more than the normal person despite their high body weight, possibly because of the load distributing characteristics of fat and their increased support areas.

From the above, it can be seen that the disabled exhibit wide variations in body sizes and proportions. Statistical information is lacking, possibly because such variability requires the use of large sample sizes to produce meaningful statistical results. One study in the USA has produced anthropometric information on cerebral palsy subjects (Hobson *et al.*, 1987). At present, the most useful general anthropometric information for the orthotist or bioengineer is available from ergonomic literature based on the normal population such as in Humanscale (Diffrient *et al.*, 1974).

(b) Shape

Body shape abnormalities particularly of the spine and pelvis can cause severe seating problems. These may disturb the balance of the body and may also constrain the positioning of supporting forces. Most problems result from scoliosis or kyphoscoliosis which are often associated with pelvic obliquity and rib deformities. The 'windswept' configuration of some cerebral palsied people combines all these features with hip contractures or dislocation to produce the characteristic Z-shaped body (Bleck, 1987). The cause of such deformities is thought to be a combination of muscle imbalance affecting the spine in conjunction with the habitual adoption of asymmetrical postures. The latter may predispose to or aggravate hip subluxation or dislocation as a result of pelvic obliquity.

Seating can do little more than accommodate such deformities in the hope that their progression can be slowed down. In most cases, only orthotic solutions are likely to result in some correction of the deformity (see Chapter 13). The early provision of good seating in conjunction with careful orthopaedic care and therapy may subsequently prevent or reduce the severity of these deformities. Other pathologies such as muscular dystrophy, particularly in its later stages, spina bifida, arthrogryposis and osteogenesis imperfecta may all produce similar severe deformities which will present a challenge to the provision of suitable seating.

14.2.3 Physiological considerations

A wide variety of physiological considerations resulting from these different pathologies can constrain and influence the means by which a seat supports the disabled user.

(a) Pressure sores

Many pathologies such as spinal cord injury, spina bifida, cerebral palsy and ageing increase susceptibility to pressure sores through a variety of mechanisms. These may range through reduced tissue viability, tissue anaesthesia, inability to relieve tissue loading, high pressure levels from bony prominences, asymmetrical body shape increasing pressure, etc. A detailed description of the intrinsic factors associated with the development of pressure sores is found in Chapter 5.

(b) Pain

A small number of pathologies are characterized by pain during sitting. These include rheumatoid arthritis, mutliple sclerosis and back pain. The cause may be an inability to move to change posture which appears to be an inherent need for avoiding discomfort. In addition, pain may arise from the continuous heavy loading of tissues, particularly under the ischial tuberosities. This pain may be a useful warning of imminent tissue damage but may arise from excessively sensitive tissues, such as the ischio-gluteal bursa (Gorman, 1988; Zacharkow, 1988).

Back pain during sitting may be postural resulting from spinal nerve roots being compressed in certain spinal configurations during sitting. In many cases, however, the cause of pain during sitting may be unknown (Nachemson, 1985). It may be possible with seating to promote postures which reduce this pain.

(c) Respiratory insufficiency

Many of the more severely disabled suffer from respiratory insufficiency. Particular examples include muscular dystrophy, cerebral palsy and quadriplegic spinal injury. This may often preclude the use of spinal jackets as a postural support. Such individuals may be sensitive to their seated posture which can hinder or facilitate lung expansion (Stewart, 1991).

(d) Abdominal function

Abdominal function, like respiration, can be influenced by posture, despite it apparently functioning normally in severely deformed individuals. Swallowing ability and gastric reflux, especially for those with a hiatus hernia, can be influenced by posture. Cerebral palsy is the pathology which most frequently exhibits such problems.

(e) Oedema

Prolonged sitting results in venous pooling, especially in the legs, as the venous pump from muscle action is not operative (Zacharkow, 1988) nor is lymphatic flow stimulated when there is no muscle action. The impaired circulation associated with ageing aggravates this condition and often results in postural oedema of the legs. Elevation of the legs while seated can help to control this problem.

(f) Other factors

Many other physiological considerations from a variety of pathologies can give rise to seating problems. They are less frequently encountered than the above and are not expanded in this chapter, but the reader is directed to Stewart (1991) for further details.

14.2.4 Functional considerations

Mobility is obviously a major problem for patients with the pathologies outlined above as they usually involve locomotor disability. The wheelchair is intended to provide mobility but it is necessary to ensure that its seat provides the optimum position relative to the wheels to facilitate propulsion. Many wheelchairs fail to do this.

For those still able to walk, the process of sitting down and rising from sitting can be extremely demanding. This problem is particularly apparent in the elderly and accounts for a major proportion of their accidents in the home (Loud and Gladwin, 1981.). Incontinence can result when difficulties in rising delay reaching the toilet.

Many activities of daily living such as eating, toileting and washing, essential to independence, are performed from a seated position, and hence require an appropriate posture. In addition other activities, such as school work and recreation involving the use of a table or work surface require freedom of movement for the arms above the surface and the head. The competence of performance of these activities is often influenced by seating which can have major impact upon the individual's independence, and quality of life.

14.2.5 Comfort

Comfort (or lack of discomfort) is a priority requirement of any seat (Zacharkow, 1988). Lack of comfort probably accounts for the majority of rejected seats. Comfort is difficult to define and may involve a number of factors. The restriction of function either by obstruction or by inappropriate posture may be percevied as discomfort. Restriction of movement by too much postural support is often perceived as discomfort because of the sustained loading of soft tissues and because the body has an inherent habit of movement. Conversely, inadequate support requires more muscle action and associated 'effort' to maintain a desired posture. All these factors may contribute to 'discomfort'.

Conditions of pressure, temperature and humidity at the supporting surfaces also play a major part in comfort. These may be perceived as 'discomfort' and may act as early warnings of imminent pressure sores (see Chapter 5).

Finally, disabled people and their parents or carers are often extremely sensitive to the appearance of the seating. So much time is spent in a seat that it becomes closely related to body image in the same way as clothes are for able-bodied people. Hence an appropriate seat may need to reflect the personality of the individual. No matter how well a seat performs, it should also be as attractive as possible to the user.

14.3 Biomechanics of sitting

The following section begins with a brief summary of general postural objectives. It then describes some of the anatomical considerations and the methods by which the individual elements of the body maintain stability during sitting and hence contribute to the postural objectives.

14.3.1 Postural objectives

Figures 14.2 and 14.3 show the generally accepted concept of the ideal sitting posture. It represents a balanced posture which, in theory, reduces muscle effort, evenly distributes supporting forces, and facilitates activities whilst optimizing the physiological functioning of the body. People, however, have an inherent need for movement and change of posture (Branton, 1969). Hence this posture is rarely maintained and may in fact never be exactly achieved, as there are other factors which may conflict with it. Nevertheless it is a useful objective, at least initially, to attempt to achieve.

In the frontal view (Figure 14.2) symmetry about the midline is a primary objective to ensure optimum weight bearing evenly spread under the two ischial tuberosities and a vertical spine. The most useful landmarks to ascertain symmetry are first the iliac crests followed by the knees, shoulders and eyes. The sagittal view (Figure 14.3) of this posture is usually characterized by the hips, knees and ankles at 90° of flexion with the spine following its normal 'S'-shaped curve. Viewed from below, the hips are at neutral ab/adduction. Abduction would improve lateral stability but is limited by a socially acceptable posture.

14.3.2 Pelvis

The pelvis is the 'foundation stone' of the body during sitting, upon which all other body segments are largely dependent for their position. The ischial tuberosities are the two bony projections at the base of the pelvis and are primarily responsible for providing support in the seated position. The iliac crests are formed from the upper flares of the pelvis and are useful landmarks to indicate the orientation of the pelvis. They may however be difficult to palpate in obese subjects and may be distorted in patients with severe deformities.

The patellae form useful landmarks to indicate rotation of the pelvis. An anteriorly positioned patella normally indicates that the pelvis is rotated anteriorly on that side. In a few

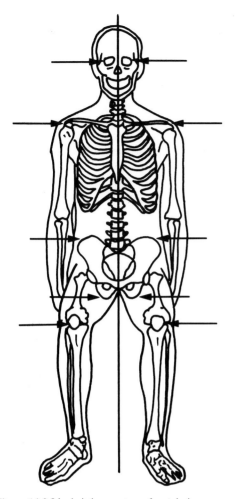

Figure 14.2 Ideal sitting posture, frontal view

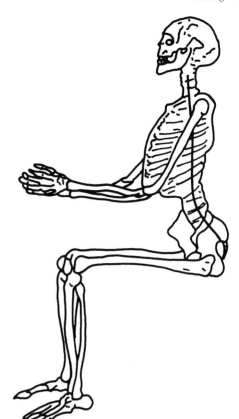

Figure 14.3 Ideal sitting posture, lateral view

instances, this patella position can be the result of a leg-length discrepancy or hip dislocation.

The sacrum completes the bony ring of the pelvis and forms the base of the spine. Any displacement of the pelvis directly affects the spine and generally the whole upper body. Hence a major priority of seating is to control and stabilize the posture of the pelvis.

During sitting approximately 80% of the weight of the trunk is supported by the pelvis (Zacharkow, 1988). Virtually all this load is transmitted through the ischial tuberosities through their underlying soft tissues to the seat. These soft tissues consist of a thin covering of skin and subcutaneous tissues usually comprised of muscle and the ischiogluteal bursa. Normally during sitting, the gluteus maximus slides laterally away from the ischial tuberosities and provides little weight-bearing assistance. The ischial tuberosities are shaped like small rockers measuring approximately 5 cm long by 2.5 cm wide. Their weight-bearing area is less than 10 cm^2 and consequently some of the highest pressures experienced by the body during sitting are generated in this area. Hence discomfort and, eventually, pressure sores are frequent problems.

The pelvis is inherently unstable viewed in the sagittal plane as it is balanced precariously on the ischial tuberosities. For optimum stability and minimum muscle effort, the centre of gravity (C of G) of the trunk should be directly over these tuberosities (Figure 14.4) (Zacharkow, 1988).

The inherent continuous movement of the sitting individual prevents this position being maintained over significant periods of time. Movement usually shifts the trunk C of G

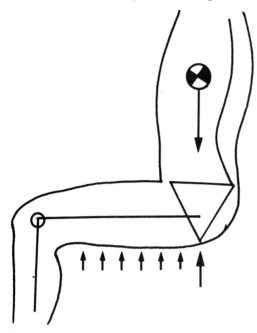

Figure 14.4 Optimum sitting stability with trunk centre of gravity directly above ischial tuberosities

increased muscle action particularly of hip extensors and the erector spinae muscles to maintain stability, but this demand can be reduced by the use of arm supports to prop up the shoulder girdle. It has significant benefits in enhancing the lumbar lordosis and distributes supporting pressures more evenly under the thighs and away from the ischial tuberosities. It is usually associated with table or desk activities where the patient's arms may provide additional support.

The pelvis is more stable in the frontal plane as it is supported over a wider base by the separation of the two ischial tuberosities. This distance varies from approximately 12 to 14.5 cm with a mean of 13 cm and is larger for females than males (Zacharkow, 1988). It is particularly important that the ischial tuberosities are as horizontal as possible to maintain the vertical linear alignment of the spine above. Many seats such as wheelchair canvasses have lateral curvatures which do not encourage a horizontal pelvis.

anteriorly or posteriorly from the ischial tuberosities. This effect is encouraged by the rocker shape of the ischial tuberosities.

If the C of G lies posterior to the ischial tuberosities, the pelvis will tend to rotate posteriorly, encouraging the body to slump down and slide forwards on the chair. This movement is seen as one of the most frequent postural habits of seated people (Branton and Grayson, 1967). This compromises the spine, which loses its lumbar lordosis and in addition reduces the sitting support area. The resulting lordotic posture compromises the spine by increasing intervertebral disc deformation whilst reducing the load carrying areas of the intervertebral joints (Zacharkow, 1988). The sitting support areas are decreased resulting in increases in surface pressures whilst high shear forces are generated by friction between the person and the seat surface. Both these effects increase discomfort and may eventually generate pressure sores.

Clearly, this pattern of posterior pelvic rotation is undesirable. A prime objective of seating for the disabled is to provide support to prevent this pattern.

Movement of the trunk C of G forwards from the ischial tuberosities is less frequently observed and less problematical. It requires

14.3.3 Femora

Together with the pelvis, the femora form the main supporting base of the seated body. Their major influence in seating is in controlling the orientation of the pelvis. The femora project laterally at the hip joint to form the greater trochanters which can contribute to weight bearing.

Ideally the femora should be horizontal. This will ensure a more uniform distribution of load under the supporting surfaces of the thighs. If lifted above the horizontal distally, then part of their weight is transmitted through the hip joint to the ischial tuberosities. This increases pressures over an area which is already overloaded and prone to pressure damage.

If the femora are dropped below the horizontal distally, there is a tendency for a component of their weight to pull forwards at the hip pulling the lower pelvis out of the seat. This also encourages the pelvis to rotate posteriorly. Hip extensor muscles tend to be more powerful than the flexors. This imbalance exacerbates the tendency for posterior rotation of the pelvis.

The habit of crossing the legs at the knees during sitting has been cited as a mechanism which reduces the tendency to posteriorly rotate the pelvis (Branton, 1969). This position forms a closed three-bar linkage of the two femurs with the pelvis and it has been suggested that this forms a more stable base with the uppermost femur being 'locked' in a position near the end of its flexion-adduction range. This in turn locks the lower femur and increases the loading on the lower leg to resist the forward slide. However it is felt that this posture should not be encouraged as it generates rotation in the spine and asymmetrical loading of muscles and ischial tuberosities.

Similar habits to form more stable closed linkages may be seen in other parts of the body such as in ankle crossing (Branton, 1969) or supporting the chin on the forearms (Zacharkow, 1988).

14.3.4 Lower legs (shanks)

It is essential that the lower legs are supported through the feet and independently of the femora. If not supported in this way, components of their weight are transmitted to the femurs resulting in high pressures under the thighs at the edge of the seat. This is quickly perceived as discomfort and may stimulate reflex activity.

Ideally, a 90° knee angle is used to minimize shear forces at the ground. Most normal people tend however to adopt a more extended knee position. This is often not possible in the disabled population, particularly for cerebral palsy patients who tend to have tight hamstrings. The hamstrings are two-joint muscles, thus if the knee is extended then the hip will be caused to flex and will produce posterior rotation at the pelvis. It is more desirable to accept a flexed knee position than a posteriorly rotated pelvis (Trefler and Taylor, 1991).

14.3.5 Feet

The importance of appropriate foot position and support is often neglected. This importance lies in the need to support the lower leg which in turn affects load distributions and configurations of the femurs and pelvis. A 90° ankle position is felt to be ideal but this angle is not critical. More important is the need to provide a support for the foot and the full load of the lower leg.

14.3.6 Spine

The spine is a highly complex structure consisting of a series of vertebral bodies interconnected by ligaments and controlled by a system of muscles. This arrangement provides considerable flexibility with a surprisingly good load carrying ability. It is, however, vulnerable to damage and requires careful consideration when supported during sitting. Chapter 13 has described the main structural elements of the spine. The following section relates this information to the configuration and function of the spine during sitting.

The 'S' shape of the spine is acknowledged as desirable for sitting, despite the fact that it is rarely accurately adopted by most people. It would appear that this position provides some shock absorbing properties whilst generally aligning the vertebral bodies under the C of G of the trunk. This reduces the muscle activity required to maintain stability. Also, it permits a kyphotic thorax which may facilitate chest expansion for respiration.

This shape also appears to correspond to the position in which the minimum intervertebral disc pressures occur and best utilizes the load bearing capabilities of the facet joints. The muscles mainly responsible for maintaining this shape are the erector spinae (extension), the rectus abdominus (flexion) and the oblique abdominals (lateral flexion).

At birth, lumbar lordosis is absent. It develops in parallel with the child's neuromuscular development for postural control. Normally lumbar lordosis is present at an early age but does not mature until 12 years of age (Zacharkow, 1988). It can be delayed, sometimes indefinitely, in the disabled child. Hence seating should not always attempt to promote a lordosis in individuals who have not reached the stage of developing a lordosis.

Rotation of the spine is known to be particularly undesirable as it predisposes the intervertebral discs to damage. In addition, if the spinal column as a whole is regarded as a column with an asymmetrical cross-section, any rotation increases its tendency to buckle into scoliosis under loading (Dickson and Archer, 1986).

The spine can be divided into four different regions, each with very different functions, characteristics and loading conditions:

1. The cervical spine has a wide range of mobility to give maximum flexibility to the

head position. It benefits from carrying only the load of the head and neck and consequently is only at risk of acute injury in extreme conditions such as in high deceleration car accidents.

Except for reclined, relaxing postures, the head and neck does not normally need external support as this may impede movement. It is, however, important to align the spine under the C of G of the head to minimize muscle effort and to maintain stability. This is a priority for most people and will occur often independently of the position the seat is providing.

2. The thoracic spine forms part of the rib cage. This is a relatively rigidly jointed structure which helps to stiffen the thoracic spine. Hence a seat does little to affect the configuration of this section of the spine. Normally, some support is necessary but forces tend to be small.

3. The lumbar area is where the major spinal movement occurs. This corresponds to the area of maximum loads and consequently is a particularly vulnerable part of the spine. Some stabilization is provided by the pressure from the abdominal cavity but this effect is not great, especially when seated.

   Lordosis in the lumbar region is thought to be particularly beneficial to stability of the spine. It aligns the C of G of the trunk through the heavily loaded lumbar vertebra and over the ischial tuberosities. More interestingly, lordosis brings the facet joints of the lumbar spinous processes more closely together. This increases the weight-bearing areas of the vertebra and locks them together to resist rotation more effectively (Gorman, 1988; Zacharkow, 1988).

4. The sacrum forms the base of the spine which is connected directly to the supporting pelvis. Hence any tendency for the pelvis to rotate posteriorly as described in 14.3.2 immediately affects the configuration of the whole spine, especially in the lumbar region which becomes flattened or even kyphotic.

   The junction of the sacrum with the rest of the spine at L5/S1 may be angulated up to 40° to the horizontal and carries the large majority of body weight. This joint therefore experiences prolonged high shear forces and is vulnerable to damage. Excessive lumbar lordosis does increase these shear forces and should not be encouraged.

14.3.7 Shoulder/arms

The positions of the shoulder girdle and arms are largely dependent upon the rest of the body, particularly the spine. Ideally, the shoulders should be horizontal with the elbows at 90° flexion and the forearms horizontal. Often, priorities for seating lie in movement of the arms and shoulders when activity is taking place. In such instances, support in unnecessary or may even be undesirable.

Less active situations require arm support to reduce the loading on the shoulder and spine. This avoids the inevitable depression (slump) of the shoulders. It may also assist in maintaining a good position of the spine and avoiding the downward slide of the trunk.

14.4 Biomechanics of seats

A wide variety of supporting elements can be incorporated into a seating system to meet the seating needs of the disabled. Depending upon the needs of the user, these needs may vary in extent or complexity from the simple flat surface of a stool to the total support provided by a whole body mould. Figures 14.5 and 14.6 illustrate the different elements which may be used.

Ideally the support elements should have as large a surface area as possible and should be contoured approximately to follow body shape. This will ensure interface pressures are

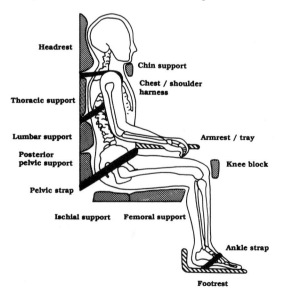

Figure 14.5 Potential seating support elements, lateral view

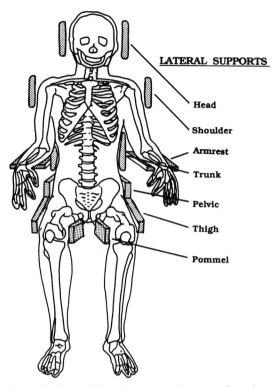

LATERAL SUPPORTS

Head

Shoulder

Armrest

Trunk

Pelvic

Thigh

Pommel

Figure 14.6 Potential seating support elements, frontal view

kept to a minimum. This ideal is not always possible to achieve and may not be important for some areas such as around the higher levels of the trunk where loads are smaller.

Care however should be taken to avoid generating shear forces in all areas as these are known to be particularly effective in creating pressure sores.

Seating elements can be divided into two groups relating to their predominant action in either the sagittal or lateral directions. General considerations of seating configurations will be discussed at the end of this section.

14.4.1 Sagittal support

The one feature common to all seats is a seat base which supports the pelvis and femora. In most cases, the loads and their distributions under the ischial tuberosities are very different to those under the femora. Hence it is useful to consider a seat base to be composed of two separate elements, the ischial support and the femoral support, despite there being no distinction between these areas in the design structure in many seating systems. From cli-

nical experience, the femoral support is usually twice the length of the ischial support.

(a) Ischial support

Ideally the ischial support surface should be horizontal to ensure that a horizontal pelvis is achieved in the frontal plane and to maintain an upright pelvis in the sagittal plane (Green and Nelham, 1991). The highest supporting pressures are encountered in this area and may require special consideration to avoid pressure sores. Foam, gel or air filled materials may be used to minimize peak pressures or shaping may be incorporated to transfer loads from the ischial tuberosities.

Contouring may be used to improve pressure distribution. This shaping may be contoured to the extent of raising the surface under the greater trochanters to transfer loads from the ischial tuberosities.

(b) Femoral support

The femoral support carries much lower loads than the ischial support but is of importance in governing the hip angle and subsequent orientation of the femora. The proximal end of the femur is supported through the hip joints by the pelvis. The undersurface of the femur, however, is supported only by soft tissues which compress under load. Hence to achieve the ideal position of a horizontal femur, the femoral support needs to be angled higher distally than proximally. Usually this angle is approximately 15° to the horizontal, beginning just forwards of the pubis.

Other hip angles may be dictated by a variety of postural objectives. These angles may be achieved by varying the angle of the femoral support from a point distal to the ischial tuberosities. It should not involve the ischial support as this would upset pelvic orientation.

(c) Posterior pelvic support

The support posterior to the pelvis is responsible for maintaining an upright pelvis in the sagittal plane. As in all back supporting elements, loads are relatively low and hence pressure distribution is not usually a problem. The surface of this support should be perpendicular to the ischial platform to achieve this position (Green and Nelham, 1991).

(d) Pelvic strap or bar

Pelvic straps may be used as shown in Figure 14.5 as a safety precaution to prevent people falling out of their seat. Alternatively they may be used more actively to hold the pelvis in the desired position. This reduces the tendency for posterior rotation of the pelvis to occur and thus subsequent sliding out of the chair. Such straps should be placed low over the iliac crests and at an angle bisecting the angle between the ischial and posterior pelvic supports. Waist straps positioned higher and horizontally tend to be ineffective.

The most effective support of this nature can be provided by a padded metal bar locked into position across the anterior superior iliac spine, (termed 'sub ASIS bar') (Margolis *et al.*, 1988). This bar is fixed on an axis parallel to the plane of the seat/backrest and in contact with each ASIS. It should be curved out over the abdomen. Accurate location is critical to achieve the desired stability whilst avoiding discomfort and tissue damage. Obviously, a detachable location system is necessary.

(e) Knee blocks

Knee blocks although considered by some to be the 'last resort' to lock a pelvis in position do act very efficiently in preventing forward motion of the femurs which in turn prevent forward motion of the pelvis. They are often combined with adduction blocks and can fulfil a valuable role in controlling windswept deformities (Green and Nelham, 1991). Knee blocks should be positioned over the distal end of the femur and the patella. They should not be located lower down over the tibia as this may result in damaging shear forces across the knee joint. Hips should be carefully examined before knee blocks are used as problems such as dislocation or subluxation may be exacerbated by the resultant forces they produce.

(f) Foot support

The importance of adequate foot support is often underrated. If positioned incorrectly, loads under the pelvis and thighs may be adversely affected and reflex activity may be increased. Conversely good foot support may reduce elevated muscle tone and reflex activity. It can assist considerably in stabilizing the whole body.

Normally a flat surface such as the floor or a footplate is adequate. A rear stop or heel loops may be added to maintain the required knee angle and to prevent the feet fouling the castors of a wheelchair. Ankle straps can be surprisingly effective in maintaining ankle angle and inhibiting athetoid or extensor movement. However they are not always effective and their use can result in exaggerated movement in other parts of the body.

Foot support usually aims at providing a plantagrade foot position but deformities may prevent this position from being achieved. Alternatively a dorsiflexed position may be required to reduce muscle tone. This objective, however, is best achieved by an orthosis with the foot support simply accommodating the resulting foot position.

(g) Lumbar support

The practice of including a forward curve in backrests is widely used to encourage a lumbar lordosis. This curve may not be necessary if the pelvis is held sufficiently vertically by the posterior pelvic support. The spinous processes may be prominent in this region and contouring of the lumbar support may be required to avoid pressure sores. Ideally the lumbar support should not be used alone to maintain the pelvis in an upright position as this increases the loads over the vulnerable L5/S1 joint. It should extend to include the pelvis and the lower thorax.

(h) Thoracic support

Loads at the thoracic level are much lower and less demanding in terms of support configuration. For vertical postures, loads may be zero and this element may be unnecessary. It becomes more important as the angle of back recline (or backward tilt of the trunk) increases and loads across the whole of the backrest subsequently increase.

Activities involving significant movement such as wheelchair propulsion may limit the extent of this support as it can restrict shoulder and subsequent arm function.

(i) Headrest

Head support, if required, is often difficult to provide satisfactorily. Ideally the head should be balanced over the cervical spine to minimize the need for support. However kyphoses and similar spinal problems often prevent this ideal. Flexor patterns or neck muscle weakness can present insuperable problems with the head falling forwards and away from the head support.

Some patients have extensor reflexes which are triggered by pressure on the occiput and consequently this has to be avoided in any head support supplied for them. If this reflex is not present, headrests can be contoured to give a component of vertical support under the occiput.

Head support should be kept to a minimum to avoid restricting head movement. Normally, the support does not need to extend above the most posterior aspect of the skull. More extensive head support is required as the angle of recline increases.

(j) Chin support

Persistent flexion of the neck from weakness or flexor patterns can be tackled by the addition of a chin support. This may be as simple as a soft foam collar under the chin or may be a structural element of the headrest. The latter requires to be removable to allow access. An orthosis can be more effective in this area to give the necessary support. No ideal chin support exists as they tend to be socially unpleasant, restrictive to movement and can upset dentition.

(k) Chest/shoulder harness

Chest or shoulder harnesses may be used to prevent excessive forward flexion of the trunk. Shoulder harnesses tend to be most effective but are more complex to fit. Chest harnesses tend to slip down the chest and become less effective. Both approaches suffer from being restrictive to movement and should be regarded as 'last resort' solutions.

(l) Arm support

Arm support is normally provided by an armrest simply to support the weight of the arm. Armrests play a critical role in the process of rising from the seated position. They should project forwards of the seat and be of appropriate height and separation for the individual.

Trays can provide a more extensive arm support and are less critical in their positioning. They can be used at the appropriate height to prop up the trunk using the arms as supports. Obviously this may restrict arm function. Grab bars can be useful if fitted to trays because they help sitters reposition themselves and provide a grip for stabilizing their bodies.

14.4.2 Lateral support

In general, the extent and number of lateral elements provided in a seat should be kept to a minimum as they limit freedom of movement, restrict function and make access to the chair difficult. Lateral curvature can help stability and improve comfort by giving a more uniform pressure distribution and by increasing lateral support. However significant numbers of patients require additional lateral support to maintain an upright posture. Unless removable, lateral supports should not curve round in front of the sitter as this prevents access to the chair.

Lateral supports normally need to be used in combinations of two or three elements on opposite sides of the body. Use of a single element will merely push the whole body to the opposite side. A counteracting force needs to be provided on the opposite, even if provided by existing structures such as armrests or armrest panels.

(a) Lateral pelvic support

For lateral trunk support, the most effective element is at pelvic level. Many problems of stability may be solved merely by the addition of a lateral pelvic support as this may be sufficient on its own to give a stable base to the spine. The individual may then have sufficient muscle power and control to maintain an upright posture.

(b) Spinal support

With decreasing stability there is a need to extend lateral supports above the pelvis and up the trunk. The maximum height of support is limited to 2 cm below the axilla where nerves are near the surface of the skin and vulnerable to compression.

For symmetrical trunks, lateral supports should be used in pairs only to ensure stability. Used singly, there would be no counteracting

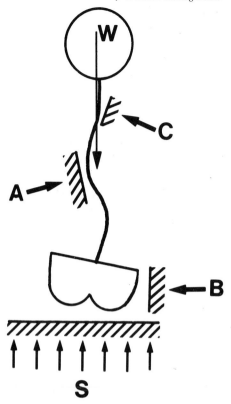

Figure 14.7 Simplified force system for supporting a scoliotic spine

force to prevent the body moving away in the direction opposite to the support. For asymmetrical trunks such as those with a scoliosis, it is useful to consider lateral supports acting in a three-point loading system (Figure 14.7) (Nelham, 1984). One support (A) applies a force just below the apex of the major curve acting medially and upwards. This force is counteracted on the opposite side of the trunk by two forces at B and C acting medially and also upwards at C. Supports B and C should have the maximum possible vertical separation for maximum effectiveness. This is a highly simplified analysis of supporting a scoliotic spine. It takes no account of the inevitably associated rotation of the spine.

Rotation can be such a problem that the planar surfaces of a seat are inadequate to provide the required support in three dimensions. Such problems may be exacerbated by voluntary or involuntary movements which may rotate the spine out of any support system.

It is unlikely that any significant correction of a scoliosis can be achieved by a seating

system. The closed support of a spinal orthosis is required for this purpose (see Chapter 13). Many patients, however, cannot tolerate the forces of an orthosis, particularly if they have respiratory insufficiency. At best, scoliosis can be managed with special seating only with the hope that further collapse of the spine is retarded. In severe cases, the lower ribs begin to rest on the pelvis and restrict respiration. Seating can be effective in separating the ribs and pelvis to help respiration and reduce impingement pain.

(c) Armrests

Lateral trunk support of an approximate nature is often provided by the armrests of a seat, particularly in a wheelchair. The support is provided through the arms to the upper trunk. This is not ideal for intimate support as armrests tend to be too narrow and also restrict arm function.

More specific support may be provided by extending the medial surfaces of the armrests down to the seat to act as lateral pelvic supports. Some armrests include a vertical element on their lateral side to prevent arms falling outside the width of a wheelchair and catching in doorways.

(d) Shoulder support

In extreme cases of trunk stability problems, lateral supports may be positioned outside the shoulder. This approach is rarely used as it limits arm movement and produces a very cumbersome, unwieldy seat.

(e) Headrests

Lateral instability of the head is a frequent problem which can be very difficult to solve. Lateral head supports may be included but any forward motion of the head enables it to clear the support and fall laterally, often to be trapped underneath the headrest. These supports may be extended forwards but then limit the visual field of the sitter.

(f) Adduction blocks (pommels)

Adduction blocks, or pommels as they are often known, are used frequently to maintain the hips in an abducted position and to prevent adduction. Adduction forms part of the extension reflex pattern and often needs to be controlled. Positioning hips in abduction has the benefit of reducing extensor tone and inhibiting the extension pattern.

Adduction blocks should provide a large surface area positioned distally along the femurs where they will be mechanically most effective. They require careful padding at their proximal end to prevent high pressure occurring over the genitalia if the sitter slides down the seat. For this reason adduction blocks should not be used to prevent sliding out of seats.

(g) Abduction blocks

Hypotonic individuals characteristically adopt a posture with hips in wide abduction and externally rotated. As a consequence femoral and foot support is compromised with resulting contractures at the hips and ankles. It also increases the overall width of the seat. Abduction blocks extending from the pelvis to the distal femur may be added to prevent this problem occurring.

(h) Ab/Ad-duction and kneeblock combinations

All the above elements of seating support may be used in any combinations. The combination of adduction, abduction and a knee block can be very successful in the control of windswept deformities of the pelvis. In this condition both hips have contractures which direct the femurs towards the same side of the body. The adducted hip may sublux or dislocate.

It is particularly important to attempt to correct this deformity as it prevents the achievement of a horizontal pelvis and subsequently encourages the progression of scoliosis (Rang *et al.*, 1981). It may be corrected as shown in Figure 14.8 by an adducting force and a posteriorly directed force applied to the abducted knee. These may be applied by a knee block and an abduction block. They are counteracted by reaction forces from the backrest to produce a correcting moment at this hip. The tendency for the pelvis to escape laterally is prevented by a lateral block applied to the opposite hip.

At the same time the adducted hip should be abducted to neutral by a pommel or adduction block. Care should be taken to avoid excessive

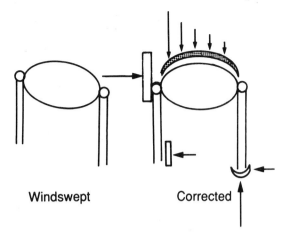

Figure 14.8 Force system for correcting windswept hips

axial loading of the adducted femur as it is usually vulnerable to dislocation.

14.4.3 General considerations of seating configurations

Having considered the individual supporting elements which may comprise a seat, their overall configuration may be varied in their position in space in the following ways:

(a) Recline

The angle of recline of a seat may have a dramatic effect upon the sitter and his functional ability. Ideally, a seat should support an upright posture as described in 14.3.1. This provides a balanced posture which is optimum for function. However, this position may be demanding to maintain especially over long periods of time. Reclining a seat may be less demanding as more support is then provided by the backrest and headrest. This increase in comfort however is nearly always achieved at the expense of a loss of functional ability. Also, rising from a reclined seat for a disabled person can be particularly difficult.

The optimum angle of recline for any individual may be quite variable during the day as they tire or when different activities are carried out. Seats with variable angles of recline are beneficial for this purpose. This variation, however, should retain the same back to seat angle to prevent the tendency to slide out of the seat as happens when the back alone is reclined.

Typical backrest angles with respect to the horizontal are 5–10° for functional postures, increasing to 20° for relaxation. For an ideal seat, the ischial support section should be horizontal with a 15° ramp rising under the thighs. The more usual, simpler designs of seat are flat and raked backwards at approximately 5–10° to the horizontal. Completely flat horizontal seats are best avoided as these encourage forward sliding out of the seat.

(b) *Lateral tilt*

Lateral tilt of a seat should only be used for people with asymmetrical postures in the frontal plane and even then should be used with considerable caution. However some deformities reach extremes where some tilt is required. The level of tilt is inevitably a compromise between the conflicting objectives of maintaining a horizontal pelvis and balancing the C of G of the head and trunk over the average centre line of the spine. There are no clear guidelines to achieve this compromise, only the practical experience of the orthotist/bioengineer, but care should be taken to observe the resulting head position and spinal configuration whilst monitoring the tissue responses under the lower ischial tuberosity (see Chapter 5).

(c) *Height*

The height of the seat influences the functional abilities of the sitter, especially for rising from the seated position. Increased height of the seat usually facilitates standing as the distance the sitter is required to move is reduced. However stability, foot support and comfort are compromised when following this philosophy to extreme.

Seat height must also be considered in conjunction with associated furniture such as tables, footstools, etc. Obviously, the heights of each must be selected for compatibility.

(d) *Seat dimensions*

The dimensions of a seat need to be matched to those of the individual in order to provide the appropriate support. Methods for determining the basic dimensions of the individual and subsequently translating them into seat dimensions are described by Wilson (1986) and ICE (1983).

14.5 Types of seating

After many years of neglect, seating has recently become a subject of increased interest resulting in the development of a wide variety of seating systems. A detailed description of every individual seating system is beyond the scope of this article. It is, however, possible to divide seating systems into a few broad categories. These are described in the following section beginning with the simplest and finishing with the more complex designs. Some indications of the applications of the different types of seating are included. These categories will be illustrated with specific examples. In general, the simplest solution should always be chosen to avoid unnecessary complexity and cost. However, the demands of increasingly difficult problems and the consequent seating requirements often lead to the need for more complex solutions.

14.5.1 Fixed format seats

An enormous range of fixed format seating is available in a wide variety of sizes. These meet the needs of a large proportion of disabled people who simply require an accurately fitting chair. The majority provide a horizontal seat with an upright backrest. Armrests are sometimes included and may be useful as reminders to maintain an upright posture but usually give little lateral support. Their prime role lies in assisting rising from the seated position.

The majority of these designs are intended primarily for the able-bodied but may be applicable to the disabled. Mass-produced plastic shell seats are widely used for normal babies before they are capableee of sitting and can be very appropriate for some younger disabled children. Similarly, school furniture is produced in incremental sizes for normal children and consequently may allow the accurate matching of size which is required by the disabled (Figure 14.9).

Adults, however, tend to be poorly served with fixed format seating as fashion, rather than function, appears to dictate size and shape. Most domestic furniture for relaxation tends to be low and too deep. Ergonomists have tended to focus their attention in seating on the two areas of office and car seats. The designs of typists' chairs have been particularly innovative and provide shaping with size adjustability to suit a range of individuals. Many

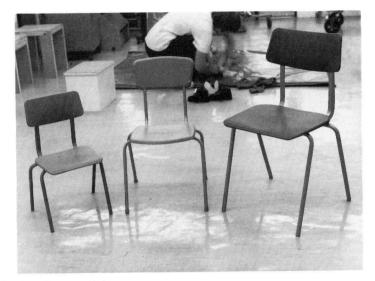

Figure 14.9 School furniture in range of sizes

are easily adjustable for height. Some designs have developed to the extent of allowing changes of postural support. One notable development has been that of the Balans type of chair which permits the extended hip position described in 2.2.1 (Figure 14.10). Difficulties of getting in and out of this chair have

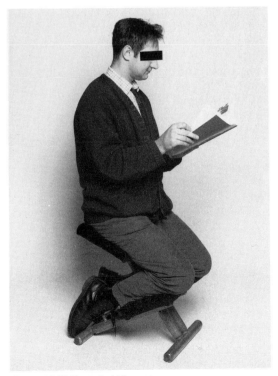

Figure 14.10 Extended hip seat

tended to limit its application to the disabled but variations of the design incorporating saddle-type seats have been used successfully (Pope *et al.*, 1988).

Modern office furniture holds much potential for seating for the disabled in the future and is worthy of investigation. Their applications, however, tend to be limited to the more functionally oriented uses.

Ergonomists have also expended considerable efforts in the design of seating for cars, probably because this is the chair in which the able-bodied are constrained for the longest periods of time. Specific contouring has been built into designs to provide stability whilst accommodating a wide variety of body sizes (Bulstrode and Harrison, 1985). Most current designs provide adjustability, at least for seat to backrest angle. The numbers of adjustments seem to increase in direct proportion to the cost of the car. Top range luxury models may include powered adjustment of seat height, recline, backrest angle and lumbar lordosis.

The application of car seating to the disabled in situations other than a car may hold significant potential benefit. Early experience at the Dundee Limb Fitting Centre has shown that car seats can be located on wheelchairs and have proved successful where other designs have failed.

A large number of fixed format 'easy chairs' or 'orthopaedic chairs' are produced for the elderly population, often resident in nursing homes or hospitals (ICE, 1983). They are usually deficient in their range of sizes and tend to have minimal contouring giving a very upright posture. Often they have a high seat height to facilitate rising. Many designs have small wheels for ease of movement and trays may be added for eating or leisure activities. These trays also sometimes provide a form of restraint for confused patients. In the past these types of chairs have been poorly designed for the occupant, producing upright postures with inappropriate sizing. New designs are becoming available and providing much needed improvements.

The majority of wheelchairs have a fixed format seat and are designed in incremental sizes to give the necessary dimensional matching. Wheelchair seating, however, particularly of the buggy type suffers because of the use of sling-seats (Figure 14.11). This is helpful for folding but gives poor support as it sags and hammocks to encourage a flexed posture and pelvic obliquity.

Recent developments in children's push-chairs have resulted in considerable improve-ments in their seating. The sling seats have been stiffened by wooden slats to provide better support. Their major drawback is that they tend to be very expensive, heavier and more difficult to fold.

(a) Modifications

The intimacy of support provided by fixed designs is limited. However simple modifi-cations can extend their applicability conside-rably and solve mild instability problems. Layers of foam may be added to adjust dimen-sions to provide lateral support where re-quired. This may be achieved rapidly with minimal resources such as a knife and pot of glue.

A simple pelvic strap can be added to pre-vent forward sliding. Care should be taken to locate such straps to pull *down* over the iliac crests of the pelvis, bisecting the angle between the seat and backrest (Figure 14.5 and Section 4.1.4). Cushions with firm bases or sag com-pensators (see section 3.2) may be added to sling seats to give a horizontal surface which helps maintain the pelvis horizontally in the midline. Ramping may be added under the cushion to help maintain horizontal femurs and to inhibit forward sliding (Figure 14.4).

Some elegant hardware is becoming avail-able as additional components for seating. These include lateral supports and headrests which can be bolted to existing wheelchair frameworks and can be detached when not required. (Figure 14.12). Complete backrests and seat sections can now be fitted to give adjustability comparable with purpose-built adjustable systems (Figure 14.13).

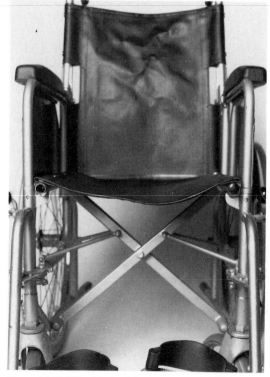

Figure 14.11 Wheelchair with sling seat (note sag)

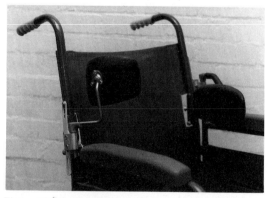

Figure 14.12 Adjustable lateral supports which can be swung away or detached

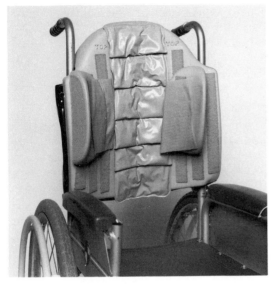

Figure 14.13 Adjustable backrest

The approach of using simple modifications frequently suffers from poor appearance as the modifications are often glaringly obvious. Also these modifications are limited in the extent of problems they can handle.

14.5.2 Adjustable seating

A number of seating designs incorporate adjustable features which permit more matching to individuals' requirements than is possible with a fixed format (Figure 14.14). This adjustability may allow changes to match the changing needs of the child either in the short term during the day or in the longer term as their sitting abilities develop. Angle of recline is the most common adjustable feature and may affect the whole seat or the backrest alone. Further features such as lateral supports, leg supports, armrests and head supports may be incorporated to give variability. Nearly all wheelchairs incorporate adjustable footrests to accommodate the variations in leg lengths. Clearly there are benefits from adjustable types of seating systems, but usually the extent of adjustability and hence the severity of problems they can accommodate is limited. Some highly adjustable systems have been developed for this reason but can become complex in design and adjustment. Recent developments have produced more elegant designs (Figure 14.15).

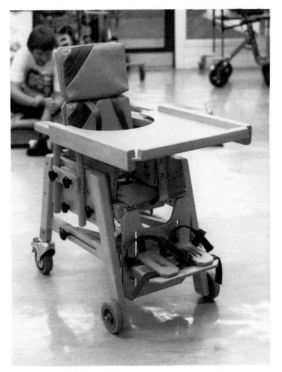

Figure 14.14 Adjustable seating system, wooden construction

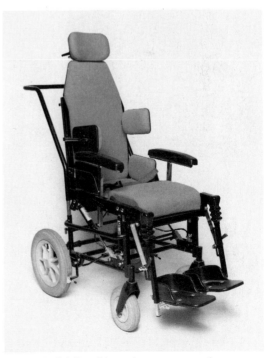

Figure 14.15 Adjustable seating system, metal construction

14.5.3 Modular seating

A number of recent developments have concentrated on a modular approach to seating design. This involves assembling a seat from a standard kit of components to give the desired size and configuration. Usually some adjustability is retained in the assembled seat which consequently can accommodate changing needs. The advantages of this approach is that it provides a wide range of adjustability without excessive complexity and avoids the expensive fabrication involved in customized seating. The versatility of this approach can be appreciated through the ability to combine different types of 'module' in one seat. For example, individually contoured elements and special pressure distribution cushions can be combined with standard components to produce a hybrid seat.

Some modular systems rely on a tubular framework onto which a variety of supporting elements are clamped in the required format and position (Figure 14.16) (Mulcahy *et al.*, 1988). Some rely on a plastic shell with velcro fastenings to locate support pads in a variable format (Figure 14.17) (Harrison *et al.*, 1986).

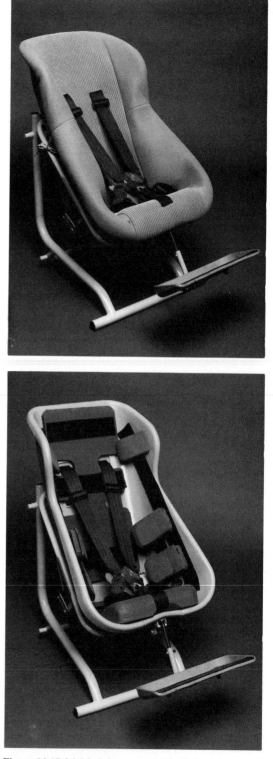

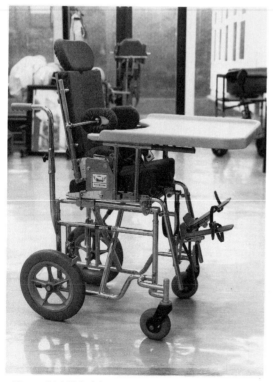

Figure 14.16 Modular seat, tubular metal frame

Figure 14.17 (a) Modular seat, plastic shell with pads.
(b) Modular seat, plastic shell with pads

Most of these systems attempt to fulfil a variety of functions by being interchangeable on a range of support structures such as a wheelchair, a static frame or a car seat.

14.5.4 Customized seating

Customized seating involves fabrication of a seat specifically for the individual. It is used only for the most difficult seating problems as it is usually expensive, has a limited life and tends to 'lock' the occupant into one posture. However, it is sometimes the only applicable solution, particularly for those with no sitting ability or severe skeletal deformities. A wide variety of different types are available, as described below.

(a) Foam and wood

This is probably the most versatile type of customized seating and requires a minimum of special equipment. It involves production of a wooden structure which is approximately the shape of the desired seat. This is padded with foam to give the required precision of support and then upholstered (Figure 14.18).

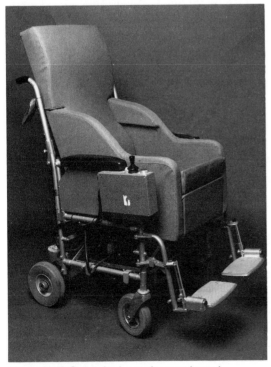

Figure 14.18 Customized seat, foam and wood construction

The technique suffers from being time-consuming and requires highly skilled technicians to achieve an acceptable quality of finish. Also, errors in configuration occur easily and it is difficult to modify the seat once it has been completed. The use of a simulator greatly assists in producing an accurate seat (see Section 14.7.3).

Despite its problems, this approach is often provided as a 'last-resort' solution for some people because of the comfort and the freedom of movement it can provide. Typical applications would be for multiple sclerosis, rheumatoid arthritis and some types of cerebral palsy.

(b) Shapeable surface systems

These systems rely on a series of small interlocking components which can be released to produce a flexible surface (Figure 14.19) (Cousins *et al.*, 1983). These may be shaped to follow body contours and subsequently can be locked into the desired shape. Normally, a metal tubular framework is constructed specifically to support the resulting shape. Also, a thin cover is produced for padding and appearance.

These systems have considerable advantages as they are able to follow a wide variety of shapes and allow adjustment as the individual's needs change. They require only the minimum of tools and facilities and usually have an open structure which provides good ventilation to

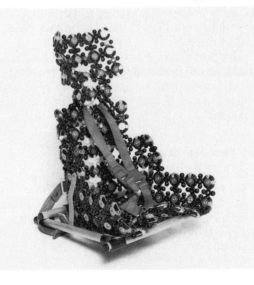

Figure 14.19 Shapeable surface seat, matrix construction

the seating surface. They suffer from being heavier than other designs of seat and can be difficult to manipulate into the required shape. They require a cooperative patient while the seat is being set up but can be contoured using a cast if patient cooperation is a problem. Their facility to be re-used is a major attraction but can be limited by the supporting framework.

(c) Moulded foam

Polyurethane foam may be obtained in two or three liquid components which, when mixed together, release gas to produce foam which subsequently sets to form the characteristic honeycomb structure of foam. If during this 'foaming' process the foam is contained within an enclosed space, it sets according to the shape of the container.

Customized seats can be made using this technique by using the individual's body in a sitting posture as part of the moulding container (Tooms and Hobson, 1981). The liquid is poured into a plastic bag underneath and around the subject. The foam then expands around the individual and sets in the form of a negative impression of their body shape. This can produce a comfortable customized seat very rapidly but difficulties may be experienced in maintaining the required posture during the foaming process. Also, it cannot be adjusted other than by cutting away undesired areas of foam. The technique can be improved by using a bead bag system to determine the seat shape and then foaming around a plaster cast of the bag.

The potential softness of the resulting seat shape gives some flexibility of movement which may be beneficial to muscular dystrophy patients who dislike being confined to one position.

(d) Bead bag vacuum consolidation

This technique relies on the use of plastic bags filled with small polystyrene beads. These conform to the shape of the individual. When vacuum is applied to the bag, it consolidates in a rigid form which follows the shape of the individual.

Considerable skill is required to manipulate the bead bags and position the individual in the required posture. This process can be facili-

tated by supporting the bead bags in an adjustable simulator (see Section 14.7.3). It may also be enhanced by using several separate bead bags to position different body segments independently and thus save having to control the entire body at the same time.

Some systems use this approach as the final seat for day to day use by the individual. It needs to be reshaped as required or when vacuum is lost through the inevitable leaks. This is particularly attractive as an adjustable customized seat but requires skilled operators available at all times.

Other systems introduce adhesive to the beads just prior to the time of moulding. This sets after moulding to hold the seat in a fixed form without the need for a continuous vacuum. It is then covered and fixed into a seat frame.

(e) Moulded plastic

The most elaborate development from the vacuum consolidation technique involves copying the seat shape in plaster which subsequently forms the mould for a vacuum-formed plastic shell lined with foam. Again a framework is required to support the seat in a wheelchair or other similar structure (Figure 14.20) (Ring *et al.*, 1978). Normally, these seats do not require covering.

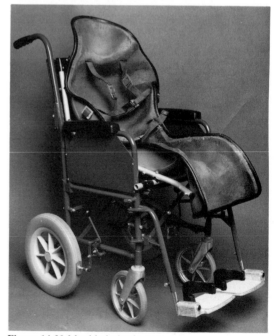

Figure 14.20 Moulded plastic seat

14.5.5 Associated devices

A number of devices can be used in association with a seat to improve its supporting characteristics and to extend its usefulness as follows:

(a) Wheelchairs

Many disabled people require a wheelchair to provide mobility whilst seated. This article does not attempt to cover the wide subject of wheelchairs. However, several seating systems have been specifically designed to fit into wheelchairs which were not originally designed for this purpose. This is most frequently provided by the customized forms of seating. Special care is required to ensure that the configuration of seat, wheelchair and occupant is stable over the likely range of slopes which the wheelchair will negotiate, and that the occupant is positioned within easy reach of the propelling wheels if he is to self-propel the chair. These objectives can often be difficult to achieve.

(b) Cushions

A wide variety of cushions are available to control pressure distributions under the buttocks. They are intended to improve comfort and prevent or help treat pressure sores. Normally, high quality foam with an appropriate stretch cover is sufficient for most people. More vulnerable buttocks require the use of gel- or air-filled cushions to achieve the required pressure distribution. A wide-ranging summary of the various types of cushions and their applications has been reported by Tuttiett (1990).

The use of a firm base or convex shape of bottom surface to the cushion is beneficial to negate the effects of the inevitable sagging wheelchair canvas. The latter are often referred to as 'sag compensators'.

(c) Straps and harnesses

Ideally these should be avoided because of the restraint they impose on the individual. However, they may be required as a simple safety precaution in a wheelchair or where forward flexion or sliding is a problem. Lap straps may hold the pelvis back at the desired upright position but must be located low over the iliac crests and should bisect the angle between the seat and the backrest (see Section 14.4.1, (d) Pelvic strap or bar above). More extensive support can be achieved for the upper body by chest harnesses located by shoulder and chest straps.

Foot straps may provide anchorage for wayward feet and can have surprising effects in stabilizing the lower part of the body. Alternatively they can occasionally aggravate instability by converting foot movement to whole body movement and consequently should be used with caution.

(d) Trays and tables

Nearly all seats are intended to facilitate function. This consideration often extends to incorporating trays to allow activities such as feeding, writing, play, etc. It is essential that this surface is in an optimum position relative to the individual to ensure maximum function. Trays can usually be fitted to wheelchairs for this purpose without too many problems. Trays may fulfil a dual function for some individuals by providing arm support thus inhibiting flexion at the trunk.

Tables often present difficulties in compatibility with seating systems and associated wheelchairs. These should be selected with care to ensure accessibility by the wheelchair and optimum height relative to the seat.

14.6 Alternative approaches

Some seating problems of the disabled may be tackled more effectively using alternative approaches to seating. Usually, they do not provide a complete solution in themselves and are likely to require some special consideration in subsequent seating provision.

14.6.1 Surgery

Problems of abnormal shape create many difficulties for seating and may be alleviated best by surgical correction of the patient. This is particularly relevant for hip and pelvic abnormalities which prevent horizontal support to the ischial and femoral areas. Soft tissue releases of hip contractures can simplify problems dramatically, with minimal surgery (Bleck, 1987). More extensive problems involving fixed deformities require more radical surgery and involve greater risk of failure but can sometimes present the only practical solution.

Early intervention using surgery may prevent the development of more severe seating problems at a later stage. Hip dislocation, for example, has been associated with spinal deformity through its influence on pelvic orientation (Rang *et al.*, 1981).

Early correction of dislocation may help maintain spinal alignment. Muscular dystrophy patients are prone to developing severe kyphoscoliosis in their later stages, despite careful positioning by seating. Surgical intervention with internal fixation of the spine has been recommended for the early management of these patients before significant spinal deformity is evident (Miller *et al.*, 1985).

14.6.2 Orthoses

Orthoses sometimes present the only solution to the problem of supporting parts of the body. Spinal orthoses in the form of rigid jackets worn close to the skin are the most effective spinal support (see Chapter 13). These devices, however, are not tolerated by many people and may be contraindicated for people with respiratory problems. Softer jackets made from more flexible foam (e.g. plastazote) are tolerated more readily but give less support. Neck orthoses made from a sheet or tubular form may be the only solution to the collapse into flexion of the cervical spine. Ankle–foot orthoses are essential to control foot position accurately and may also be used in dorsiflexion to reduce extensor patterns of movement (Meadows *et al.*, 1980).

14.7 Provision of seating

A 'system' of provision is required to ensure that each individual receives the seat which is most appropriate for their needs. The system involves the sequence of events detailed below.

14.7.1 Assessment

The characteristics and the needs of the patient are determined at this important stage. Seating can be involved in many aspects of the life of the disabled and assessment has to be correspondingly wide-ranging. Ideally it should involve a multidisciplinary team including medical, physical, functional and technical elements. Where possible, it should be a quantified process as prescribed by Mulcahy *et al.* (1988) in their assessment of sitting ability. This is rarely practical for all elements in view of the subjective nature of seating.

The results of the assessment should be recorded and should end with a clear specification of the objectives which the seat should fulfil. The use of routine procedures guided and recorded by standard documentation can assist this process.

14.7.2 Prescription

The type of seat is selected in this stage. Correct selection of the type is dependent upon knowledge of the available range of seats, their indications and contraindications. Some guidance can be obtained from literature (Trefler and Taylor, 1991) and catalogues but at present, practical experience is the primary source of knowledge.

14.7.3 Positioning

Selection of the appropriate configuration of seat requires positioning the individual in their optimum posture (or range of postures) and determining the support required from the seat to maintain that posture (Ward, 1984; Trefler and Taylor, 1991). This is a critical part of the provision of seating. In particular, 'positioning the disabled' is a subject in its own right and beyond the scope of this article. A trial and error approach is often adopted by holding the patient in different positions and observing their response. Care should be taken not to rush this process as the effects of different positions can take time to become apparent.

This process is helped considerably by the use of 'simulators' which are sufficiently adjustable to simulate a range of different seating configurations (Figure 14.21) (Bardsley and Taylor, 1982). They permit controlled variations over a wide range of adjustments for indefinite periods of time. The required seat is then selected or manufactured to provide this optimum configuration.

Lightweight portable simulators are available commercially and can be particularly use-

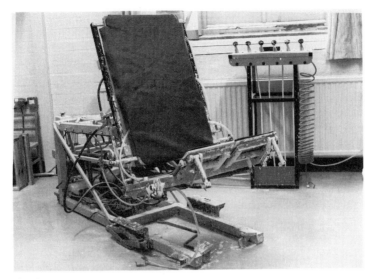

Figure 14.21 Seating simulator

ful when there is a need to travel to clients. These, however, can be limited in variability and size. Some seating systems are sufficiently adjustable to be considered as incorporating their own simulator.

The process of positioning tends to follow a routine sequence corresponding to the priorities for stabilizing the different body segments. Normally, this process commences with the pelvis as this forms the foundation for the body. Feet and thighs are positioned next to complete the base of support. The spine and head are then supported, finishing with the arms. The process is usually iterative, being repeated through the same order to check positions and make adjustments as necessary. Positioning procedures vary considerably depending upon the objectives for the individual patient and on the therapeutic regimen employed.

14.7.4 Fabrication

Ideally, all seats should be provided instantly on an 'off-the-shelf' basis. This avoids delays in provision during which time the patient's needs may change. It may also reduce the costs associated with fabrication. Modular and adjustable seats have considerable potential advantages for this reason.

The more customized seats, however, inevitably need fabrication. An intermediate 'fitting' stage is often necessary as part of this process. This has the benefit of allowing fine tuning of the seat and is a useful check that the prescription is appropriate.

Materials used in seating systems are quite varied as highlighted in the discussion of the different types of seating. Older designs tend to use upholstery, foam and wood, whereas more modern designs use plastics and lightweight metals.

Foam of various types is used extensively in the vast majority of systems to distribute loads. Strict legislation applies to the fire retardancy of foam used in furniture and must be observed in all seating systems (HMSO, 1988). This legislation varies between different countries. Only seating systems which comply with these regulations should be used. Similarly, systems which are fabricated 'in house' must use certified fire retardant materials and must be labelled accordingly. Samples of appropriate combinations of materials require to be tested.

Polyurethane foam with a density of 50 kg m^{-3} is used where considerable redistribution of loads is required, such as in seat cushions. This potentially is the most dangerous foam for flammability as it releases toxic fumes during burning. Ethylene foam (e.g. Evazote, Plastazote) 50 kg m^{-3} tends to be used for postural control where accurate positioning of forces is required such as for lateral supports. High density grades 70 kg m^3 are used for adjustments in dimensions where deformation is not desirable, such as on footrests or in sag compensators.

Upholstery coverings are required for most polyurethane foams both for aesthetic and comfort reasons. It is important that these do not impair the foam characteristics and they should be highly elastic. Knitted stretch cotton is ideal but is not waterproof. For incontinent patients knitted nylon with a polyurethane film can be obtained to give the necessary 'waterproofing' whilst permitting some 'breathe-ability'. Conventional vinyl upholstery tends to be inelastic and uncomfortable but benefits from being more durable.

14.7.5 Delivery

The definitive seat is handed over at the delivery stage. It is important to check that the seat fulfils the objectives set out at the initial assessment and that it is of an adequate technical standard. Modifications to wheelchairs such as the addition of seat inserts can affect the stability of the wheelchair which has to be tested. The Department of Health recommends such systems, when occupied, should be stable on slopes up to 16° for attendant-propelled wheelchairs and 12° for occupant-propelled wheelchairs (DHSS, 1980).

The patient and/or attendant also require instructions in the use and maintenance of the seat. Placing the patient in the seat can be difficult, especially in close-fitting systems, and may require special techniques. It is essential that this technique is taught properly otherwise the benefits of the seat will not be realized and either pressure sores or failure to use the seat may result.

Finally, problems frequently arise from incorrect adjustment and fitting of seats in wheelchairs. Again this can lead to dangerous situations with the patient at risk of, for instance, falling out of the wheelchair. Careful instruction of the users is required to prevent such problems.

14.7.6 Review

Regular reviews of patients and their seating are essential to ensure that the seating continues to be appropriate and that it continues to function satisfactorily. Consequently, a delivery system must ensure that the appropriate reviews occur at regular intervals.

Time between reviews is variable depending upon the individual patient, but should not normally exceed 12 months.

14.8 Research and development

The large majority of development work for seating has concentrated on producing new designs of seating systems. The recent proliferation of seating improvements have been mostly of a modular nature, probably because of the versatility these systems provide. Examples are described in Section 14.5.3.

The most innovative developments currently in progress utilize CADCAM technology (computer-aided design and manufacturing). The seated shape of the individual is detected using displacement transducers in a seating simulator. Alternatively plaster casts derived as for a moulded seat may be scanned using optical or electromechanical transducers. The shape information may then be manipulated by computer to produce the required seat shape. This is then produced by a computer controlling a carving machine to cut out the seat shape from a block of material such as foam (Inigo and Kwiatkowski, 1991).

The attractions of this approach are that, potentially, it may produce seats rapidly and identical copies of the seat can be produced very easily. It produces a quantified record of the seat which may assist improvements for subsequent seats for the individual. Initially, there is a heavy capital cost for the equipment but leasing arrangements and central fabrication facilities may reduce this drawback. Commercial systems using this technology are just starting to become available as, for example, in the Silhouette Seat by Pin Dot Products.

Cushions are always the subject of R&D interest. Rarely a year passes without several new designs becoming available. The stimulus in this work is partly financial to save costs on the more expensive but most effective cushions. CADCAM may have its earliest contributions to cushions in its ability to control pressure distribution by contouring.

The more fundamental areas of research in seating have tended to be ignored in the past, probably because they have been considered less important than the development of new systems and because they are difficult to carry out.

Posture and positioning have been the subjects of significant research programmes (Hobson, 1988). This work is hampered by the difficulties encountered in measuring the effects of seating and posture. Pressure is most readily measured (Bar, 1991) and a number of systems are currently available for this purpose. They vary from very simple, crude but clinically useful systems (e.g. Talley pressure evaluator) to expensive sensor mats which can be used also as a research tool. Other measurements which have been investigated include muscle tone (Nwaobi, 1986) and body shape.

Without such measurements, procedures such as assessment, positioning and review are restricted to a subjective nature and inherently limit the understanding of the process of seating provision. There is evidence of increasing interest in the more fundamental research into seating, which hopefully will elevate the subject from an art form into a more science-based skill.

References

Bardsley G.I. and Taylor P.M. (1982) The development of an assessment chair. *Prosthet. Orthot. Int.* **6**, 75–78

Bar C. (1991) Evaluation of cushions. *Prosthet. Orthot. Int.* **15**, 232–240

Bleck E.E. (1987) *Orthopaedic Management in Cerebral Palsy.* Lavenham Press, Lavenham, Suffolk.

Branton P. (1969) Behaviour, body mechanics and discomfort. In: Grandjean E. (ed.), *Proceedings of a Symposium on Sitting Posture 1969.* Taylor and Francis, London

Branton P. and Grayson G. (1967) An evaluation of train seats by observation of sitting behaviour. *Ergonomics* **10**, 35–51

Bridger R.S., von Eisenhart-Rothe C. and Henneberg M. (1989) Effects of seat slope and hip flexion on spinal angles in sitting. *Hum. Factors* **31**, 679–688

Bulstrode S.J. and Harrison R.A. (1985) *Assessment of Replacement Car Seats. DHSS Aids Assessment Programme.* HMSO, London

Cousins S.J., Jones K. and Akerley K. (1983) The matrix body support system. In: *Proceedings of ISPO 4th World Congress, London*

Dickson R.A., and Archer I.A. (1986) Biomechanics of spinal deformity. *J. Bone Joint Surg.* **68B**, 682

DHSS (1980) General Specification for Moulded Seat Supports and their Attachments to Wheelchairs, TB/SA/6 Department of Health and Social Security.

Diffrient N., Tilley A.R. and Bardagjy J.C. (1974) *Humanscale 1/2/3.* MIT Press, London

Gorman J. (1988) *The Cause of Lumbar Back Pain – and the Solution.* J. Gorman, Eversley, UK

Green E.M. and Nelham R.L. (1991) Development of sitting ability, assessment of children with a motor handicap and prescription of appropriate seating systems

Harrison D.W., Bardsley G.I., Fairgrieve E.M. *et al.* (1986) A modular nursery seat for disabled children. In: *Proceedings of ISPO UKNMS Annual Meeting, Glasgow*

HMSO (1988) *Consumer Protection: Furniture and Furnishings (Fire) (Safety) Regulations 1988.* No. 1324. HMSO, London

Hobson D. (1988) Contributions of Posture and Deformity to the Body–Seat Interface Conditions of a Person with Spinal Cord Injuries. PhD thesis, University of Strathclyde

Hobson D., Shaw C.G., Monahan L.C. *et al.* (1987) *Anthropometric Studies for the Physically Disabled Population.* University of Tennessee, Rehabilitation Engineering Centre

ICE (1983) *Seating for Elderly and Disabled People.* Institute for Consumer Ergonomics, Loughborough

Inigo R.M. and Kwiatkowski R.J. CAD/CAM for Custom Seating Measurements and Body Positioning. University of Virginia, Charlotsville.

Loud P. and Gladwin J. (1981) *Domestic Accidents Involving Easy Chairs.* Report. Institute for Consumer Ergonomics, Loughborough

Margolis S.A., Wengert M.E. and Kobar K.A. (1988) The subasis bar. In: *Proceedings of 4th International Seating Symposium, February.* University of Vancouver

Meadows C.B., Anderson D.M., Duncan L.M. *et al.* (1980) *The Use of Polypropylene Ankle–foot Orthoses in the Management of the Young Cerebral Palsied Child.* Report. Tayside Rehabilitation Engineering Services, Dundee

Miller F., Moseley C. and Koreska J. (1985) Treatment of spinal deformity in Duchenne muscular dystrophy. *Orthop. Trans.* **9**, 125

Mulcahy C.M., Putney T.E., Nelham R.L. *et al.* (1988) Adaptive seating for motor handicap. *Br. J. Occup. Ther.* **51**, 347–352

Nachemson A.L. (1985) Advances in low-back pain. *Clin. Orthop. Rel. Res.* **200**, 266–278

Nelham R. (1984) Principle and practice in the manufacturing of seating for the handicapped. *Physiotherapy* **70**, 54–58

Nwaobi O.M. (1986) Effects of body orientation in space on tonic muscle activity of patients with cerebral palsy. *Dev. Med. Child Neurol.* **28**, 41–44

Pope M.P., Boath E. and Gosling G. (1988) The development of alternative seating and mobility systems. *Physiother. Pract.* **4**, 78–93

Rang M., Douglas G., Bennet G.C. *et al.* (1981) Seating for children with cerebral palsy. *J. Pediat. Orthop.* **1**, 279–287

Ring N., Nelham R.L. and Pearson F.A. (1978) Moulded supportive seating for the disabled. *Prosthet. Orthot. Int.* **2**, 30–34

Scrutton D. (1991) The courses of developmental deformity and their implication for seating. *Prosthet. Orthot. Int.* **15**, 199–202

Stewart C.P.U.S., (1991) Physiological consideration in seating. *Prosthet. Orthot. Int.* **15**, 193–198

Tooms R. and Hobson D. (1981) *A Preliminary Report on Foam-in-place Seating for the Severely Disabled.* Annual report. University of Tennessee Rehabilitation Engineering Centre, Memphis

Tortora G.J. and Anagnostakos N.P. (1984) *Principles of Anatomy and Physiology* 4th ed. Harper & Row, New York.

Trefler E. and Taylor S.J. (1991) Prescription and positioning: evaluating the physically disabled individual for wheelchair seating. *Prosthet. Orthot. Int.* **15**, 217–224

TRES (1981) *Body Support Systems for the Severely Disabled Patient.* Final Report to SHHD. K/RED/14/47

Tuttiett S. (1990) *Wheelchair Cushions – Summary Report,* 2nd edn. Department of Health, London

Ward D.E. (1984) *Positioning the Handicapped Child for Function.* Phoenix Press, Missouri

Wilson A.B. Jr (1986) *Wheelchairs, A Prescription Guide.* Rehabilitation Press, Charlottesville, VA

Zacharkow D. (1988) *Posture, Sitting, Standing, Chair Design and Exercise.* Thomas, Illinois

Index